Hematologic Malignancies

Series Editor

Martin Dreyling
München, Germany

This series of professional books provides in-depth information on all aspects of the diagnosis and treatment of different hematologic cancers, including clinical evaluation, imaging diagnosis, staging, current treatment strategies, novel targeted approaches, and evaluation of treatment response. Readers will also find coverage of methodological and research issues and factors that influence treatment outcome. Each volume is designed to serve both as a quick reference and as a comprehensive source of knowledge that will be invaluable in improving management of the malignancy under consideration. The volume editors and authors have been selected for their international reputations and acknowledged expertise. The series will appeal to hematologists and oncologists in hospitals or private practices, residents, and others with an interest in the field.

More information about this series at http://www.springer.com/series/5416

Martin Dreyling • Marco Ladetto
Editors

Indolent Lymphomas

Springer

Editors
Martin Dreyling
Department of Medicine III
LMU Hospital
München, Bayern
Germany

Marco Ladetto
Azienda Ospedaliera Nazionale
SS Antonio e Biagio e Cesare Arrigo
Alessandria
Italy

ISSN 2197-9766 ISSN 2197-9774 (electronic)
Hematologic Malignancies
ISBN 978-3-030-55988-5 ISBN 978-3-030-55989-2 (eBook)
https://doi.org/10.1007/978-3-030-55989-2

This Springer imprint is published by the registered company Springer Nature Switzerland AG
The registered company address is: Gewerbestrasse 11, 6330 Cham, Switzerland

Contents

Part II T-Cell Lymphoma

1 The General Pathology

Giorgio Alberto Croci, Elias Campo, and Wolfram Klapper

1.1 Introduction

1.1.1 What Are Indolent Lymphomas?

The current WHO classification of lymphomas basically contains the overruling categories of Hodgkin lymphoma, B-cell lymphoma, and T-cell lymphoma, the latter two separated in precursor cell and mature neoplasms [1]. A categorization into indolent and aggressive lymphomas is not an integral part of the classification. Historically, classifications of Non-Hodgkin Lymphoma (NHL) grouped entities according to the cytologic appearance of the lymphoma cells and correlated them to the stages of differentiation of normal lymphocytes. This ultimately led to the pathologic/morphologic concept of "low" (small mature cells) and "high" (blastic cells) grades of malignancy, which actually proved to correlate, to a certain degree, with the clinical behavior of each given subtype: "low" grade with indolent and "high" grade with aggressive clinical behavior. The absence of such categories like indolent/aggressive and "low"/"high" grade in the current classification of WHO is based on several observations and biologic considerations. Indolent behavior implies a clinical course that is characterized by low growth dynamics, frequent relapses, and lack of curability despite chemosensitivity. These clinical features correlate only imperfectly with pathologic features, for example, small-cell morphology and low amounts of blasts. Examples are follicular lymphoma, which may show considerable number of blasts in cases of follicular lymphoma grade 3A but an indolent clinical course (low growth dynamics, frequent relapses). In contrast, mantle cell lymphoma may show aggressive clinical behavior with fast progression despite non-blastic (small cell) morphology. Moreover, the clinical course is heavily influenced by clinical management, which is not reflected by the classification of diseases. Finally, the identification of molecular and clinico-pathological subgroubs within lymphoma entities explains to some extent the variability in clinical behavior but prevents the assignment of an entity to the category of indolent lymphomas with certainty. Nevertheless, the distinction of lymphomas with an indolent course from those with an aggressive course is still a frequent although arbitrary process in daily practice.

G. A. Croci
Department of Pathophysiology and Transplantation, Pathology Unit, University of Milan, Milan, Italy
e-mail: giorgio.croci@unimi.it

E. Campo
Institute for Biomedical Research August Pi i Sunyer (IDIBAPS), University of Barcelona, Barcelona, Spain

W. Klapper (✉)
Department: Department of Pathology, Hematopathology Section, University Hospital Schleswig-Holstein, Kiel, Germany
e-mail: wklapper@path.uni-kiel.de

M. Dreyling, M. Ladetto (eds.), *Indolent Lymphomas*, Hematologic Malignancies,
https://doi.org/10.1007/978-3-030-55989-2_1

The diagnostic workup of indolent NHL as it is considered in this book roughly deals with two basic clinical–biologic scenarios. The first one, and vastly most common, is that of a lymphoid proliferation composed of cells that resemble one of the mature stages of lymphocyte differentiation, typically as small- to medium-sized cells and, in fact, mostly show features of an indolent clinical course (Table 1.1). This group of lymphomas contains very frequent diseases, such as chronic lymphocytic leukemia/small lymphocyte lymphoma and follicular lymphoma (FL). NHL with marginal zone and lymphoplasmacytoid differentiation follows next in the list, plus mycosis fungoides as a T-cell neoplasia. In clinical practice, mantle cell lymphoma (MCL) is usually still considered part of this arbitrary group despite the fact that the disease may present with an aggressive clinical behavior. In fact, the recognition of the distinct, indolent "leukemic/non-nodal" subset of MCL, on the one hand, and aggressive variants, on the other hand, exemplifies the heterogeneity in respect to indolent and aggressive clinical courses that may be observed within a biologically well defined entity.

Table 1.1 List of non-Hodgkin lymphoma subtypes with indolent course

B-cell phenotype
"Low grade" histology, B-cell
• Follicular lymphoma
• Chronic lymphocytic leukemia/small lymphocyte lymphoma
• Mantle cell lymphoma (leukemic/non-nodal variant)
• Extranodal marginal zone lymphoma
• Nodal marginal zone lymphoma
• Splenic marginal zone lymphoma
• Lymphoplasmacytic lymphoma
• Hairy cell leukemia
• Splenic B-cell leukemia/lymphoma, unclassifiable (splenic diffuse red pulp small-B-cell lymphoma, hairy cell leukemia variant)
"High grade" histology
• Lymphomatoid granulomatosis (grade 1–2 histology)
• Epstein-Barr-Virus-positive mucocutaneous ulcer
• Fibrin-associated diffuse large-B-cell lymphoma
T/NK-cell phenotype
"Low grade" histology
• Mycosis fungoides
• Primary cutaneous peripheral T-cell lymphomas, rare subtypes (primary cutaneous CD4+ small/medium T-cell lymphoproliferative disorder, primary cutaneous acral CD8+ T-cell lymphoma)
• T-Cell large granular lymphocytic leukemia
• Chronic lymphoproliferative disorder of NK cells
"High grade" histology
• Primary cutaneous CD30-positive T-cell lymphoproliferative disorders (lymphomatoid papulosis, primary cutaneous anaplastic large-cell lymphoma)
• Breast implant-associated anaplastic large-cell lymphoma
• Subcutaneous panniculitis-like T-cell lymphoma

The second, less-common scenario is that of NHL that presents as localized and often curable diseases. NHL may resemble either a subgroup of otherwise indolent lymphomas (e.g., FL of pediatric type) or independent entities, such as primary cutaneous CD30-positive T-cell lymphoproliferative disorders. The latter may also be considered as rather benign variants of aggressive lymphomas since they frequently present with a "high grade" histology (Table 1.1).

1.1.2 General Considerations on Indolent NHL Diagnostics

1.1.2.1 Technical Issues

As the label of "indolent" for a given case is based on proper clinical evaluation and follow-up, the importance of the dialogue between pathologists and hematologists to achieve a fruitful clinic-pathologic correlation cannot be overstressed. Indolent NHL is mostly seen in adult patients; thus, great caution should be taken in the pediatric setting, in which atypical reactive processes may mimic neoplastic processes.

In the precision medicine era, cytology of lymphoma cells still acts as the prime discriminator, particularly with regard to the aggressive subtypes. Thus, morphologic assessment of smears and histologic slides (May–Grünwald–Giemsa, hematoxylin-eosin, and Giemsa stains), coupled with immunohistochemistry, constitutes the gold standard for guiding the diagnosis of indolent NHL and allows the prognostic stratification and the detection of therapeutic targets.

This task requires the availability of representative specimens of good quality and proper size, to render the cytologic detail and the architecture of the lesion. Molecular-genetic analysis may help the diagnosis in challenging cases but, most promisingly, can add valuable information both to predict the clinical behavior and to guide the therapeutic approach.

1.1.2.2 Anatomic Issues

There is no anatomic compartment specifically associated with indolent NHL; however, it should be underscored that non-nodal modality of presentation is predominant in certain subtypes and is of prognostic significance in others. A consequence of the diagnostic ground is that pathologists are often required to deal with specimens from peripheral blood and bone marrow, which allow to collect and integrate a wide array of morphologic, phenotypic (either by flow or by immunohistochemistry), histologic, and molecular parameters.

Reference

1. Swerdlow SH, Campo E, Harris NL, Jaffe ES, Pileri SA, Stein H, Thiele J, editors. WHO classification of tumours of haematopoietic and lymphoid tissues (revised). 4th ed. IARC: Lyon; 2017.

Molecular Genetics in Indolent Lymphomas

2

Jude Fitzgibbon and Oliver Weigert

2.1 Introduction

The earliest genetic maps of indolent lymphomas appear quite rudimentary today and for the most part relied almost exclusively on conventional cytogenetics and array-based profiling to document chromosomal translocations and copy number aberrations. These observations have served as an important framework upon which next-generation sequencing (NGS) tools are delivering additional insights into the genomes of these malignancies. Certainly, we have moved away from thinking of a genetic lesion as simply the presence or absence of mutation, and there is a growing emphasis now on the longitudinal and spatial profiling of these indolent lymphomas, the early and late occurrences of mutations in lymphoma evolution, the complex reciprocal interactions of lymphoma cells with components of the tumor microenvironment, and the importance of dynamic monitoring of diseases. The growing body of knowledge is providing us with an unprecedented understanding of the biology of this group of lymphomas, and with each additional layer, there remains the ever-present challenge to translate these new insights into meaningful interventions for the benefit of lymphoma patients.

2.2 The Molecular Biology of Indolent Lymphomas: Follicular Lymphoma as a Prototypical Example

2.2.1 The Translocation t (14;18) in FL

The primary genetic event in the classical model of FL pathogenesis is the reciprocal translocation t (14;18) (q32;q21) that is detected in approximately 90% patients [1]. This rearrangement relocates the immunoglobulin heavy chain (IGH) enhancer region adjacent to the anti-apoptotic *BCL2* gene, resulting in aberrant constitutive overexpression of *BCL2*. This critical early step in the pathogenesis of FL occurs in the bone marrow in response to faulty VDJ recombination early during B-cell maturation, though the occurrence of the rearrangement in 30–50% of normal, healthy individuals supports the notion that upregulation of *BCL2* alone is not sufficient for FL development. These t (14;18) B cells are long-lived IgD$^+$ or IgM$^+$ CD27$^+$ memory B cells, which have experienced the germinal center while bypassing the usual

J. Fitzgibbon
Centre for Haemato-Oncology, Barts Cancer Institute, Queen Mary University of London, London, UK
e-mail: j.fitzgibbon@qmul.ac.uk

O. Weigert (✉)
Department of Medicine III, LMU Hospital, Munich, Germany
e-mail: oliver.weigert@med.uni-muenchen.de

M. Dreyling, M. Ladetto (eds.), *Indolent Lymphomas*, Hematologic Malignancies,
https://doi.org/10.1007/978-3-030-55989-2_2

physiological cell-death signaling that occurs in non-antigen-stimulated B cells, enabling repeated reentry into the GC reaction to acquire the necessary secondary hits. In a landmark study, [2]. demonstrated a clonal relationship between paired pre-diagnostic blood samples and their corresponding subsequent tumor samples, suggesting that circulating t (14;18) positive cells does indeed represent a low-risk pre-malignant precursor cell [2, 3] that can predate the disease by several years.

The reason why some individuals with t (14;18) positive circulating cells go on to develop FL while the majority do not is still debated, and while predisposing (epi-)genetic factors may offer one explanation [4, 5], it is plausible that cell intrinsic (secondary genetic hits) and extrinsic (immune microenvironmental) factors may also be of greater significance. These variables may in part explain the diversity of FL-related conditions, which include in situ follicular neoplasia [6], the highly curable pediatric-type follicular lymphoma that is typically t (14;18) negative [7], and duodenal-type FL, which bears a similar mutational profile to classical FL, yet possesses a distinctive tumor microenvironment and follows a benign clinical course [8].

2.2.2 Recurrent Genetic Alterations in FL

Molecular profiling has become synonymous with the documentation of gene mutations. Rapid advancements in the field of DNA sequencing have led to the development of cost-effective technologies capable of profiling a large series of malignancies, fueling initiatives like the Cancer Genome Atlas (TCGA) and the International Cancer Genome Consortium [9], and databases like COSMIC cataloguing somatic mutations in cancer [10]. These programs, in conjunction with stand-alone studies by single centers, have collectively succeeded in creating an encyclopedic knowledge around the coding landscape of cancers, including indolent lymphoma.

With >1000 FL tumors subjected to whole exome (WES), genome (WGS), or targeted resequencing, the coding genome and knowledge of the mutations that work in concert with the t (14;18) are nearing completion (Table 2.1). Prior to NGS, cytogenetic studies demonstrated chromosomal alterations in nearly all cases of FL with changes including translocation of *BCL2*; deletions of 1p36, 6q, and 17p; gains in chromosomes 2, 7, 8, 12, 18, and X; and copy neutral loss of heterozygosity (cnLOH) of 16p, 1p36, and 6p [45–52]. We can now point to many target genes residing within these chromosomal regions (*CREBBP, TNFRSF14, TP53,*) and throughout the genome, informed both by NGS and by functional studies confirming their role in lymphoma pathogenesis [14–16, 18, 20–22, 25, 36, 53–56].

The landscape of recurrently mutated genes in follicular lymphoma shows significant overlap with those found in other lymphoid malignancies, especially the Germinal Centre B cell (GCB) subtype of the aggressive diffuse large B-cell lymphoma (DLBCL). The FL mutational profile is most notable for the occurrence of multiple gene mutations encoding components of the epigenome, while other core processes recurrently disrupted in cancer are also affected, including B-cell receptor (BCR)-Nf-κB, (*CARD11*, *TNFAIP3*), JAK-STAT (*STAT6*), and mTOR signaling [13, 14, 17, 27, 34, 35, 57–60]. While mTORC1 signaling is usually restrained by a scarcity of amino acids, this natural brake on cell metabolism is abrogated in ~20% of FL, by mutations in *RRAGC* and related lysosomal components *ATP6V1B2* and *ATP6AP1*, with these mutations being conspicuously unique to FL [34].

2.2.3 Mutations in Epigenetic Regulators

From the earliest NGS studies, it was apparent that mutations in genes that regulate the epigenome, particularly histone modifiers, were a hallmark of the genetic features of FL and to a lesser extent many of the other indolent lymphomas. The term *epigenetics* refers to (heritable) mechanisms involved in regulating gene expression that do not alter the underlying DNA sequence. These typically involve the dynamic

Table 2.1 Gene mutations affecting >10% of classical follicular lymphoma

Gene	Effect	Frequency (%)	Mutation	Function	Lymphoma biology
KMT2D	↓	80–90	Pastore et al. (2015) [11], Karube et al. (2018) [12], Morin et al. (2011) [13] and Green et al. (2013) [14]	Histone K4me3 methytransferase	Zhang et al. (2015) [15] and Ortega-Molina et al. (2015) [16]
CREBBP	↓	33–70	Pastore et al. (2015) [11], Pasqualucci et al. (2011) [17], Karube et al. (2018) [12], Morin et al. (2011) [13] and Green et al. (2013) [14]	Histone acetylation	Zhang et al. (2017) [18], Hashwah et al. (2017) [19], Ennishi et al. (2019) [20, 21] and Mondello et al. (2020) [22]
TNFRSF14	↓	18–50	Launay et al. (2012) [23], Cheung et al. (2010) [24], Karube et al. (2018) [12] and Green et al. (2013) [14]	Regulator inflammatory and inhibitory T-cell immune response	Boice et al. (2016) [25]
Histone linkers	↓	40	Okosun et al. (2014) [26, 27] and Karube et al. (2018) [12]	Chromatin remodeling	–
EZH2	↑	25	Pastore et al. (2015) [11], Karube et al. (2018) [12] and Bodor et al. (2013) [28]	Histone K27me3 metyltransferase	Caganova et al. (2013) [29], Béguelin et al. (2013, 2016) [30, 31] and Berg (2014) [32]
EP300	↓	10–20	Pastore et al. (2015) [11], Okosun et al. (2014) [26, 27], Pasqualucci et al. (2011) [17] and Morin et al. (2011) [13]	Histone acetyltransferase	Meyer et al. (2019) [33]
ARID1A	↓	15	Pastore et al. (2015) [11], Karube et al. (2018) [12] and Morin et al. (2011) [13]	SWI/SNF family, transcriptional regulator	–
RRAGC *ATP6V1B2,ATP6AP1*	↑	20	Okosun et al. (2016) [34] and Green et al. (2015) [35]	mTORC1 regulators	Ortega-Molina et al. (2019) [36]
MEF2B	↓	10	Pastore et al. (2015) [11], Karube et al. (2018) [12] and Morin et al. (2011) [13]	Transcription factor	Brescia et al. (2018) [37]
GNA13	↓	10	Pastore et al. (2015) [11], Karube et al. (2018) [12], Morin et al. (2011) [13] and Green et al. (2013) [14]	B-cell growth and lymphoma cell dissemination	Muppidi et al. (2014) [38]
FOXO1	↑	10	Karube et al. (2018) [12]	Transcription factor	Szydlowski et al. (2016) [39] and Kabrani et al. (2018) [40]
CARD11	↑	10	Pastore et al. (2015) [11], Okosun et al. (2014) [26, 27], Karube et al. (2018) [12] and Morin et al. (2011) [13]	NF-κB regulator	Compagno et al. (2009) [41] and Davis et al. (2010) [42]
STAT6	↑	10	Pastore et al. (2015) [11], Yildiz et al. (2015) [43] and Okosun et al. (2014) [26, 27]	JAK-STAT signalling	Yildiz et al. (2015) [43]

↑ Gain, ↓ loss of function (Table modified from Carbone et al. [44])

addition or removal of chemical groups to histones or DNA by enzymes known as writers or erasers, thereby altering the access of transcription factors and the expression levels of affected genes [61, 62]. In FL, the most prevalent mutations affect histone methyltransferases (*KMT2D, EZH2*), acetyltransferases (*CREBBP, EP300*), and chromatin structure (*ARID1A,* histone linkers, e.g., *HIST1H1E*) [13, 17, 26, 57, 63, 64], with these "epimutations" co-occurring in up to 80% cases [65, 66]. These somatic mutations are predominantly inactivating, with the exception of *EZH2,* and alter chromatin state to condensed transcriptionally repressed heterochromatin. These lesions are well established as early, disease-initiating events in low-grade FL [14, 26, 35, 57, 60], and their lymphoma-promoting functional consequences have emerged, such as the GC expansion and terminal differentiation block induced by KMT2D loss [15, 16] and immune evasion through MHC class I/II downregulation seen with *CREBBP* [35], and *EZH2* mutations [21]. Critically, we are lacking an understanding of why FL (and other indolent lymphomas to a lesser extent) are addicted to mutations affecting components of the epi-machinery and how coexisting epi-mutations may cooperate over the course of lymphomagenesis.

2.2.4 Molecular Genetics and the Role of the Tumor Microenvironment

The importance of the immune microenvironment in FL is highlighted by the fact that in vitro growth of tumors is challenging [67]. Molecular studies employing gene expression profiling of bulk tumor samples have played an important role in characterizing the tumor microenvironment, complementing efforts to enumerate immune cell populations by immunohistochemistry or flow cytometry [68] seminal study described two prognostic gene expression signatures that were crucially defined not by tumor cell characteristics but by the dominant cellular composition of the microenvironment. Although these signatures appear to lose prognostic significance in cohorts treated with rituximab-containing therapy (thus highlighting the changing fortunes of such prognostic markers as therapy evolves), the importance of the immune microenvironment composition to outcome constituted a core principle for subsequent studies [69].

An important new area of study is an understanding of how specific genetic lesions enable FL tumor cells to co-opt the microenvironment for their benefit, with several individual examples emerging. One early link was the observation that unusually high numbers (~80%) of FL cases carry novel sites for immunoglobulin N-glycosylation, as a result of activation-induced cytidine deaminase (AID)–driven somatic hypermutation affecting heavy chain variable (V_H) genes [70] and with functional studies showing the ability of the resulting glycosylated immunoglobulin to bind dendritic cell and macrophage-expressed lectins, thus stimulating BCR signaling [71, 72]. TNFRSF14, a cell surface receptor involved in T-cell signaling and loss of *TNFRSF14* through mutations, deletions (1p36), and cnLOH in approximately 20–40% FL cases, has been linked to a tumor-supportive microenvironment with an increase in stroma-activating cytokines and T follicular helper (T_{FH}) cells. Intriguingly, TNFRSF14 function could be restored after the administration of soluble TNFRSF14 protein via specifically engineered chimeric antigen receptor T cells in a mouse xenograft model [25].

The impact of epimutations on the immune microenvironment is likely to proceed by multiple mechanisms. *CREBBP* and *EZH2* mutation likely contribute to immune evasion through class I/II downregulation [21, 35], while recent functional work showed that activating, *EZH2* mutations skewed GC B-cell dependence away from the normal T_{FH} cell signal support and toward lymphotoxin β-mediated dendritic cell (DC) support, with *EZH2*-mutant FL pathology samples intriguingly showing increased follicular dendritic cell networks [56]. It is likely that we are only scratching the surface of the microenvironmental effects of the epimutations and that novel approaches such as single-cell transcriptomics combined with improved disease models will constitute fertile ground for further discovery.

2.2.5 Histological Transformation of Follicular Lymphoma

There is considerable interest in understanding the biology of histological transformation (HT) of indolent lymphoma to an aggressive subtype, usually DLBCL, with HT representing the leading cause of follicular lymphoma-related mortality [73]. While the examination of serial FL–HT biopsies has been invaluable, research programs have been hampered by the paucity of available biopsies, leading to all cases of HT being combined together to adequately power genetic observations. It would be preferable to examine the genetics of HT in discrete subgroups, whereby distinctions may exist between transformations following chemotherapy relative to treatment-naïve HT [74, 75], differing time to HT, number of preceding episodes of FL, and prior therapies. We also need to be mindful that most genetic studies predate the use of anti-CD20 therapy rituximab, which has reduced HT rate and undoubtably impacted tumor evolution and will need renewed validation.

Accepting these limitations, studies have described an increased genomic complexity and mutational burden accompanying HT [57, 60], while recurrent events associated with transformation include disruption to DNA damage response and cell cycle regulation through *CDKN2A/B* loss and *TP53* mutation/deletion, and increased activity of key GC cell cycle regulator MYC through translocation, amplification, and/or mutation [26, 57, 60, 76, 77]. The molecular heterogeneity between HT cases is considerable however, and indeed most HT-associated events occur in pre-transformation samples at lower incidence. These obstacles to curating a discrete genetic signature for HT emphasizes the importance of pursuing parallel investigative approaches, including gene expression profiling and immune microenvironment characterization.

2.2.6 Classifying Mutations

The application of NGS tools has facilitated the sequencing of each unique DNA position hundreds and thousands of times, improving the sensitivity for detecting low-variant allele frequency (VAF) variants that may reflect either a low proportion of tumor cells within a biopsy sample or a "subclonal" variant that is present in only a fraction of tumor cells. It is worth emphasizing that several important variables, including depth of sequencing, the biopsy tumor content, and the occurrence of sequencing artifacts, impact the confidence in detecting subclonal variants. Mutations can also be defined by their computationally modeled or experimentally validated pathogenic potential (Table 2.1), with driver events viewed as mutations that confer a fitness advantage to the tumor cell within the context of a given microenvironment, while passenger mutations seemingly play no pathogenic role [78, 79]. Thus, it is important to note that defining a driver mutation is often inferred from surrogate factors, such as its clonal prevalence and postulated biologic effect, and not always confirmed by experimental evidence, although many of the landscape mutations in FL have indeed been shown to drive lymphomagenesis (Table 2.1). Driver mutations, somewhat surprisingly, may occur both clonally and in rare subclones in tumors with patterns varying according to the tumor type; *TP53* mutations, for example, are predominantly clonal in follicular lymphoma [80], but may be subclonal in chronic lymphocytic leukaemia (CLL), with a shift toward clonality over time [81]. Strikingly, the impact of a mutation may vary depending on when it arises during development, with studies by [15] demonstrating that conditional deletion of *Kmt2d* early during B-cell development, but not after the initiation of the GC reaction, results in an increase in GC B cells and enhances B-cell proliferation.

2.2.7 Temporal and Spatial Evolution in FL and Evidence for a Common Progenitor Cell (CPC)

Concepts of tumour evolution stem from the seminal work in the 1970s by Peter Nowell and John Cairns [82, 83], with early theories focussed on the linear acquisition of mutations, each providing a growth and proliferation advantage driving malignant transformation. In recent years, high-throughput sequencing of sequential and spatial biopsies and more recently cell-free DNA studies have led to a much greater appreciation of the clonal and subclonal structure of tumors, revealing a previously underappreciated degree of genetic and evolutionary complexity [84, 85]. The multiple relapsing indolent haematologic malignancies, including CLL [81, 86], and FL [14, 26, 35, 57, 60] have provided some of the earliest models for examining tumor heterogeneity and clonal evolution, revealing both patterns of early and late divergence at relapse and evidence of intraclonal competition within the unique ecosystem of the tumor microenvironment.

In GC lymphomas the most comprehensive analysis of temporal clonal evolution has been performed in FL. Initial studies in paired FL and HT cases analyzed somatic hypermutation patterns in the immunoglobulin heavy-chain variable region (*IGH-VH*), which uniquely tag each clone [87–89]. Although both linear (evolved directly from the diagnostic sample) and branching (evolved separately from an earlier CPC) evolutionary patterns were described, the predominant mechanism was one of early branching evolution. Moreover, the molecular analysis of donor-derived examples of FL offers further support for this notion of a progenitor cell population occurring many years prior to clinically detectable disease, reminiscent of work on comparisons of paired pre-diagnostic peripheral blood and subsequent FL tumor discussed previously [2]. In both published donor-derived cases, the patients underwent a bone marrow transplant for another hematological malignancy, after which both the donor and the recipient developed a clonally related FL, between 3 and 11 years posttransplant [87, 90].

In more recent studies, NGS has been leveraged to better characterize the CPC and the genetic changes driving transformation and progression [14, 26, 35, 57, 58, 60]. Described phylogenetic trees comprising a predominant branched evolutionary pattern, where truncal mutations shared between separate disease episodes were enriched for the epigenetic regulators *CREBBP* and *KMT2D* and allowed inference that these genetic events are likely to characterize this CPC population of cells. These findings have been built on by other groups, most notably by [57], who performed a similar temporal study in a larger cohort of FL–HT and FL–FL cases and undertook a detailed analysis of clonal dynamics. Using ultra-deep sequencing, they demonstrated that HT events were predominantly composed of clones that were not detectable even at low levels at diagnosis, suggesting later acquisition and selection, while cases with relapsed or progressive FL were characterized by the expansion of preexisting subclones, pointing to markedly different evolutionary mechanisms underpinning both these processes. Indeed, it is now apparent that virtually all tumor types, including FL, comprise a mixture of subclones, each with a distinct mutation profile, driven by their inherent genetic instability and providing a rich substrate for Darwinian natural selection. Tumor progression and treatment resistance are reliant on this genetic plasticity, with evidence to suggest that increased intratumor heterogeneity at diagnosis predicts a more aggressive disease course and poorer prognosis. Meanwhile, spatial profiling of FL biopsies has demonstrated the marked genetic heterogeneity that may coexist within the same patient at the same timepoint [91].

Together, these models may have significant implications for treatment, raising pertinent questions regarding the appropriateness of tailoring therapy to the molecular profile of a single biopsy, the need to target subclonal mutations, the possible role of chemotherapy in driving the selection of more aggressive subclones, and critically the nature of the CPC B cells that potentially serve as a reservoir for subsequent disease episodes. These challenges are not unique to FL but indeed all forms of indolent lymphomas, discussed in this book.

2.3 Molecular Genetics in Indolent Lymphomas: A Clinical Perspective

Despite our increasing understanding of the molecular biology of these lymphomas, translation into clinical practice is still lagging.

Ultimately, the biggest challenge for any genetic test is to demonstrate clinical utility. The revised WHO classification acknowledges the evolving role of genetics in the classification of lymphoid malignancies, complementing clinical, morphologic, and immunophenotypic features [92, 93]. The field is rapidly evolving, and genetics holds great promise to improve diagnostic accuracy, to serve as robust prognostic and predictive biomarkers, and ultimately to guide and personalize treatment.

Methods used in clinical practice include karyotyping (conventional and metaphase cytogenetics), fluorescent in situ hybridization (FISH), polymerase chain reaction (genomic and reverse transcriptase (RT) PCR), array technology (comparative genomic hybridization, single-nucleotide polymorphism, and gene expression arrays), massive-parallel sequencing of DNA and RNA (often referred to as next-generation sequencing, NGS), and analysis of circulating tumor cells and cell-free DNA (often referred to as liquid biopsies). Appropriate molecular workup is best performed in specialized centers and laboratories, with expertise in deciding if, when, and what assay to perform for which patient and sample; by understanding the benefits but also limitations of each test; and through interpretation of the data. As of today, only few tests are mandatory, but an increasing number is optional or recommended, and numerous promising assays are in development and clinical evaluation. The following section will briefly describe current and evolving standards for genetic testing in patients with different subtypes of indolent lymphoma.

2.3.1 Follicular Lymphoma

Clonality tests (immunoglobulin rearrangements) are usually not required to make the diagnosis and should be restricted to samples with diagnostic difficulties, such as inconclusive morphology or suspected lymphoma despite reactive morphology. The EuroClonality (BIOMED-2) consortium has developed a standardized multiplex PCR assay, which detects most but not all clonal *IGH* rearrangements. False negative results may result from rare rearrangements, which are not covered, and from sequence variants interfering with primer binding in regions affected by somatic hypermutation.

Molecular genetics can help confirm the presence of clonal *BCL2* rearrangements, a hallmark of FL (see the previous section). Karyotype analysis is capable of detecting the prototypical t (14;18) (q32;q21) [*IGH*/*BCL2*] translocations as well as other less-common translocations. More commonly, the FISH technology with *BCL2* break-apart or fusion probes is used to detect 18q21/*BCL2* rearrangements irrespective of their translocation partners [94]. However, this is rarely needed to make the diagnosis of FL in routine practice. Of note, most FL negative for the *BCL2* rearrangements still aberrantly express BCL2 protein by immunohistochemistry (IHC). Furthermore, despite distinct differences in their molecular profiles, the absence of the BCL2 translocation has not yet been shown to impact outcome of patients with grade 1, 2, and 3A FL who received standard treatment [95]. Rare variants, such as pediatric-type FL—a clinically highly indolent subtype—typically lack *BCL2* rearrangements [7].

The clinical impact of gene mutations in FL is a rapidly evolving research field [96]. Mutations in few individual genes have been associated with outcome in patients with FL. Most notably, *TP53* mutations (present in <5% of newly diagnosed FL) predicted inferior outcome both in pre-rituximab and rituximab eras [11, 80]. Gain-of-function mutations in *EZH2* (seen in up to 25% of newly diagnosed FL; also see the previous section) have been consistently associated with favorable treatment outcome in studies of homogenously treated patients who received frontline cyclophosphamide, hydroxydaunorubicin (doxorubicin), oncovin (vincristine), and prednisone- and cyclophosphamide, vincristine, and prednisone-based immunochemotherapy for advanced, symptomatic FL [97, 98]. Accordingly, *EZH2* mutations hold promise to serve both as a biomarker and as a therapeutic target.

Prognostic risk models integrating gene mutations [11, 99], copy number alterations [100], and gene expression data have shown promising results, but further optimization, standardization, validation, and exploration in additional cohorts is needed before they can be recommended for routine clinical use.

Finally, minimal residual disease (MRD) assessments hold promise to increasingly personalize patient management in FL, but also in other lymphomas. Clonal markers, such as chromosomal rearrangements and/or somatic mutations, can be identified in many (but not all) lymphomas and quantified in circulating tumor cells and/or cell-free DNA from peripheral blood and bone marrow samples (or other patient materials) by various techniques, including polymerase chain reaction–based methods and NGS [101]. MRD results can provide real-time information about tumor burden and response to therapy, noninvasive genomic profiling, and monitoring of clonal dynamics. However, MRD assessment is not (yet) a clinical standard and should be further validated in clinical trials to determine how to best incorporate MRD testing into routine practice and whether MRD-directed therapies improve treatment outcome.

2.3.2 Marginal Zone Lymphoma (MZL)

The detection of *IgH* gene rearrangements (e.g., by PCR) can be helpful in distinguishing extranodal MZL of mucosa-associated lymphoid tissue (MALT lymphoma) from reactive proliferations. Although not diagnostic, the detection of recurrent chromosomal translocations involving *MALT1* (t (11;18) (q21;q21)), *BCL10* (t (1;14) (p22;q32)), or *FOXP1* (t (3;14) (p13;q32)) strongly supports the diagnosis of MALT lymphoma. Furthermore, approximately half of the cases show trisomies of 3/3q or 18/18q or deletions of 6q23 [102]. All these alterations can be detected by karyotyping or FISH testing. Chromosomal studies may be useful to identify patients with gastric MALT lymphoma who are less likely to benefit from *H. pylori* eradication, including presence of a t (11;18) translocation or trisomy 3/3q [103, 104]. Furthermore, MALT lymphomas harboring a t (3;14) translocation seem to have a higher risk of histologic transformation to high-grade tumors.

Nodal marginal zone lymphomas (NMZL) typically lack recurrent chromosomal translocations, but often harbor numerical abnormalities similar to those seen in MALT lymphomas, such as trisomies 3/3q, 18/18q, as well as deletions of 6q23. Likewise, splenic marginal zone lymphomas (SMZL) also usually do not carry chromosomal translocations, but often have abnormal karyotype, including deletion of 7q31 or 8p, or complex chromosomal alterations [105]. Molecular studies have identified recurrent mutations in *NOTCH2* and *KLF2* (in up to 40% of cases of SMZL) and in genes of the NF-KB pathway (including *MALT1*, *CARD11*, *TNFAIP3*, and *MYD88*); however, the data on their clinical impact is still controversial and an area of active research [106–108].

2.3.3 Waldenström's Macroglobulinemia

Waldenström's macroglobulinemia (WM) or lymphoplasmocytic lymphoma (LPL) with IgM paraprotein carries highly recurrent somatic mutations, including activating mutations in MYD88 (>90% of cases [109]) and in CXCR4 (approximately 30% of cases [110]). As these mutations virtually all cluster in hotspots (MYD88 L265P point mutations and nonsense (NS) or frameshift (FS) mutations within the C-terminus of CXCR4 (so-called "warts, hypogammaglobulinemia, infections, myelokathexis (WHIM) syndrome-like" mutations), they can easily be detected by PCR-based assays [111]. Determining the MYD88 and CXCR4 mutation status is not only helpful in distinguishing WM from other B-cell lymphomas with indolent morphology, but also provides important prognostic and predictive information. Patients with $MYD88^{L265P}/CXCR4^{WHIM/NS}$ often present with more aggressive disease and high tumor burden. $CXCR4^{WHIM/FS}$ mutation status has been associated with high IgM levels, including hyperviscosity crisis [112]. Importantly, response to the BTK inhibition is adversely impacted by $MYD88^{wild\text{-}type}$ and $CXCR4^{WHIM}$; hence, determining the mutation status of these genes before the initiation of ibrutinib treatment should now be considered the standard of care [111]. Whether mutations in other genes like *BTK* or downstream *CARD11* or *PLCG2* are also involved in mediating treatment resistance is an area of active research. In that regard, WM can serve as a prime example, illustrating that response to molecular targeting treatments may be particularly predictable by gene mutation status. As the field is increasingly shifting toward cytotoxic-free therapies, a broader mutational analysis will probably be required to personalize treatment approaches in the very near future. Other aberrations have also been shown to be associated with poor outcome in patients with WM, including deletions of 6q and 11q, as well as 17p/*TP53*, but validation of these results with modern therapies is pending [113].

2.3.4 Mantle Cell Lymphoma (MCL)

Almost all cases of MCL harbor the t (11;14) [*IGH*/*CCND1*] translocation, which can easily be detected by FISH or, with a lower sensitivity, by PCR. However, similar to FL, the detection of this hallmark translocation is required to make the diagnosis only if routine morphological workup (including IHC for CCND1 (cyclin D1)) yields inconclusive results. In cyclin D1-negative MCL, *CCND2* and, rarely, *CCND3* translocations have been described [114]. Most MCLs have a pre-germinal center phenotype with unmuted *IGVH* regions and aggressive clinical course. However, a subset of MCLs have mutated *IGVH* genes and a more indolent clinical course, including non-nodal/leukemic presentation and splenomegaly. Chromosomal abnormalities, such as tetraploidy or complex karyotype, and deletions/losses of 17p13/*TP53* and 9p21/*CDKN2A* have been associated with inferior treatment outcome, even in the context of dose-intensified regimens [115]. Similarly, mutations in *TP53* as well as *NOTCH1* and *NOTCH2* have been shown to be associated with blastoid morphology, highly aggressive clinical course, and dismal treatment outcome [116, 117]. Similar to FL, prognostic and predictive models integrating gene mutations [118], gene expression data [119, 120], or miRNA profiles [121] have been proposed but require further validation in additional cohorts.

2.3.5 Hairy Cell Leukemia (HCL)

More than 95% of cases of hairy cell leukemia (HCL) carry the somatic, activating BRAF mutation V600E [122]. As the HCL clone can be small, sensitive molecular assays, such as allele-specific oligonucleotide (ASO)-PCR, digital droplet PCR (ddPCR), or NGS, are required to detect the mutation in peripheral blood and/or bone marrow samples. Although not specific, the presence of the mutation can be helpful in distinguishing HCL from other B-cell lymphoproliferative disorders [123]. Rare variants of HCL lack the BRAF V600E mutation (HZL-v), many of which haboring mutations in *MAP2K2* instead [124], particularly cases with IGHV4–34 immunoglobulin rearrangements. With the availability of BRAF inhibitors and other molecular-targeting therapeutics, testing for these mutations is expected to be increasingly relevant in the clinical setting. Numerous other genetic and karyotypic abnormalities (e.g., chromosome 5 abnormalities in approximately 40% cases) have been described [125]; however, none of these have been incorporated into the diagnostic criteria for HCL yet.

2.3.6 Chronic Lymphocytic Leukemia

Understanding the prognostic and predictive value of specific cytogenetic and molecular findings in CLL is increasingly guiding treatment decisions in clinical practice (see Chap. 13). Briefly, interphase FISH (e.g., for del (17p), del (11q), and del (13q)) and determining the mutation status of *IGVH* and *TP53* are widely considered standard clinical tests [126, 127]. Unmutated *IGVH* regions are found in approximately half of CLL and have invariably been linked with inferior treatment outcome, including higher risk of relapse and shorter overall survival [128, 129].

Cytogenetic abnormalities are present in >80% of CLL. The single most common alteration is deletion of 13q (present in up to 50% of CLL), which has historically been associated with a favorable clinical course [130]. Deletions of 11q22–23 occur in up to 20% CLL, typically involve *ATM* and sometimes *BIRC3*, and are often linked to refractoriness to chemotherapy [131]. Patients with deletions of 17p and/or inactivating mutations in *TP53* often have complex karyotype, aggressive clinical course, and poor response to standard chemotherapy and should be prioritized for TP53-independent therapies, such as ibrutinib, idelalisib, and venetoclax [132] (and *ESMO guidelines eUpdate from June 27, 2017: Chronic Lymphocytic Leukaemia Treatment Recommendations*). Interestingly, the mutation frequency of *TP53* increases over time, from approximately 5% at initial diagnosis to about 40% at the time of refractory disease [133]. Hence, testing for *TP53* mutations is recommended for all patients before the start of any new therapy. Also, deep sequencing rather than Sanger sequencing is recommended (capturing at least exons 4–9), as subclonal *TP53* mutations (i.e., <1%) seem to have the same unfavorable clinical impact as *TP53* mutations present in the major clone. Emerging data indicates that other recurrent gene mutations, such as *SF3B1* and *NOTCH1* mutations, are associated with more aggressive disease [131], but further validation in additional cohorts is needed, especially in the context of novel therapies. Furthermore, screening for genetic treatment resistance is a rapidly developing field, as exemplified by ibrutinib resistance mediated by the C481S point mutation in *BTK* or activating mutations in downstream *PLCG2* [134].

2.3.7 Indolent T-Cell Lymphomas

T-cell lymphomas (TCL) are much less common and—with the exception of cutaneous TCL (see Chap. 14) and large granular lymphocytic (LGL) lymphoma (see Chap. 15)—mostly have an aggressive clinical course. Rearrangements of T-cell receptor (*TCR*) genes are frequently seen and can be diagnostically helpful [135]. The aforementioned BIOMED-2 multiplex PCR assay captures the most common *TCR* rearrangements (mostly *TCRγ* and *TCRβ*, less commonly *TCRα*). However, clinicians should be aware of false positive results, as clonal T-cell clones can be detected with increasing frequency in elderly subjects [136]. Translocations affecting the *TCR* genes are much less common compared to B-cell lymphomas. Other genetic tests are not routinely performed in indolent TCL, but defining the molecular landscapes of these diseases is an area of highly active research.

2.4 Perspective

At the time of writing, genetics has become synonymous with coding mutations, and we have an unparalleled understanding of the coding genome and genes that are subject to recurring gene mutation in indolent lymphomas. This is in contrast with the relatively scant information gleaned thus far on how individual gene mutations work together, if all mutations in the same genes behave the same, and if the impact of specific mutation is maintained throughout the course of the disease. The portrait of these indolent lymphomas will change significantly as we incorporate knowledge on genetic susceptibility, the non-coding (epi) genome, and decide whether collectively these can unlock insights into the personalities of these lymphoma that will pave the way to improvements in the overall management of our patients, for their life both with and after lymphoma.

References

1. Tsujimoto Y, Cossman J, Jaffe E, Croce CM. Involvement of the bcl-2 gene in human follicular lymphoma. Science. 1985;228(4706):1440–3.
2. Roulland S, Kelly RS, Morgado E, Sungalee S, Solal-Celigny P, Colombat P, et al. T (14;18) translocation: a predictive blood biomarker for follicular lymphoma. J Clin Oncol. 2014;32(13):1347–55.
3. Hirt C, Camargo MC, Yu KJ, Hewitt SM, Dolken G, Rabkin CS. Risk of follicular lymphoma associated with BCL2 translocations in peripheral blood. Leuk Lymphoma. 2015;56(9):2625–9.

4. Skibola CF, Bracci PM, Halperin E, Conde L, Craig DW, Agana L, et al. Genetic variants at 6p21.33 are associated with susceptibility to follicular lymphoma. Nat Genet. 2009;41(8):873–5.
5. Conde L, Halperin E, Akers NK, Brown KM, Smedby KE, Rothman N, et al. Genome-wide association study of follicular lymphoma identifies a risk locus at 6p21.32. Nat Genet. 2010;42(8):661–4.
6. Schmidt J, Ramis-Zaldivar JE, Bonzheim I, Steinhilber J, Muller I, Haake A, et al. CREBBP gene mutations are frequently detected in in situ follicular neoplasia. Blood. 2018;132(25):2687–90.
7. Louissaint A Jr, Schafernak KT, Geyer JT, Kovach AE, Ghandi M, Gratzinger D, et al. Pediatric-type nodal follicular lymphoma: a biologically distinct lymphoma with frequent MAPK pathway mutations. Blood. 2016;128(8):1093–100.
8. Hellmuth JC, Louissaint A Jr, Szczepanowski M, Haebe S, Pastore A, Alig S, et al. Duodenal-type and nodal follicular lymphomas differ by their immune microenvironment rather than their mutation profiles. Blood. 2018;132(16):1695–702.
9. International Cancer Genome C, Hudson TJ, Anderson W, Artez A, Barker AD, Bell C, et al. International network of cancer genome projects. Nature. 2010;464(7291):993–8.
10. Forbes SA, Bindal N, Bamford S, Cole C, Kok CY, Beare D, et al. COSMIC: mining complete cancer genomes in the catalogue of somatic mutations in Cancer. Nucleic Acids Res. 2011;39(Database issue):D945–50.
11. Pastore A, Jurinovic V, Kridel R, Hoster E, Staiger AM, Szczepanowski M, et al. Integration of gene mutations in risk prognostication for patients receiving first-line immunochemotherapy for follicular lymphoma: a retrospective analysis of a prospective clinical trial and validation in a population-based registry. Lancet Oncol. 2015;16(9):1111–22.
12. Karube K, Enjuanes A, Dlouhy I, Jares P, Martin-Garcia D, Nadeu F, et al. Integrating genomic alterations in diffuse large B-cell lymphoma identifies new relevant pathways and potential therapeutic targets. Leukemia. 2018;32(3):675–84.
13. Morin RD, Mendez-Lago M, Mungall AJ, Goya R, Mungall KL, Corbett RD, et al. Frequent mutation of histone-modifying genes in non-Hodgkin lymphoma. Nature. 2011;476(7360):298–303.
14. Green MR, Gentles AJ, Nair RV, Irish JM, Kihira S, Liu CL, et al. Hierarchy in somatic mutations arising during genomic evolution and progression of follicular lymphoma. Blood. 2013;121(9):1604–11.
15. Zhang J, Dominguez-Sola D, Hussein S, Lee JE, Holmes AB, Bansal M, et al. Disruption of KMT2D perturbs germinal center B cell development and promotes lymphomagenesis. Nat Med. 2015;21(10):1190–8.
16. Ortega-Molina A, Boss IW, Canela A, Pan H, Jiang Y, Zhao C, et al. The histone lysine methyltransferase KMT2D sustains a gene expression program that represses B cell lymphoma development. Nat Med. 2015;21(10):1199–208.
17. Pasqualucci L, Trifonov V, Fabbri G, Ma J, Rossi D, Chiarenza A, et al. Analysis of the coding genome of diffuse large B-cell lymphoma. Nat Genet. 2011;43(9):830–7.
18. Zhang J, Vlasevska S, Wells VA, Nataraj S, Holmes AB, Duval R, et al. The CREBBP acetyltransferase is a haploinsufficient tumor suppressor in B-cell lymphoma. Cancer Discov. 2017;7(3):322–37.
19. Hashwah H, Schmid CA, Kasser S, Bertram K, Stelling A, Manz MG, et al. Inactivation of CREBBP expands the germinal center B cell compartment, down-regulates MHCII expression and promotes DLBCL growth. Proc Natl Acad Sci U S A. 2017;114(36):9701–6.
20. Ennishi D, Jiang A, Boyle M, Collinge B, Grande BM, Ben-Neriah S, et al. Double-hit gene expression signature defines a distinct subgroup of germinal center B-cell-like diffuse large B-cell lymphoma. J Clin Oncol. 2019;37(3):190–201.
21. Ennishi D, Takata K, Beguelin W, Duns G, Mottok A, Farinha P, et al. Molecular and genetic characterization of MHC deficiency identifies EZH2 as therapeutic target for enhancing immune recognition. Cancer Discov. 2019;9(4):546–63.
22. Mondello P, Tadros S, Teater M, Fontan L, Chang AY, Jain N, et al. Selective inhibition of HDAC3 targets synthetic vulnerabilities and activates immune surveillance in lymphoma. Cancer Discov. 2020;10(3):440–59.
23. Launay E, Pangault C, Bertrand P, Jardin F, Lamy T, Tilly H, et al. High rate of TNFRSF14 gene alterations related to 1p36 region in de novo follicular lymphoma and impact on prognosis. Leukemia. 2012;26(3):559–62.
24. Cheung KJ, Johnson NA, Affleck JG, Severson T, Steidl C, Ben-Neriah S, et al. Acquired TNFRSF14 mutations in follicular lymphoma are associated with worse prognosis. Cancer Res. 2010;70(22):9166–74.
25. Boice M, Salloum D, Mourcin F, Sanghvi V, Amin R, Oricchio E, et al. Loss of the HVEM tumor suppressor in lymphoma and restoration by modified CAR-T cells. Cell. 2016;167(2):405–18 e13.
26. Okosun J, Bodor C, Wang J, Araf S, Yang CY, Pan C, et al. Integrated genomic analysis identifies recurrent mutations and evolution patterns driving the initiation and progression of follicular lymphoma. Nat Genet. 2014;46(2):176–81.
27. Okosun J, Packham G, Fitzgibbon J. Investigational epigenetically targeted drugs in early phase trials for the treatment of haematological malignancies. Expert Opin Investig Drugs. 2014;23(10):1321–32.
28. Bodor C, Grossmann V, Popov N, Okosun J, O'Riain C, Tan K, et al. EZH2 mutations are frequent and represent an early event in follicular lymphoma. Blood. 2013;122(18):3165–8.
29. Caganova M, Carrisi C, Varano G, Mainoldi F, Zanardi F, Germain PL, et al. Germinal center dysregulation by histone methyltransferase

EZH2 promotes lymphomagenesis. J Clin Invest. 2013;123(12):5009–22.
30. Beguelin W, Popovic R, Teater M, Jiang Y, Bunting KL, Rosen M, et al. EZH2 is required for germinal center formation and somatic EZH2 mutations promote lymphoid transformation. Cancer Cell. 2013;23(5):677–92.
31. Beguelin W, Teater M, Gearhart MD, Calvo Fernandez MT, Goldstein RL, Cardenas MG, et al. EZH2 and BCL6 cooperate to assemble CBX8-BCOR complex to repress bivalent promoters, mediate germinal center formation and lymphomagenesis. Cancer Cell. 2016;30(2):197–213.
32. Berg T, Thoene S, Yap D, Wee T, Schoeler N, Rosten P, et al. A transgenic mouse model demonstrating the oncogenic role of mutations in the polycomb-group gene EZH2 in lymphomagenesis. Blood. 2014;123(25):3914–24.
33. Meyer SN, Scuoppo C, Vlasevska S, Bal E, Holmes AB, Holloman M, et al. Unique and shared epigenetic programs of the CREBBP and EP300 acetyltransferases in germinal center B cells reveal targetable dependencies in lymphoma. Immunity. 2019;51(3):535–47. e9
34. Okosun J, Wolfson RL, Wang J, Araf S, Wilkins L, Castellano BM, et al. Recurrent mTORC1-activating RRAGC mutations in follicular lymphoma. Nat Genet. 2016;48(2):183–8.
35. Green MR, Kihira S, Liu CL, Nair RV, Salari R, Gentles AJ, et al. Mutations in early follicular lymphoma progenitors are associated with suppressed antigen presentation. Proc Natl Acad Sci U S A. 2015;112(10):E1116–25.
36. Ortega-Molina A, Deleyto-Seldas N, Carreras J, Sanz A, Lebrero-Fernandez C, Menendez C, et al. Oncogenic rag GTPase signaling enhances B cell activation and drives follicular lymphoma sensitive to pharmacological inhibition of mTOR. Nat Metab. 2019;1(8):775–89.
37. Brescia P, Schneider C, Holmes AB, Shen Q, Hussein S, Pasqualucci L, et al. MEF2B instructs germinal center development and acts as an oncogene in B cell lymphomagenesis. Cancer Cell. 2018;34(3):453–65. e9
38. Muppidi JR, Schmitz R, Green JA, Xiao W, Larsen AB, Braun SE, et al. Loss of signalling via Galpha13 in germinal centre B-cell-derived lymphoma. Nature. 2014;516(7530):254–8.
39. Szydlowski M, Kiliszek P, Sewastianik T, Jablonska E, Bialopiotrowicz E, Gorniak P, et al. FOXO1 activation is an effector of SYK and AKT inhibition in tonic BCR signal-dependent diffuse large B-cell lymphomas. Blood. 2016;127(6):739–48.
40. Kabrani E, Chu VT, Tasouri E, Sommermann T, Bassler K, Ulas T, et al. Nuclear FOXO1 promotes lymphomagenesis in germinal center B cells. Blood. 2018;132(25):2670–83.
41. Compagno M, Lim WK, Grunn A, Nandula SV, Brahmachary M, Shen Q, et al. Mutations of multiple genes cause deregulation of NF-kappaB in diffuse large B-cell lymphoma. Nature. 2009;459(7247):717–21.
42. Davis RE, Ngo VN, Lenz G, Tolar P, Young RM, Romesser PB, et al. Chronic active B-cell-receptor signalling in diffuse large B-cell lymphoma. Nature. 2010;463(7277):88–92.
43. Yildiz M, Li H, Bernard D, Amin NA, Ouillette P, Jones S, et al. Activating STAT6 mutations in follicular lymphoma. Blood. 2015;125(4):668–79.
44. Carbone A, Roulland S, Gloghini A, Younes A, von Keudell G, López-Guillermo A, Fitzgibbon J. Follicular lymphoma. Nat Rev Dis Primers. 2019;5(1):83. PMID 31831752.
45. Cheung KJ, Shah SP, Steidl C, Johnson N, Relander T, Telenius A, et al. Genome-wide profiling of follicular lymphoma by array comparative genomic hybridization reveals prognostically significant DNA copy number imbalances. Blood. 2009;113(1):137–48.
46. Cheung MC, Bailey D, Pennell N, Imrie KR, Berinstein NL, Amato D, et al. In situ localization of follicular lymphoma: evidence for subclinical systemic disease with detection of an identical BCL-2/IGH fusion gene in blood and lymph node. Leukemia. 2009;23(6):1176–9.
47. Johnson NA, Al-Tourah A, Brown CJ, Connors JM, Gascoyne RD, Horsman DE. Prognostic significance of secondary cytogenetic alterations in follicular lymphomas. Genes Chromosomes Cancer. 2008;47(12):1038–48.
48. Fitzgibbon J, Iqbal S, Davies A, O'Shea D, Carlotti E, Chaplin T, et al. Genome-wide detection of recurring sites of uniparental disomy in follicular and transformed follicular lymphoma. Leukemia. 2007;21(7):1514–20.
49. Katzenberger T, Ott G, Klein T, Kalla J, Muller-Hermelink HK, Ott MM. Cytogenetic alterations affecting BCL6 are predominantly found in follicular lymphomas grade 3B with a diffuse large B-cell component. Am J Pathol. 2004;165(2):481–90.
50. O'Shea D, O'Riain C, Gupta M, Waters R, Yang Y, Wrench D, et al. Regions of acquired uniparental disomy at diagnosis of follicular lymphoma are associated with both overall survival and risk of transformation. Blood. 2009;113(10):2298–301.
51. Schwaenen C, Viardot A, Berger H, Barth TF, Bentink S, Dohner H, et al. Microarray-based genomic profiling reveals novel genomic aberrations in follicular lymphoma which associate with patient survival and gene expression status. Genes Chromosomes Cancer. 2009;48(1):39–54.
52. Viardot A, Moller P, Hogel J, Werner K, Mechtersheimer G, Ho AD, et al. Clinicopathologic correlations of genomic gains and losses in follicular lymphoma. J Clin Oncol. 2002;20(23):4523–30.
53. Yap DB, Chu J, Berg T, Schapira M, Cheng SW, Moradian A, et al. Somatic mutations at EZH2 Y641 act dominantly through a mechanism of selectively altered PRC2 catalytic activity, to increase H3K27 trimethylation. Blood. 2011;117(8):2451–9.

54. Jiang Y, Ortega-Molina A, Geng H, Ying HY, Hatzi K, Parsa S, et al. CREBBP inactivation promotes the development of HDAC3-dependent lymphomas. Cancer Discov. 2017;7(1):38–53.
55. Garcia-Ramirez I, Tadros S, Gonzalez-Herrero I, Martin-Lorenzo A, Rodriguez-Hernandez G, Moore D, et al. Crebbp loss cooperates with Bcl2 over-expression to promote lymphoma in mice. Blood. 2017;129(19):2645–56.
56. Beguelin W, Teater M, Meydan C, Hoehn KB, Phillip JM, Soshnev AA, et al. Mutant EZH2 induces a pre-malignant lymphoma niche by reprogramming the immune response. Cancer Cell. 2020;37(5):655–73 e11.
57. Kridel R, Chan FC, Mottok A, Boyle M, Farinha P, Tan K, et al. Histological transformation and progression in follicular lymphoma: a clonal evolution study. PLoS Med. 2016;13(12):e1002197.
58. Bouska A, Zhang W, Gong Q, Iqbal J, Scuto A, Vose J, et al. Combined copy number and mutation analysis identifies oncogenic pathways associated with transformation of follicular lymphoma. Leukemia. 2017;31(1):83–91.
59. Krysiak K, Gomez F, White BS, Matlock M, Miller CA, Trani L, et al. Recurrent somatic mutations affecting B-cell receptor signaling pathway genes in follicular lymphoma. Blood. 2017;129(4):473–83.
60. Pasqualucci L, Khiabanian H, Fangazio M, Vasishtha M, Messina M, Holmes AB, et al. Genetics of follicular lymphoma transformation. Cell Rep. 2014;6(1):130–40.
61. Bannister AJ, Kouzarides T. Regulation of chromatin by histone modifications. Cell Res. 2011;21(3):381–95.
62. Plass C, Pfister SM, Lindroth AM, Bogatyrova O, Claus R, Lichter P. Mutations in regulators of the epigenome and their connections to global chromatin patterns in cancer. Nat Rev Genet. 2013;14(11):765–80.
63. Pasqualucci L. The genetic basis of diffuse large B-cell lymphoma. Curr Opin Hematol. 2013;20(4):336–44.
64. Green MR, Vicente-Duenas C, Romero-Camarero I, Long Liu C, Dai B, Gonzalez-Herrero I, et al. Transient expression of Bcl6 is sufficient for oncogenic function and induction of mature B-cell lymphoma. Nat Commun. 2014;5:3904.
65. Araf S, Okosun J, Koniali L, Fitzgibbon J, Heward J. Epigenetic dysregulation in follicular lymphoma. Epigenomics. 2016;8(1):77–84.
66. Lunning MA, Green MR. Mutation of chromatin modifiers; an emerging hallmark of germinal center B-cell lymphomas. Blood Cancer J. 2015;5:e361.
67. Johnson PW, Watt SM, Betts DR, Davies D, Jordan S, Norton AJ, et al. Isolated follicular lymphoma cells are resistant to apoptosis and can be grown in vitro in the CD40/stromal cell system. Blood. 1993;82(6):1848–57.
68. Dave SS, Wright G, Tan B, Rosenwald A, Gascoyne RD, Chan WC, et al. Prediction of survival in follicular lymphoma based on molecular features of tumor-infiltrating immune cells. N Engl J Med. 2004;351(21):2159–69.
69. Huet S, Tesson B, Jais JP, Feldman AL, Magnano L, Thomas E, et al. A gene-expression profiling score for prediction of outcome in patients with follicular lymphoma: a retrospective training and validation analysis in three international cohorts. Lancet Oncol. 2018;19(4):549–61.
70. Zhu D, McCarthy H, Ottensmeier CH, Johnson P, Hamblin TJ, Stevenson FK. Acquisition of potential N-glycosylation sites in the immunoglobulin variable region by somatic mutation is a distinctive feature of follicular lymphoma. Blood. 2002;99(7):2562–8.
71. Coelho V, Krysov S, Ghaemmaghami AM, Emara M, Potter KN, Johnson P, et al. Glycosylation of surface Ig creates a functional bridge between human follicular lymphoma and microenvironmental lectins. Proc Natl Acad Sci U S A. 2010;107(43):18587–92.
72. Amin R, Mourcin F, Uhel F, Pangault C, Ruminy P, Dupre L, et al. DC-SIGN-expressing macrophages trigger activation of mannosylated IgM B-cell receptor in follicular lymphoma. Blood. 2015;126(16):1911–20.
73. Sarkozy C, Maurer MJ, Link BK, Ghesquieres H, Nicolas E, Thompson CA, et al. Cause of death in follicular lymphoma in the first decade of the rituximab era: a pooled analysis of French and US cohorts. J Clin Oncol. 2019;37(2):144–52.
74. Link BK, Maurer MJ, Nowakowski GS, Ansell SM, Macon WR, Syrbu SI, et al. Rates and outcomes of follicular lymphoma transformation in the immunochemotherapy era: a report from the University of Iowa/MayoClinic specialized program of research excellence molecular epidemiology resource. J Clin Oncol. 2013;31(26):3272–8.
75. Rusconi C, Anastasia A, Chiarenza A, Marcheselli L, Cavallo F, Rattotti S, et al. Outcome of transformed follicular lymphoma worsens according to the timing of transformation and to the number of previous therapies. A retrospective multicenter study on behalf of Fondazione Italiana Linfomi (FIL). Br J Haematol. 2019;185(4):713–7.
76. Elenitoba-Johnson KS, Gascoyne RD, Lim MS, Chhanabai M, Jaffe ES, Raffeld M. Homozygous deletions at chromosome 9p21 involving p16 and p15 are associated with histologic progression in follicle center lymphoma. Blood. 1998;91(12):4677–85.
77. Sander CA, Yano T, Clark HM, Harris C, Longo DL, Jaffe ES, et al. p53 mutation is associated with progression in follicular lymphomas. Blood. 1993;82(7):1994–2004.
78. Stratton MR, Campbell PJ, Futreal PA. The cancer genome. Nature. 2009;458(7239):719–24.
79. Vogelstein B, Papadopoulos N, Velculescu VE, Zhou S, Diaz LA Jr, Kinzler KW. Cancer genome landscapes. Science. 2013;339(6127):1546–58.
80. O'Shea D, O'Riain C, Taylor C, Waters R, Carlotti E, Macdougall F, et al. The presence of TP53 mutation at diagnosis of follicular lymphoma identifies

a high-risk group of patients with shortened time to disease progression and poorer overall survival. Blood. 2008;112(8):3126–9.
81. Landau DA, Carter SL, Stojanov P, McKenna A, Stevenson K, Lawrence MS, et al. Evolution and impact of subclonal mutations in chronic lymphocytic leukemia. Cell. 2013;152(4):714–26.
82. Cairns J. Mutation selection and the natural history of cancer. Nature. 1975;255(5505):197–200.
83. Nowell PC. The clonal evolution of tumor cell populations. Science. 1976;194(4260):23–8.
84. Gerlinger M, Rowan AJ, Horswell S, Math M, Larkin J, Endesfelder D, et al. Intratumor heterogeneity and branched evolution revealed by multiregion sequencing. N Engl J Med. 2012;366(10):883–92.
85. McGranahan N, Swanton C. Clonal heterogeneity and tumor evolution: past, present, and the future. Cell. 2017;168(4):613–28.
86. Schuh A, Becq J, Humphray S, Alexa A, Burns A, Clifford R, et al. Monitoring chronic lymphocytic leukemia progression by whole genome sequencing reveals heterogeneous clonal evolution patterns. Blood. 2012;120(20):4191–6.
87. Carlotti E, Wrench D, Matthews J, Iqbal S, Davies A, Norton A, et al. Transformation of follicular lymphoma to diffuse large B-cell lymphoma may occur by divergent evolution from a common progenitor cell or by direct evolution from the follicular lymphoma clone. Blood. 2009;113(15):3553–7.
88. Eide MB, Liestol K, Lingjaerde OC, Hystad ME, Kresse SH, Meza-Zepeda L, et al. Genomic alterations reveal potential for higher grade transformation in follicular lymphoma and confirm parallel evolution of tumor cell clones. Blood. 2010;116(9):1489–97.
89. Ruminy P, Jardin F, Picquenot JM, Parmentier F, Contentin N, Buchonnet G, et al. S (mu) mutation patterns suggest different progression pathways in follicular lymphoma: early direct or late from FL progenitor cells. Blood. 2008;112(5):1951–9.
90. Weigert O, Kopp N, Lane AA, Yoda A, Dahlberg SE, Neuberg D, et al. Molecular ontogeny of donor-derived follicular lymphomas occurring after hematopoietic cell transplantation. Cancer Discov. 2012;2(1):47–55.
91. Araf S, Wang J, Korfi K, Pangault C, Kotsiou E, Rio-Machin A, et al. Genomic profiling reveals spatial intra-tumor heterogeneity in follicular lymphoma. Leukemia. 2018;32(5):1261–5.
92. Swerdlow SH, Campo E, Harris NL, Jaffe ES, Pileri SA, Stein H, Thiele J, Vardiman JW. In: IARC, editor. WHO classification of tumours of haematopoietic and lymphoid tissues. Lyon: WHO Press; 2008.
93. Swerdlow SH, Campo E, Pileri SA, Harris NL, Stein H, Siebert R, et al. The 2016 revision of the World Health Organization classification of lymphoid neoplasms. Blood. 2016;127(20):2375–90.
94. Dreyling M, Ghielmini M, Rule S, Salles G, Vitolo U, Ladetto M, et al. Newly diagnosed and relapsed follicular lymphoma: ESMO clinical practice guidelines for diagnosis, treatment and follow-up. Ann Oncol. 2016;27(suppl 5):v83–90.
95. Leich E, Hoster E, Wartenberg M, Unterhalt M, Siebert R, Koch K, et al. Similar clinical features in follicular lymphomas with and without breaks in the BCL2 locus. Leukemia. 2016;30(4):854–60.
96. Weigert O, Weinstock DM. The promises and challenges of using gene mutations for patient stratification in follicular lymphoma. Blood. 2017;130(13):1491–8.
97. Huet S, Xerri L, Tesson B, Mareschal S, Taix S, Mescam-Mancini L, et al. EZH2 alterations in follicular lymphoma: biological and clinical correlations. Blood Cancer J. 2017;7(4):e555.
98. Stevens WBC, Mendeville M, Redd R, Clear AJ, Bladergroen R, Calaminici M, et al. Prognostic relevance of CD163 and CD8 combined with EZH2 and gain of chromosome 18 in follicular lymphoma: a study by the Lunenburg lymphoma biomarker consortium. Haematologica. 2017;102(8):1413–23.
99. Jurinovic V, Kridel R, Staiger AM, Szczepanowski M, Horn H, Dreyling MH, et al. Clinicogenetic risk models predict early progression of follicular lymphoma after first-line immunochemotherapy. Blood. 2016;128(8):1112–20.
100. Qu X, Li H, Braziel RM, Passerini V, Rimsza LM, Hsi ED, et al. Genomic alterations important for the prognosis in patients with follicular lymphoma treated in SWOG study S0016. Blood. 2019;133(1):81–93.
101. Herrera AF, Armand P. Minimal residual disease assessment in lymphoma: methods and applications. J Clin Oncol. 2017;35(34):3877–87.
102. Zucca E, Bertoni F. The spectrum of MALT lymphoma at different sites: biological and therapeutic relevance. Blood. 2016;127(17):2082–92.
103. Taji S, Nomura K, Matsumoto Y, Sakabe H, Yoshida N, Mitsufuji S, et al. Trisomy 3 may predict a poor response of gastric MALT lymphoma to helicobacter pylori eradication therapy. World J Gastroenterol. 2005;11(1):89–93.
104. Liu H, Ruskon-Fourmestraux A, Lavergne-Slove A, Ye H, Molina T, Bouhnik Y, et al. Resistance of t (11;18) positive gastric mucosa-associated lymphoid tissue lymphoma to helicobacter pylori eradication therapy. Lancet. 2001;357(9249):39–40.
105. Rinaldi A, Mian M, Chigrinova E, Arcaini L, Bhagat G, Novak U, et al. Genome-wide DNA profiling of marginal zone lymphomas identifies subtype-specific lesions with an impact on the clinical outcome. Blood. 2011;117(5):1595–604.
106. Rossi D, Trifonov V, Fangazio M, Bruscaggin A, Rasi S, Spina V, et al. The coding genome of splenic marginal zone lymphoma: activation of NOTCH2 and other pathways regulating marginal zone development. J Exp Med. 2012;209(9):1537–51.
107. Clipson A, Wang M, de Leval L, Ashton-Key M, Wotherspoon A, Vassiliou G, et al. KLF2 mutation is the most frequent somatic change in splenic marginal zone lymphoma and identifies a subset with distinct genotype. Leukemia. 2015;29(5):1177–85.
108. Parry M, Rose-Zerilli MJ, Ljungstrom V, Gibson J, Wang J, Walewska R, et al. Genetics and prognos-

tication in splenic marginal zone lymphoma: revelations from deep sequencing. Clin Cancer Res. 2015;21(18):4174–83.
109. Treon SP, Xu L, Yang G, Zhou Y, Liu X, Cao Y, et al. MYD88 L265P somatic mutation in Waldenstrom's macroglobulinemia. N Engl J Med. 2012;367(9):826–33.
110. Hunter ZR, Xu L, Yang G, Zhou Y, Liu X, Cao Y, et al. The genomic landscape of Waldenstrom macroglobulinemia is characterized by highly recurring MYD88 and WHIM-like CXCR4 mutations, and small somatic deletions associated with B-cell lymphomagenesis. Blood. 2014;123(11):1637–46.
111. Kastritis E, Leblond V, Dimopoulos MA, Kimby E, Staber P, Kersten MJ, et al. Waldenstrom's macroglobulinaemia: ESMO Clinical Practice Guidelines for diagnosis, treatment and follow-up. Ann Oncol. 2018;29(Suppl 4):iv270.
112. Schmidt J, Federmann B, Schindler N, Steinhilber J, Bonzheim I, Fend F, et al. MYD88 L265P and CXCR4 mutations in lymphoplasmacytic lymphoma identify cases with high disease activity. Br J Haematol. 2015;169(6):795–803.
113. Nguyen-Khac F, Lambert J, Chapiro E, Grelier A, Mould S, Barin C, et al. Chromosomal aberrations and their prognostic value in a series of 174 untreated patients with Waldenstrom's macroglobulinemia. Haematologica. 2013;98(4):649–54.
114. Jares P, Colomer D, Campo E. Molecular pathogenesis of mantle cell lymphoma. J Clin Invest. 2012;122(10):3416–23.
115. Delfau-Larue MH, Klapper W, Berger F, Jardin F, Briere J, Salles G, et al. High-dose cytarabine does not overcome the adverse prognostic value of CDKN2A and TP53 deletions in mantle cell lymphoma. Blood. 2015;126(5):604–11.
116. Bea S, Valdes-Mas R, Navarro A, Salaverria I, Martin-Garcia D, Jares P, et al. Landscape of somatic mutations and clonal evolution in mantle cell lymphoma. Proc Natl Acad Sci U S A. 2013;110(45):18250–5.
117. Dreyling M, Klapper W, Rule S. Blastoid and pleomorphic mantle cell lymphoma: still a diagnostic and therapeutic challenge! Blood. 2018;132(26):2722–9.
118. Ferrero S, et al. *KMT2D* mutations and *TP53* disruptions are poor prognostic biomarkers in mantle cell lymphoma receiving high-dose therapy: a FIL study. Haematologica. 2020;105(6):1604–12. https://doi.org/10.3324/haematol.2018.214056.
119. Holte H, Beiske K, Boyle M, Troen G, Blaker YN, Myklebust J, et al. The MCL35 gene expression proliferation assay predicts high-risk MCL patients in a Norwegian cohort of younger patients given intensive first line therapy. Br J Haematol. 2018;183(2):225–34.
120. D'Agaro T, Zucchetto A, Vit F, Bittolo T, Tissino E, Rossi FM, et al. A B-cell receptor-related gene signature predicts response to ibrutinib treatment in mantle cell lymphoma cell lines. Haematologica. 2019;104(9):e410–e4.
121. Iqbal J, Shen Y, Liu Y, Fu K, Jaffe ES, Liu C, et al. Genome-wide miRNA profiling of mantle cell lymphoma reveals a distinct subgroup with poor prognosis. Blood. 2012;119(21):4939–48.
122. Tiacci E, Trifonov V, Schiavoni G, Holmes A, Kern W, Martelli MP, et al. BRAF mutations in hairy-cell leukemia. N Engl J Med. 2011;364(24):2305–15.
123. Grever MR, Abdel-Wahab O, Andritsos LA, Banerji V, Barrientos J, Blachly JS, et al. Consensus guidelines for the diagnosis and management of patients with classic hairy cell leukemia. Blood. 2017;129(5):553–60.
124. Waterfall JJ, Arons E, Walker RL, Pineda M, Roth L, Killian JK, et al. High prevalence of MAP 2K1 mutations in variant and IGHV4-34-expressing hairy-cell leukemias. Nat Genet. 2014;46(1):8–10.
125. Haglund U, Juliusson G, Stellan B, Gahrton G. Hairy cell leukemia is characterized by clonal chromosome abnormalities clustered to specific regions. Blood. 1994;83(9):2637–45.
126. Parikh SA, Strati P, Tsang M, West CP, Shanafelt TD. Should IGHV status and FISH testing be performed in all CLL patients at diagnosis? A systematic review and meta-analysis. Blood. 2016;127(14):1752–60.
127. International CLLIPIwg. An international prognostic index for patients with chronic lymphocytic leukaemia (CLL-IPI): a meta-analysis of individual patient data. Lancet Oncol. 2016;17(6):779–90.
128. Hamblin TJ, Davis Z, Gardiner A, Oscier DG, Stevenson FK. Unmutated Ig V (H) genes are associated with a more aggressive form of chronic lymphocytic leukemia. Blood. 1999;94(6):1848–54.
129. Ritgen M, Lange A, Stilgenbauer S, Dohner H, Bretscher C, Bosse H, et al. Unmutated immunoglobulin variable heavy-chain gene status remains an adverse prognostic factor after autologous stem cell transplantation for chronic lymphocytic leukemia. Blood. 2003;101(5):2049–53.
130. Dohner H, Stilgenbauer S, Benner A, Leupolt E, Krober A, Bullinger L, et al. Genomic aberrations and survival in chronic lymphocytic leukemia. N Engl J Med. 2000;343(26):1910–6.
131. Hallek M. Chronic lymphocytic leukemia: 2017 update on diagnosis, risk stratification, and treatment. Am J Hematol. 2017;92(9):946–65.
132. Eichhorst B, Robak T, Montserrat E, Ghia P, Hillmen P, Hallek M, et al. Chronic lymphocytic leukaemia: ESMO clinical practice guidelines for diagnosis, treatment and follow-up. Ann Oncol. 2015;26(Suppl 5):v78–84.
133. Campo E, Cymbalista F, Ghia P, Jager U, Pospisilova S, Rosenquist R, et al. TP53 aberrations in chronic lymphocytic leukemia: an overview of the clinical implications of improved diagnostics. Haematologica. 2018;103(12):1956–68.
134. Woyach JA, Furman RR, Liu TM, Ozer HG, Zapatka M, Ruppert AS, et al. Resistance mechanisms for the Bruton's tyrosine kinase inhibitor ibrutinib. N Engl J Med. 2014;370(24):2286–94.

135. Aisenberg AC, Krontiris TG, Mak TW, Wilkes BM. Rearrangement of the gene for the beta chain of the T-cell receptor in T-cell chronic lymphocytic leukemia and related disorders. N Engl J Med. 1985;313(9):529–33.
136. van Dongen JJ, Langerak AW, Bruggemann M, Evans PA, Hummel M, Lavender FL, et al. Design and standardization of PCR primers and protocols for detection of clonal immunoglobulin and T-cell receptor gene recombinations in suspect lymphoproliferations: report of the BIOMED-2 concerted action BMH4-CT98-3936. Leukemia. 2003;17(12):2257–317.

Minimal Residual Disease (MRD) in Indolent Lymphomas

3

Marco Ladetto, Christiane Coll, Martina Ferrante, Daniele Grimaldi, and Pott Christiane

3.1 Introduction

One leading concept in the management of most tumors, particularly those in which highly effective therapeutic options are available, is that a marked reduction of the tumor burden is an important preliminary step to ensure long-term disease control. This concept is not novel and is the basis also for posttreatment clinical response assessment by conventional imaging and histologic tools. The rather intuitive notion that "less tumor is better than more" should not lead to underestimate the simplistic nature of such a concept. Most recent research has indeed stressed the heterogeneity of the tumor clone rather than its homogeneity, suggesting that the quality of residual tumor cells might be more relevant than its number [1]. This is an intriguing concept that might lead to a more refined molecular dissection of residual tumor clones in future years. Nevertheless, the current unsophisticated crude quantification of the whole residual tumor clone below the sensitivity threshold of conventional histologic and imaging tools (i.e., MRD detection) has proven to be a valuable tool in most hematologic neoplasms and is of great interest in the field of truly indolent lymphoid neoplasms, such as follicular lymphoma (FL) (Table 3.1) and chronic lymphocytic leukemia (CLL), as well as in mantle cell lymphoma (MCL) (Table 3.2). This chapter will focus on this subject.

Several methods have proven useful for MRD monitoring in the context of indolent lymphomas. These will be described in a subsequent chapter. Different tools have been applied to different disorders, basically because of different performances in terms of applicability, accuracy, sensitivity, and specificity. Currently, there is no single tool that could be considered optimal in every disease and in every clinical context [2, 3]. However, at the present time, real-time quantitative PCR (RQ-PCR) is considered the "gold standard" for FL and MCL, while flow cytometry for CLL.

The issue of early detection of relapse is particularly important in the field of indolent non-Hodgkin lymphomas (iNHL). Clinically, these disorders are characterized by an indolent course and good response to treatment. Nevertheless, relapses occur frequently, and a proportion of

M. Ladetto (✉)
Azienda Ospedaliera Nazionale, SS Antonio e Biagio e Cesare Arrigo, Alessandria, Italy
e-mail: marco.ladetto@ospedale.al.it

C. Coll · P. Christiane
Second Medical Department, University Hospital Schleswig-Holstein, Kiel, Germany
e-mail: c.pott@med2.uni-kiel.de, cpott@mjed2.uni-kiel.de

M. Ferrante · D. Grimaldi
Sezione di Ematologia, Dipartimento di Biotecnologie Molecolari e Scienze per la Salute, Universita di Torino, Torino, Italy
e-mail: martina.ferrante@edu.unito.it; daniele.grimaldi@edu.unito.it

M. Dreyling, M. Ladetto (eds.), *Indolent Lymphomas*, Hematologic Malignancies,
https://doi.org/10.1007/978-3-030-55989-2_3

Table 3.1 Relevant literature on MRD detection in FL

Study	Disease	Patients	Therapy	Tissue analyzed	Method	Marker	Clinical impact of MRD
Gribben JG, Freedman AS, Neuberg D, et al. NEJM. N Engl J Med. 1991	FL	114	TBI + ASCT	Harvest	PCR	BCL2	24 M relapse incidence: 39% vs. 5% ($p < 0.0001$)
Lopez GA, Cabanillas F, McLaughlin P.et al. Blood 1998	FL	194	ATT, FND, CHOP+radiotherapy	BM, PB	PCR	BCL2, IGH	48 M FFS: 76% vs. 38% ($p < 0.001$)
Mandingers CM, Meijerink JP, Mensink EJ, et al. Blood 2001	FL	34	CVP + INFa	PB	qPCR	BLC2	Molecular date contrasting clinical response
Ladetto M, Corradini P, Vallet S. et al. Blood 2002	FL	37	HDT-ASCT	BM, PB	N-PCR	BCL2, IGH	36 M DFS: 85% vs. 35% ($p < 0.001$)
Rambaldi A, Lazzari M, Manzoni C. et al. Blood 2002	FL	87	R-CHOP	BM, PB	N-PCR	BLC2	36 M FFR: 64% vs. 32% ($p = 0.006$)
Corradini P, Ladetto M., Zallio F, et al. J Clin Oncol. 2004	FL, MCL	35	R-HD + ASCT	BM, PB, harvest	N-PCR	BLC2, IGH	75 M relapse incidence: 88% vs. 8% ($p < 0.005$)
Rambaldi A, Carlotti E, Oldani E, et al. Blood 2005	FL	86	R-CHOP	BM, PB	qPCR	BCL2, IGH	60 M FFR: 64% vs. 32% ($p = 0.006$)
Ladetto M, Valet S., Benedetti F. et al. Leukemia 2006	FL	42	TBI-HDT-ASCT	BM, PB	PCR	BCL2, IGH	24 M median PFS: NR vs. 24 m ($p < 0.001$)
Brown JR, Feng Y, Gribben JG, et al. Biol Blood Marrow Transplant. 2007	FL	96	CHOP+TBI/ABMT	BM	N-PCR	BLC2	144 M PFS: 66.7% vs. 26.3%
Ladetto M, De Marco F, Benedetti F. et al. Blood 2008	FL	60	R-HDS + ASCT vs. R-CHOP	BM	N-PCR	BCL2	48 M PFS: 78% vs. 25% ($p < 0.001$)
Hirt C, Schuler F, Kiefer Thomas et al. B. Journal Haemat 2008	FL	43	R-MCP vs. MCP	PB	qPCR	BCL2, IGH	PFS NR vs. 27 m ($p < 0.02$)
Paszkiewicz KE, Kulik J, Fabisiewicz A, et al. Med Oncol. 2009	FL	75	Not specified	BM, PB	N-PCR	BCL2, IGH	PCR status doesn't influence PFS
Van Oers MH, Tonnissen E, Van Glabbeke M, et al. J Clin Oncol 2010	FL R/R	238	R-CHOP	BM/PB	qPCR	BCL2, IGH	PCR status doesn't influence PFS
Morschhauser F., Recher C, Milpied N, et al. Ann Onc 2012	FL	40	R weekly × 4 after ASCT	BM, PB	PCR	BCL2, IGH	Median PFS: NR vs. 1.6 y ($P = 0.0095$)
Ladetto M, Lobetti B C, Mantoan B, et al. Blood 2013	FL	51	R-FND + R maintenance or consolidation	BM	N-PCR, qPCR	BCL2, IGH	PFS 72% vs. 39% 3 y; ($p < 0.007$)
Galimberti S, Luminari S, Ciabatti E, et al. Clin Cancer Res. 2014	FL	415	R-CHOP vs. R-FC vs. R-CVP	BM, PB	N-PCR, qPCR	BCL2, IGH	24 M PFS 84% vs. 50% ($p < 0.014$)
Zohren F, Bruns I, Pechtel S, et al. Blood, 2015	FL	173	R-CHOP vs. BR	PB	qPCR	BCl2	PFS NR vs. 8.7 m ($p < 0.002$)
Pott C, Belada D, Danesi N, et al. ASH 2015	R/R FL	93	G-B vs. B	BM, PB	qPCR	BCL2, IGH	PFS NR vs. 74% at 2 y
Pott C, Hoster E, Kehden B, et al. Blood 2016	FL	696	G chemo vs. R chemo	BM, PB	qPCR	BCL2, IGH	EOI MRD– associated with longer PFS HR 0.35 ($p < 0.0001$)

FL follicular lymphoma, *MCL* mantle cell lymphoma, *TBI* total body irradiation, *ASCT* autologous stem cell transplant, *R-CHOP* rituximab, cyclophosphamide, hydroxydaunorubicin, oncovin, prednisone, *RTX* rituximab, *HDS* high dose scheme, *MCP* mitoxantrone, chlorambucil, prednisolone, *FND* fludarabine, mitoxantrone, dexametasone, *FC* fludarabine, cyclophosphamide, *CVP* cyclophosphamide vincristine, prednisone, *BR* bendamustine, rituximab, *G* obinutuzumab, *BM* bone marrow, *PB* pheripheral blood, *qPCR* quantitative polymerase chain reaction, *N-PCR* nested-PCR, *FFR* failure free survival, *PFS* progression free survival, *CR* complete remissione, *PR* partial remission, *SD* stable disease, *PD* progression disease, *NR* not reached, *EOI* end of induction

Table 3.2 Relevant literature on MRD detection in MCL

Study	Disease	Patients	Therapy	Tissue analyzed	Method	Marker	Clinical impact of MRD
Howard OM, Gribben JG, Neuberg D et al. J Clin Oncol 2002	MCL	40	R-CHOP	BM.PB	N-PCR	BCL1, IGH	MRD status doesn't impact PFS (16.5 vs. 18.8 M, $P = 0.51$)
Corradini P, Ladetto M., Zallio F, et al. J Clin Oncol. 2004	FL, MCL	35	R-HD + ASCT	BM, PB, harvest	N-PCR	BLC2, IGH	75Mrelapseincidence:88%MRD+vs.8%MRD–
Pott C, Schrader C, Gesk S, et al. Blood 2006	MCL	29	R-HD + TBI + ASCT	BM, PB, harvest	qPCR	IGH	Median PFS 92 vs. 21 M ($p < 0.001$)
Geisler CH, Kolstad A, Laurell A, et al. Blood 2008	MCL	79	RmaxiCHOP/R-HDAraC+ASCT	BM, PB	N-PCR	BCL1, IGH	Median PFS: NR vs. 18 M ($p < 0.001$)
Andersen NS, Pedersen LB, Laurell A et al. J Clin Oncol. 2009	MCL	78	RmaxiCHOP/R-HDAraC + ASCT– + R pre-emptive	BM, PB	N-PCR, qPCR	BCL1, IGH	Median RFS 43 M after pre emptive treatment
Pott C, Hoster E, Delfau-Larue MH et al. Blood 2010 (younger/elderly)	MCL	190	R-CHOP+TBI + ASCT vs. R-CHOP/R-DHAP+R-HDAraC+TBI + ASCT(youger); R-CHOP vs. R-FC (elderly)	BM, PB, harvest	qPCR	BCL1, IGH	24 M PFS 77% MRD– vs. 34% MRD+ ($p <$ 0.021)
Liu H, Johnson JL, Koval G, et al. Haematologica 2012	MCL	39	R-HD-MTX + maxi-CHOP + ASCT + R maintenance	BM, PB	qPCR	BCL1, IgH	36 M TTP: 82% MRD+ vs.48% MRD– (MRD at EOI)
Pott C, Macintyre E, Dalfau Laure MH. Et al. Abstr. ASH 2014	MCL	406	R-CHOP+TBI + ASCT vs. R-CHOP/R-DHAP+R-HDAraC+TBI + ASCT(youger); R-CHOP vs. R-FC (elderly)	PB	qPCR	BCL1, IGH	Median PFS 12 M: 5.8 Y MRD– vs. 3 Y MRD +; at 24 M: NR MRD– vs. 3.4 YMRD+; at 36 M: NR MRD– vs. 3.8 Y MRD+ ($p < 0.0001$)
Visco C, Chiappella A, Franceschetti S, ICML 2015	MCL	46	R-BAC500	BM, PB	N-PCR	BCL1, IgH	Median PFS was 2 years for MRD negative patients
Callanan M, Delfau MH, Macintyre E, et al. ASH 2015	MCL	178	R-DHAP+ R-BEAM +ASCT + R maintenance	BM, PB	qPCR	BCL1, IGH	36 M PFS without R maintenance 61.6% MRD+ vs. 83.9 MRD– ($p = 0.01$); with R maintenance 86 0.2% MRD+ vs. 91.8% MRD– ($p = 0.01$)
Kolstad A, Pedersen LB2, Eskelund CW et al. Biol Blood Marrow Transplant. 2017	MCL	183	RmaxiCHOP+HDAraC +/–Zevalin +ASCT	BM, PB	qPCR, N-PCR	BCL1, IGH	Median PFS: 20 M MRD+ vs. 142 M MRD– post ASCT ($p = 0.0001$)
Kaplan LD, Maurer MJ, Stock W et al. Abstr ASH 2018	MCL	42	CHOP+MTX + EAR+CBV-ASCT+ bortezomib consolidation vs. maintenance	BM	PCR	BCL1, IGH	8 PFS: 80% MRD– vs. 43.2% MRD+ (post induction) ($p = 0.009$)
Ferrero, Barbero D, Lo Schirico M, et al. Abstr. ASH 2018	MCL	163	3RCHOP + HDC + ASCT +/– Lenalidomide maintenance	BM, PB	N-PCR, qPCR	BCL1, IGH	36 M PFS: 25% MRD+ vs. 66% MRD– (after ASCT) ($p = 0.037$)
Klener P, Fronkova E, Kalinova M, et al. Hematol Oncol. 2018	MCL	67	R-CHOP/R-ARAC + R maintenance	BM, PB	qPCR	BCL1, IGH	MRD status doesn't impact PFS/OS

R-HDAraC rituximab, high dose cytarabine, *DHAP* dexametasone, high dose cytarabine, cisplatin, *MTX* metotrexate, *EAR* etoposide, cytarabine, rituximab, *CBV* cyclophosphamide, carmustine, etoposide, *BEAM* carmustine, etoposide, cytarabine, melphalan, *M* month, *Y* year patients still die of their disease. Therefore, the identification of patients at high risk of relapse is a major goal of clinical and translational research in the iNHL field. MRD is one of the most efficient tools for outcome prediction. One lymphoma-specific criticism to MRD detection has been the supposed "localized nature" of most lymphomas, which could hamper a successful detection of residual tumors in "liquid" tissues, such as peripheral blood (PB) and/or bone marrow (BM). Despite its reasonability, this hypothesis has been ruled out by a large bulk of data mainly focused on MCL and FL. Many reports have demonstrated that even apparently localized relapses are often heralded by signals of disease activity in PB or BM (Tables 3.1 and 3.2) [4–6]. Of course, the integration of imaging tools, such as positron emission tomography (PET) with laboratory-based MRD tools, is a major field of interest that could allow an even more complete characterization of these complex entities [7].

From a historical perspective, it should be noted that early studies in this field date back to the last decade of the previous millennium [8–10]. The last two decades have witnessed dramatic progress in therapeutic strategies as well as a careful improvement in technical performances of methods, which have acquired greater robustness, accuracy, applicability, and standardization, due to both intrinsic technical advancement and collaborative efforts for harmonization and standardization [2, 11–13].

The present chapter will start by describing available methods for MRD monitoring in indolent lymphomas and CLL. Then, the clinical prognostic value will be described in various disease entities with special focus on FL, MCL, and CLL, which have been more extensively studied. Finally, the integration of MRD with other prognostic tools and future perspectives will be discussed.

3.2 Methods for MRD Determination

Different tools have been developed to detect the presence and quantify the amount of residual lymphoma cells below the sensitivity threshold of conventional diagnostic techniques. These methods vary in terms of sensitivity, specificity, accuracy of target quantification, potential technical biases, and level of standardization among different laboratories [11, 12, 14, 15]. In this chapter, the most widely employed tools will be discussed, that is, flow cytometry (FC) and molecularly based tools, including PCR-based approaches, as well as the more recently developed next-generation sequencing (NGS). Both FC-based and molecular tools have undergone tremendous development during the last decade, with substantial improvement in their performances [11, 12, 16, 17]. Notably while in CLL, FC is a fully established methodology [18], in indolent lymphomas, such as MCL and FL, most clinical trials have employed RQ-PCR, which is currently the most "widely employed" approach in this setting. However, comparison studies are ongoing, and a change of paradigm might potentially occur in the next 5 years with the progressive implementation of novel PCR tools, next-generation FC, and NGS in the context of large multicenter trials.

3.2.1 MRD Detection by FC

Multiparameter flow cytometry (MFC) is a well-established method to diagnose hematologic malignancies in clinical routine. Immunophenotypic aberrations and the detection of immunoglobulin light-chain restriction are the principal means to identify malignant B-cell populations. The short turnaround time of less than 1 day and less labor-intensive approach compared to PCR or sequencing-based methods make it an attractive method for MRD detection [18].

MFC is applicable for MRD detection in about 95% of all CLL patients, thus making them extremely useful in clinical practice [19, 20]. In both diseases, a comparative analysis to AntiSense Oligonucleotides (ASO) primer RQ-PCR confirmed a sensitivity of 1E-4 as well as the high specificity of the technique [21–23].

The clinical significance of sensitive MRD flow has been demonstrated in CLL, including prospective randomized trials [24–29].

Furthermore, international consensus papers have been published on the evaluation of flow cytometry MRD in CLL setting (also in multiple myeloma disease, which is outside the scope of this chapter), with the aim of standardizing antibody panels and data interpretation [20, 30].

In contrast to CLL, there are no established MFC panels for MRD quantification in FL and MCL disease. One major obstacle is their high immunophenotypic heterogeneity, requiring more extensive marker combinations for highly sensitive MRD approaches.

Sensitivities of 10^{-2} can be achieved using two-color flow assays [31]; however, this is not sufficient for sensitive MRD detection. Four-color MFC (4-MFC) assays in MCL reliably detect the dissemination of MCL cells to PB or BM, but do not exceed a detection limit of 8 × 10E-4 [32]. In MCL, a recent publication showed that a single, eight-color ten-antibody MFC tube allows specific MRD assessment with a robust sensitivity of 0.01% in all patients [33]; however, even eight-color MFC approaches rarely exceed this limit of sensitivity [34]. Furthermore, the comparability of MFC-based MRD detection with RQ-PCR-based approaches in clinical trials needs careful evaluation as using the cutoff level of 0.01%, MFC detected MRD in only 80% of the cases that were MRD positive by real-time quantitative PCR [34]. Data for MFC-based MRD detection in FL are entirely lacking.

Therefore, there is a need for optimized MFC strategies, and the discovery of novel useful antigens allows the construction of optimized multicolor antibody panels and together with automated gating strategies massively improves sensitivity and standardized evaluation by MFC [35, 36].

The EuroFlow consortium currently develops standards for instrument setup, panel composition, and data interpretation [37, 38] and a quality control program for MFC-based MRD detection in various hematologic malignancies [39, 40]. These assays must be applied in future clinical trials with respect to their applicability and their prognostic impact.

3.2.2 MRD Detection by PCR-Based Methods

Minimal residual disease analysis by PCR-based methods investigates the persistence of residual tumor cells through the amplification of one or more tumor-specific molecular marker, that is, DNA sequences, which are ideally always absent in normal cells and always detectable in tumor cells [5, 41]. These sequences are used to design primers and probes suitable for MRD detection assays. Tumor markers employed in mature lymphoid tumors belong to two different categories: tumor-specific translocations and antigen–receptor rearrangements (Fig. 3.1a–c). Both can be used to design patient-specific primers and probes. When present, chromosomal translocations are excellent targets for MRD detection. The most widely used are the t(14;18) in FL and the t(11;14) in MCL. The t(14;18) originates from the juxtaposition between chromosome 18 and chromosome 14 involving the immunoglobulin heavy-chain (IgH) genes and the *bcl-2* gene (Fig. 3.1a) [42]. It occurs most frequently at four different clusters, including the major breakpoint region (MBR), identified in at least 50% of FL patients; three less-common regions, that is, the minor cluster region (mcr); and other two more recently identified clusters defined as 3′ MBR and 5′ mcr [42]. Overall, a molecular marker derived from t(14;18) can be obtained in approximately 70–85% of patients starting from a macroscopically infiltrated sample [43, 44]. The t(11;14) involving the *bcl1* locus and the IgH genes is an MCL-associated translocation (Fig. 3.1b). Only breakpoint clustering at the major translocation cluster (MTR) can be routinely amplified for MRD purposes [45, 46] (Fig. 3.1b). These are a minority of t(11;14)-positive cases and account for approximately 30% of all MCL patients [47]. The IgH rearrangement is theoretically a universal target for MRD determination in mature B-cell tumors (Fig. 3.1c). However, amplification and sequencing of this target is relatively simple in the absence of somatic hypermutation or with a modest somatic hypermutation, load such as in the case of MCL [2, 5]. On the other hand, amplification failure is common in somatically hypermutated tumors, such as FL. Therefore, IGHV sequencing is successful in 80–90% of patients with MCL but in only approximately 50% of patients with FL. Moreover, the presence of ongoing somatic hypermutation in FL might give rise to some concerns about the predictive value of IGHV MRD in this tumor as opposed to MCL, where the rearrangement is stable. For this reason as well as modest practicability of the IgH rearrangement, the t(14;18) is the preferred amplification target in FL, while the IgH rearrangement is the most frequently used MRD target in MCL (Fig. 3.1a, c).

First approaches to PCR-based detection of MRD were based on qualitative endpoint amplification approaches and particularly on nested PCR [8, 9, 48]. One of the major technical advances in MRD detection in lymphoid tumors has been the development and standardization of real-time quantitative-PCR tools [49–51]. RQ-PCR is robust, accurate, and reproducible and reduces considerably the risk of contamination. The value of RQ-PCR has been further increased by the development of multi-laboratory standardization efforts, which allowed to reach a very high level of reproducibility among different MRD laboratories [2]. This effort was originally undertaken in Europe in the context of the Euro-MRD consortium for acute lymphoblastic leukemia patients [52]. Over the last decade, the standardization effort of Euro-MRD has been applied also to MCL and FL. Currently, several multicenter trials include MRD monitoring performed at different laboratories all performing the analysis using the same standardized MRD tools in both FL and MCL.

Despite its advantages, RQ-PCR also has some limitations. It is not an absolute quantification tool, as it relies on a standard curve of samples with known amounts of target DNA. Several samples cannot be fully quantified and are defined "positive not quantifiable" (PNQ) [2, 5, 52]. Moreover, they are sensitive to PCR inhibitors, which may affect amplification kinetics and target quantification. The newly introduced droplet digital PCR (ddPCR) assay overcomes some of these limitations [11]. ddPCR is an absolute quantification method based on Poisson's statistics, and since it is based on endpoint amplification, it is less sensitive to PCR inhibitors. ddPCR sensitivity levels are comparable to qPCR and are potentially able to quantify a substantial proportion of cases classified as PNQ by RQ-PCR [11]. Although very promising from the technical point of view, ddPCR still needs to demonstrate to be as predictive as RQ-PCR in the context of large multicenter trials in both FL and MCL.

3.2.3 MRD Detection by Next-Generation Sequencing

High-throughput sequencing (HTS) of immunoglobulin (IG) or T-cell receptor (TR) gene rearrangements has been successfully developed to quantify MRD in lymphoid malignancies. A comparative analysis of our groups addressing the potential of NGS to overcome some of the limitations of ASO-RQ-PCR has shown that both methods have comparable sensitivity and further increase sensitivity and specificity [12].

The first step is a multiplex PCR for the amplification of V-D-J rearrangements of IG or TR genes. This is followed by a second-round PCR with barcoded primers for library preparation and subsequent high-throughput sequencing. The crucial step is then the correct identification of the index sequence identifying the tumor-specific IG/TR rearrangement. In contrast to RQ-PCR, the laborious design and testing of patient-specific assays is avoided as the same multiplex approach is applied to follow-up samples, with re-identification of the index sequence, allowing for MRD quantification. However, this requires a well-established bioinformatic approach.

In most published studies, a 5% cutoff of all sequences is used for the identification of the index clone [13, 53, 54]. This can be considerably difficult in samples where BM or PB is used for marker identification due to unrelated B- and T-cell clones that, depending on the degree of lymphoma infiltration, account for a considerable background of amplified sequences.

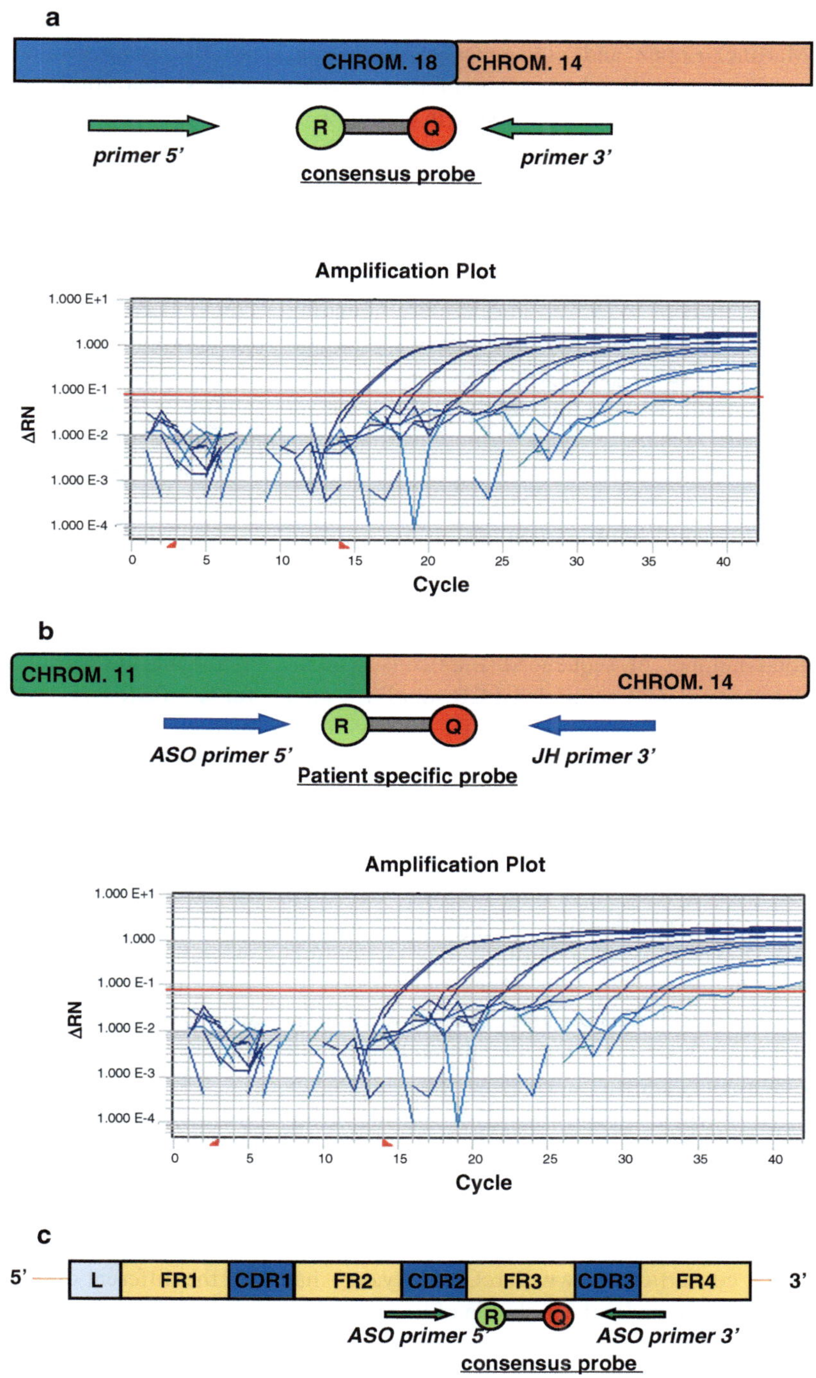

Fig. 3.1 Schematic representation of MRD detection assays by RQ-PCR. (**a**) Bcl-2/IgH translocation; (**b**) Bcl-1/IgH translocation; (**c**) IgH rearrangement (NB for this rearrangement validated assays can vary in ASO primer choice and positioning, i.e., 5′, or 3′, or both). *Chrom* chromosome, *L* leade region, *FR* framework region, *CDR* complementarity-determining region

A further issue in amplicon-based sequencing strategies is somatic mutations in primer-binding sites hampering proper primer binding. This is particularly important in mature B-cell malignancies, where the clonal IG index sequence might harbor considerable rates of somatic hypermutation (SHM) (e.g., multiple myeloma or follicular lymphoma and diffuse large B-cell lymphoma, DLBCL). This is shown in a series of Martinez-Lopez and colleagues [55] multiple myeloma patients, where a clonal IGH gene rearrangement was identified by NGS in only 63% of diagnostic BM samples, most probably due to somatic mutations of the IGH gene locus leading to mismatches at the primer-binding sites. In these cases, the addition of IGK and IGH DH-JH increases the overall identification rate of an index marker to 93%. Furthermore, ongoing SHM of the IG loci may lead to IGH clonal heterogeneity [56], resulting in a decrease of amplification efficacy and thereby to a false negative/low-MRD result.

A further aspect that has not been sufficiently addressed in recent publications is the correct MRD quantification particularly in the situation of low numbers of polyclonal background B cells. MRD quantification by counting the number of index sequences and dividing them by the total number of sequenced amplicons is error prone, as IG/TR multiplex PCR amplifies only rearranged IG/TR genes; that is, cells with the respective gene in germline configuration are not targeted. This might lead to false results particularly in situations with a low number of polyclonal background B cells, because preferential sequencing of IGH rearranged B cells might lead to a considerable overestimation of MRD. Therefore, standardized internal controls must be included in each sequencing reaction for correct MRD quantification. Currently, different approaches are proposed, like different plasmids containing known IGH gene rearrangements [54], or synthetic control templates spiked at limiting dilution into each sample and computing the average number of reads for each sequenced spiked synthetic template [57].

To address all these issues, the EuroClonality-NGS consortium (www.EuroClonality.org) has been formed under the umbrella of ESHLO, with the main objectives to develop, standardize, and validate the entire workflow of IG/TR NGS assays for (a) clonality assessment, (b) minimal residual disease detection, and (c) IG/TR gene repertoire analysis. An important section of this consortium is the development of a bioinformatic platform for standardized input processing, data selection and filtering, immunogenetic annotation of sequences, and comparative calculations and visualization. A bioinformatic pipeline (ARResT/Interrogate pipeline) has recently been published by the group and is being used for standardized MRD assessment by HTS [58].

Like all other MRD methods, the sensitivity of HTS is dependent on the number of analyzed cells and the corresponding amount of DNA. Therefore, a sensitivity of 1E-6 requires the appropriate amount of DNA for each reaction (for example, 10 μg DNA corresponding to 1.5 million cell equivalents). This is challenging and requires sequencing of several replicates as an amount of >1 μg DNA per reaction hampers proper PCR amplification.

Validated methods, standardized application, regular quality controls, and guidelines for result interpretation are a prerequisite for MRD-directed treatment in lymphoid malignancies. While this has been established since many years for RQ-PCR-based MRD detection by the Euro-MRD consortium [59–61], standards are lacking for NGS-based MRD quantification. As a consequence, the application of NGS for clinical decision making should not be performed unless data from randomized trials show a comparative validation with standard methods.

The most important aspect of any MRD assessment will require a rapid, reliable, and reproducible assay that is sensitive enough to detect disease prior to clinical relapse; HTS holds significant promise in this regard.

3.3 MRD in Follicular Lymphoma and Other Indolent Lymphomas

Of the different disease entities discussed in this review, FL was the first NHL histotype in which MRD was employed, and together with MCL, it is the NHL subtype in which MRD detection is most frequently used and where its predictive value is most clearly established (Table 3.1). The first experiences with nonstandardized qualitative tools at the Dana–Farber Cancer Institute date back to the 1990s and showed, in the autologous transplantation setting, that MRD status at the time of BM infusion and soon after transplantation has a long-term impact on the natural history of FL [9, 62]. Since then, several studies using similar or more accurate tools, such as RQ-PCR, have confirmed the major predictive value of MRD detection in FL (Table 3.1). When multivariate analysis was employed, the lack of molecular remission (MR) emerged as an independent predictor (Table 3.1). Only a minority of reports failed to demonstrate a predictive value for PCR-based MRD detection. In virtually all cases these studies investigated a very small patient series, used heterogeneous tissue sources, or contained major technical and interpretation biases, which explain why the impact of MRD on the outcome was not observed [63, 64].

From the methodological point of view, most earlier experiences were based on nonstandardized qualitative tools. However, since 2012, most high-quality studies have included the standardized RQ-PCR-based analysis. When both tools were employed, RQ-PCR usually showed a better performance in terms of outcome prediction in both FL and MCL [65]. In terms of tissue sources, both peripheral blood and bone marrow were analyzed in different studies. BM is more heavily infiltrated by FL compared to PB, both at diagnosis and in the remission phase. However, MRD on both tissues proved to be predictive for the outcome [44, 66].

The experiences accumulated thus far allow us to draw several relevant considerations:

(a) In the pre-rituximab era, autologous stem cell transplantations (ASCT)–based programs allowed a large proportion of patients with FL (up to 70%) to enter MR [9, 67]. This was in striking contrast with the nearly constant lack of molecular response in MCL patients [67, 68]. On the other hand, conventional chemotherapy achieved this goal in a minority of patients and only when used at diagnosis [9, 69].
(b) Rituximab dramatically increased the rate of MR in FL. Modern chemo-immunotherapy leads to MR rates like those observed with ASCT in the pre-rituximab age (50–80% depending on the study and schedule) [3, 44, 65, 66].
(c) Even following the introduction of rituximab, ASCT-based programs induce more MRs compared with conventional chemotherapy (70–80% vs. 0.50–60% in a Phase III study comparing the two treatments). Nevertheless, for those patients achieving MR, the outcome is similar regardless of the treatment received [70].
(d) Patients who did not achieve MR following conventional chemotherapy might achieve PCR negativity following consolidation with or without transplantation [65, 70].
(e) The use of more active monoclonal antibodies, such as obinutuzumab, ensures the achievement of higher MR rates [44, 66]. Interestingly, this benefit of obinotuzumab is particularly prominent when this agent is combined with less-intense treatments, such as CVP, indicating that a more active antibody might compensate for a less-intense chemotherapy in terms of MR achievement [44].
(f) Despite its predictive value, the first MRD-guided trial investigating whether patients achieving MRD negativity and PET negativity could skip rituximab maintenance was negative [71]. This demonstrates that even in the presence of maximal cytoreduction, rituximab maintenance remains beneficial but does not imply that MRD-based decision making could prove unsuccessful in other settings for both treatment intensification and de-intensification. This observation suggests that the optimal treatment modulation based on MRD should probably consider multiple time points in order to detect MRD reappearances rather than relying on a single time point analysis.

As previously mentioned, the great bulk of MRD data on truly indolent NHL subtypes was obtained in FL. Recently, MRD tools have been applied also in less-common subtypes. Lymphoplasmacytic lymphoma (or Waldenstrom macroglobulinemia) is an uncommon subtype characterized by the MYD88L265P point mutation in >90% cases. This mutation has been used to develop an MRD-based ddPCR, which proved suitable for MRD detection in terms of sensitivity and specificity [72]. Moreover, the applicability of MRD detection based on the IGHV rearrangement and the achievement of MR have been demonstrated in splenic marginal zone lymphoma after treatment with bendamustine and rituximab [73]. These findings are promising, but a demonstration of clinical impact on the outcome is still awaited.

3.4 MRD in Mantle Cell Lymphoma

In MCL, only in the era of combined Immunochemotherapy inducing high rates of clinical responses and in intensive treatment regimen with ASCT, the clinical relevance of MRD response could be documented.

In contrast to FL, the number of clinical trials evaluating the clinical impact of MRD in MCL is much lower (Table 3.2). cyclophosphamide, doxorubicin, vincristine, and prednisone (CHOP)-like chemotherapy without rituximab does not induce a relevant reduction of tumor load in MCL patients even among those achieving a clinical remission, indicating that CHOP monotherapy is not an optimal treatment for MCL [74].

First results from randomized trials were achieved in the European MCL Younger and Elderly trials, where combined immunochemotherapy was applied with or without ASCT in younger patients and anti-CD20 maintenance in patients ineligible for transplantation; it could be shown for the first time that relevant rates of MRD response of 40% could be achieved after R-CHOP treatment [75].

The impact of treatment on tumor load in MCL can be directly measured by MRD response after each treatment block of induction treatment. This has been convincingly demonstrated by the systematic analysis of MRD response in the context of the European MCL studies, which included a prospective MRD monitoring program.

The impact of MRD monitoring in MCL can be summarized as follows:

(a) Intensification of induction treatment by high-dose cytarabine in the alternating R-CHOP/R-DHAP arm of the European MCL Younger trial demonstrated increased MRD response rates of 66% compared to R-CHOP, with 39% occurring already at midterm induction [75], and led to a new standard for younger and fit patients. The Nordic MCL3 study provided confirmatory results to the European MCL Younger trial [76].

(b) High-dose chemotherapy and subsequent stem cell retransfusion (ASCT) have improved clinical response and long-term survival in MCL [77, 78] and is currently the standard of care in younger patients with MCL. That ASCT has still an impact on molecular response, and the outcome of MCL could be demonstrated in the European MCL studies. ASCT increases molecular remission rates after R-CHOP from 47 to 68% in PB and from 26 to 59% in BM. After R-CHOP/R-DHAP, the impact is mainly in BM, where MRD negativity is increased from 61% pre-transplant to 79% thereafter [75].

(c) MRD status after ASCT is strongly prognostic for Progression Free Survival (PFS), with 4-year PFS of about 38% (median PFS about 3 years) [75] and is also seen after adjustment for MIPI, Ki-67 index, CT status pre-ASCT, and PET status pre-ASCT. Similar results have been shown by the LYMA trial of the LYSA [79] and also in the Italian MCL0208 trial investigating a similar tumor population. In this study some pre-ASCT time points and all post-ASCT time points were highly predictive for the outcome [80].

(d) The efficiency of induction treatment prior to ASCT measured by the MRD status before ASCT impact on prognosis. Long-term follow-up of patients in clinical remission by MRD is of clinical importance, as data of the European MCL network demonstrate that reappearance of MRD in clinical remission is associated with clinical relapse.

(e) For long-term disease control, not only the achievement of MRD response but also its maintenance is a prerequisite. This is demonstrated by results of the European MCL trials, where the MRD status during the first year after ASCT of maintenance in elderly patients was strongly prognostic for subsequent PFS [75].

Overall, there is convincing evidence that MRD positivity or MRD reappearance after the currently recommended standard treatment is strongly predictive for imminent clinical relapse within 1–2 years, whereas the outcome of MCL patients in sustained molecular remission appears favorable. This observation stimulates treatment concepts adapted to MRD response independent of the preceding treatment and might include preemptive treatment approaches with novel drugs.

3.5 MRD in Chronic Lymphocytic Leukemia

In CLL, flow cytometry is the standard method for MRD detection. MRD negativity in CLL is defined as <1 CLL cell detectable per 10,000 leukocytes (0.01%). The simplest approaches to measure MRD in CLL are CD19/CD5 co-expression analysis, assessment of light-chain restriction by flow cytometry, and consensus primer PCR analysis of clonal IGHV rearrangements [81, 82]. However, these methods do not reach a sensitivity of <1% in the setting of polyclonal B cells and therefore are not suited for sensitive MRD monitoring.

Four-colour flow-cytometric approaches predominantly based on CD5, CD20, and CD79b expression have been reported, and all show a sensitivity that is tenfold higher than flow-cytometric approaches based on CD19/CD5 and κ/λ combinations. High-sensitivity quantitative PCR approaches are also available and target the IGHV rearrangement, the fingerprint of the clonal CLL population. Allele-specific quantitative PCR (ASO-RQ-PCR) has been established as the most sensitive method for the detection of residual disease reaching a sensitivity of 0.001% [22, 83]. ASO-RQ-PCR can enumerate CLL cells accurately when they represent more than 0.01% of leukocytes but can provide qualitative results only below this level [84].

Reproducible high sensitivity is also achieved by NGS-based approaches that in contrast to RQ-PCR allows quantification below the critical threshold of 0.01% [85]. However, whether sensitivity higher than 0.01% is needed at all for prognostication in CLL is currently unclear.

The key advantages of flow cytometry in comparison to ASO-RQ-PCR is that the same markers are used for all patients and that results are generated rapidly using a standard marker set in real time [81, 86].

In most of the clinical studies evaluating the impact of MRD response on outcome, four-color flow cytometry has been used and a cut-off of 0.01% has been defined as clinically relevant [87].

There is a good correlation between the level of disease in peripheral blood and bone marrow, and both sites can be used for the assessment of MRD, unless the treatment includes rituximab or alemtuzumab [27, 86]. In the setting of effective antibody treatment, bone marrow might be more informative for MRD [24]. Therapeutic antibodies preferentially deplete the peripheral blood, and therefore, peripheral blood assessment during treatment is likely to underestimate the residual tumor load but can still provide prognostic information [24, 88].

A complete MRD response is always associated with improved progression-free survival; in most studies, the improvement is highly significant and improved overall survival may also be demonstrated [24, 27, 89–92]. The clinical relevance of MRD is well established in CLL and is known to be an important predictor of outcome. Novel treatment strategies, including chemotherapy-free regimen with BCL2- or B-cell receptor (BCR) signal inhibitors, aim at more personalized approaches and guide the duration of treatment according to MRD response in bone marrow [93] in order to reduce toxicity by comparable efficiency. This change of treatment paradigm is possible by the availability of standardized MRD methods [35, 38]. Whether disease eradication at least in a subgroup of patients with early and deep MRD response and good prognostics factors will be possible by individualized treatment approaches is currently tested in modern treatment concepts.

3.6 Integrating MRD and Imaging Tools

Response assessment is very much improved by metabolic response assessment measured by 18F-fluorodeoxyglucose positron emission tomography-computed tomography (18F-FDG PET-CT). There are convincing data in follicular lymphoma showing that 18F-FDG PET-CT has become a surrogate for treatment success or failure [94]. More recently, PET has been reported to be a reliable predictor of outcome in follicular lymphoma requiring treatment [95], and prospective trials to test PET-guided therapy in this disease are anticipated.

Therefore, it is tempting to speculate whether the combination of both PET and MRD response might identify prognostic subgroups among responders who might be (a) functionally cured in the case of PET and MRD response or (b) candidates for a response-adapted treatment, including treatment escalation and de-escalation, in case of persistent PET and/or MRD positivity.

Data for the prognostic value of combining both methods for an improved response assessment emerge from a subgroup analysis of the Gallium trial in untreated primary FL. Achievement of a complete metabolic response (CMR) or MRD at EOI was prognostic for prolonged PFS and overall survival. A combined analysis of PET and MRD response was possible in 298 patients at the end of induction treatment with immunochemotherapy. CMR was achieved in 266 (89%) and MRD response in 275 (92%) of 298 evaluable patients. Of 266 patients in CMR, 250 (94%) were MRD negative in parallel. Median follow-up in the evaluable group was 44 months. In the patient group with both CMR and MRD-negative response 2.5-year PFS (from EOI) was 85% (95% CI: 80–89), compared with 69% (95% CI: 40–86) in the CMR and MRD-positive group. Patients achieving only either CMR or MRD negativity had a higher risk of progression or death (>2.1-fold) compared to patients who achieved both [96].

This suggests that for response-adapted treatment strategies, both methods for response assessment are required.

However, if MRD response is understood as a surrogate parameter for treatment efficiency and is associated with an improved outcome, treatment reduction might not be the right concept for response-adapted treatment. This is supported by results of the interim analysis of the FOLL12 trial conducted by the Fondazione Italiana Linfomi, who performed a response-adapted maintenance strategy in a Phase III randomized trial. The treatment consisted of a standard maintenance arm in comparison to an experimental treatment arm, where PET- and MRD-negative patients received no rituximab maintenance, while PET/MRD-positive patients received an intensified treatment with radioimmunotherapy and standard rituximab maintenance [71]. The 3-year PFS in the experimental arm was significantly worse with 69 months compared to 84 months for the standard maintenance. Further studies are needed to challenge the current concept of maintenance in follicular lymphomas.

3.7 Future Perspectives

MRD diagnostics has become an increasingly important tool for the measurement of treatment efficiency in clinical trials and estimation of prognosis in mature B-cell malignancies.

This also includes the evaluation of new treatment modalities, where MRD measurements can demonstrate the effectiveness of the novel treatment and can also be used as a surrogate endpoint in clinical trials.

Consequently, standardized MRD diagnostics should be available for the assessment of treatment response in each individual patient, to be used for personalized medicine and accurate risk-group assessment.

A major disadvantage of the currently used methods for MRD is their restriction to only a subset of the patient cohort due to technical reasons. Next-generation sequencing might bridge this gap and might raise the number of patients with a sensitive MRD marker in clinical trials. However, the validation of NGS as a clinical endpoint is currently lacking for all main B-cell malignancies.

Additionally, standardized technical procedures have to be established for multicenter application, including sensitivity definition, MRD cutoff levels for risk-group definition, practical application conditions, as well as result reporting.

This requires an international effort and a comparison with currently used methods as well regular quality controls, but this is highly necessary with respect to in vitro diagnostics.

In the light of plenty of novel treatment options, MRD assessment will be highly relevant as an early read-out parameter in clinical trials and study endpoint. Furthermore, MRD and metabolic response will be the best tool for risk stratification and individualized treatment.

References

1. Gascoyne RD, Nadel B, Pasqualucci L, Fitzgibbon J, Payton JE, Melnick A, Weigert O, Tarte K, Gribben JG, Friedberg JW, Seymour JF, Cavalli F, Zucca E. Follicular lymphoma: state-of-the-art ICML workshop in Lugano 2015. Hematol Oncol. 2017;35:397–407.
2. Pott C. Minimal residual disease detection in mantle cell lymphoma: technical aspects and clinical relevance. Semin Hematol. 2011;48:172–84.
3. Galimberti S, Luminari S, Ciabatti E, Grassi S, Guerrini F, Dondi A, Marcheselli L, Ladetto M, Piccaluga PP, Gazzola A, Mannu C, Monitillo L, Mantoan B, Del Giudice I, Della Starza I, Cavalli M, Arcaini L, Tucci A, Palumbo GA, Rigacci L, Pulsoni A, Vitolo U, Boccomini C, Vallisa D, Bertoldero G, Gaidano G, Musto P, Petrini M, Federico M. Minimal residual disease after conventional treatment significantly impacts on progression-free survival of patients with follicular lymphoma: the FIL FOLL05 trial. Clin Cancer Res. 2014;20:6398–405.
4. Hoster E, Pott C. Minimal residual disease in mantle cell lymphoma: insights into biology and impact on treatment. Hematology. 2016;2016:437–45.
5. Ferrero S, Drandi D, Mantoan B, Ghione P, Omedè P, Ladetto M. Minimal residual disease detection in lymphoma and multiple myeloma: impact on therapeutic paradigms. Hematol Oncol. 2011;29:167–76.
6. Gritti G, Pavoni C, Rambaldi A. Is there a role for minimal residual disease monitoring in follicular lymphoma in. Mediterr J Hematol Infect Dis. 2017;9(1): e2017010.
7. Luminari S, Galimberti S, Versari A, Biasoli I, Anastasia A, Rusconi C, Ferrari A, Petrini M, Manni M, Federico M. Positron emission tomography response and minimal residual disease impact on progression-free survival in patients with follicular lymphoma. A subset analysis from the FOLL05 trial of the Fondazione Italiana Linfomi. Haematologica. 2016;101:e66–8.
8. Gribben JG, Freedman A, Woo SD, Blake K, Shu RS, Freeman G, Longtine JA, Pinkus GS, Nadler LM. All advanced stage non-Hodgkin's lymphomas with a polymerase chain reaction amplifiable breakpoint of bcl-2 have residual cells containing the bcl-2 rearrangement at evaluation and after treatment. Blood. 1991;78:3275–80.
9. Gribben JG, Freedman AS, Neuberg D, Roy DC, Blake KW, Woo SD, Grossbard ML, Rabinowe SN, Coral F, Freeman GJ. Immunologic purging of marrow assessed by PCR before autologous bone marrow transplantation for B-cell lymphoma. N Engl J Med. 1991;325:1525–33.
10. Gribben JG, Neuberg D, Freedman AS, Gimmi CD, Pesek KW, Barber M, Saporito L, Woo SD, Coral F, Spector N. Detection by polymerase chain reaction of residual cells with the bcl-2 translocation is associated with increased risk of relapse after autologous bone marrow transplantation for B-cell lymphoma. Blood. 1993;81:3449–57.
11. Drandi D, Kubiczkova-Besse L, Ferrero S, Dani N, Passera R, Mantoan B, Gambella M, Monitillo L, Saraci E, Ghione P, Genuardi E, Barbero D, Omedè P, Barberio D, Hajek R, Vitolo U, Palumbo A, Cortelazzo S, Boccadoro M, Inghirami G, Ladetto M. Minimal residual disease detection by droplet digital PCR in multiple myeloma, mantle cell lymphoma, and follicular lymphoma: a comparison with real-time PCR. J Mol Diagn. 2015;17:652–60.
12. Ladetto M, Brüggemann M, Monitillo L, Ferrero S, Pepin F, Drandi D, Barbero D, Palumbo A, Passera R, Boccadoro M, Ritgen M, Gökbuget N, Zheng J, Carlton V, Trautmann H, Faham M, Pott C. Next-generation sequencing and real-time quantitative PCR for minimal residual disease detection in B-cell disorders. Leukemia. 2014;28:1299–307.
13. Ladetto M, Bruggemann M, Monitillo L, Ferrero S, Pepin F, Drandi D, Barbero D, Palumbo A, Passera R, Boccadoro M, Ritgen M, Gokbuget N, Zheng J, Carlton V, Trautmann H, Faham M, Pott C. Next-generation sequencing and real-time quantitative PCR for minimal residual disease detection in B-cell disorders. Leukemia. 2014;28:1299–307.
14. Pott C, Bruggemann M, Ritgen M, van der Velden VH, van Dongen JJ, Kneba M. MRD detection in B-cell non-Hodgkin lymphomas using Ig gene rearrangements and chromosomal translocations as targets for real-time quantitative PCR. Methods Mol Biol. 2013;971:175–200.
15. Rawstron AC, Hillmen P. Assessing minimal residual disease in chronic lymphocytic leukemia. Curr Hematol Malig Rep. 2008;3:47–53.
16. Brüggemann M, Kotrová M, Knecht H, Bartram J, Boudjogrha M, Bystry V, Fazio G, Froňková E, Giraud M, Grioni A, Hancock J, Herrmann D, Jiménez C, Krejci A, Moppett J, Reigl T, Salson M, Scheijen B, Schwarz M, Songia S, Svaton M, van Dongen JJM,

Villarese P, Wakeman S, Wright G, Cazzaniga G, Davi F, García-Sanz R, Gonzalez D, Groenen PJTA, Hummel M, Macintyre EA, Stamatopoulos K, Pott C, Trka J, Darzentas N, Langerak AW. Standardized next-generation sequencing of immunoglobulin and T-cell receptor gene recombinations for MRD marker identification in acute lymphoblastic leukaemia; a EuroClonality-NGS validation study. Leukemia. 2019;33:2241–53.

17. Böttcher S. Flow Cytometric MRD detection in selected mature B-cell malignancies. New York: Humana Press; 2019. p. 157–97.
18. Böttcher S, Ritgen M, Kneba M. Flow cytometric MRD detection in selected mature B-cell malignancies. Methods Mol Biol. 2013;971:149–74.
19. Rawstron AC, Orfao A, Beksac M, Bezdickova L, Brooimans RA, Bumbea H, Dalva K, Fuhler G, Gratama J, Hose D, Kovarova L, Lioznov M, Mateo G, Morilla R, Mylin AK, Omede P, Pellat-Deceunynck C, Perez AM, Petrucci M, Ruggeri M, Rymkiewicz G, Schmitz A, Schreder M, Seynaeve C, Spacek M, de Tute RM, Van VE, Weston-Bell N, Owen RG, San Miguel JF, Sonneveld P, Johnsen HE. Report of the European Myeloma Network on multiparametric flow cytometry in multiple myeloma and related disorders. Haematologica. 2008;93:431–8.
20. Rawstron AC, Villamor N, Ritgen M, Bottcher S, Ghia P, Zehnder JL, Lozanski G, Colomer D, Moreno C, Geuna M, Evans PAS, Natkunam Y, Coutre SE, Avery ED, Rassenti LZ, Kipps TJ, Caligaris-Cappio F, Kneba M, Byrd JC, Hallek MJ, Montserrat E, Hillmen P. International standardized approach for flow cytometric residual disease monitoring in chronic lymphocytic leukaemia. Leukemia. 2007;21:956–64.
21. Bö Ttcher S, Stilgenbauer S, Busch R, Brü Ggemann M, Raff T, Pott C, Fischer K, Fingerle-Rowson G, Dö Hner H, Hallek M, Kneba M, Ritgen M. Standardized MRD flow and ASO IGH RQ-PCR for MRD quantification in CLL patients after rituximab-containing immunochemotherapy: a comparative analysis. Leukemia. 2009;23:2007–17.
22. Bottcher S, Ritgen M, Pott C, Bruggemann M, Raff T, Stilgenbauer S, Dohner H, Dreger P, Kneba M, Böttcher S, Ritgen M, Pott C, Brüggemann M, Raff T, Stilgenbauer S, Döhner H, Dreger P, Kneba M. Comparative analysis of minimal residual disease detection using four-color flow cytometry, consensus IgH-PCR, and quantitative IgH PCR in CLL after allogeneic and autologous stem cell transplantation. Leukemia. 2004;18:1637–45.
23. Sarasquete ME, García-Sanz R, González D, Martínez J, Mateo G, Martínez P, Ribera JM, Hernández JM, Lahuerta JJ, Orfão A, González M, San Miguel JF. Minimal residual disease monitoring in multiple myeloma: a comparison between allelic-specific oligonucleotide real-time quantitative polymerase chain reaction and flow cytometry. Haematologica. 2005;90:1365–72.
24. Böttcher S, Ritgen M, Fischer K, Stilgenbauer S, Busch RM, Fingerle-Rowson G, Fink AM, Buhler A, Zenz T, Wenger MK, Mendila M, Wendtner CM, Eichhorst BF, Dohner H, Hallek MJ, Kneba M. Minimal residual disease quantification is an independent predictor of progression-free and overall survival in chronic lymphocytic leukemia: a multivariate analysis from the randomized GCLLSG CLL8 trial. J Clin Oncol. 2012;30:980–8.
25. Fink AM, Böttcher S, Ritgen M, Fischer K, Pflug N, Eichhorst B, Wendtner C-M, Winkler D, Bühler A, Zenz T, Staib P, Mayer J, Hensel M, Hopfinger G, Wenger M, Fingerle-Rowson G, Döhner H, Kneba M, Stilgenbauer S, Busch R, Hallek M. Prediction of poor outcome in CLL patients following first-line treatment with fludarabine, cyclophosphamide and rituximab. Leukemia. 2013;27:1949–52.
26. Dreger P, Ritgen M, Bottcher S, Schmitz N, Kneba M. The prognostic impact of minimal residual disease assessment after stem cell transplantation for chronic lymphocytic leukemia: is achievement of molecular remission worthwhile? Leukemia. 2005;19:1135–8.
27. Moreton P, Kennedy B, Lucas G, Leach M, Rassam SMB, Haynes A, Tighe J, Oscier D, Fegan C, Rawstron A, Hillmen P. Eradication of minimal residual disease in B-cell chronic lymphocytic leukemia after Alemtuzumab therapy is associated with prolonged survival. J Clin Oncol. 2005;23:2971–9.
28. Varghese AM, Rawstron AC, Hillmen P. Eradicating minimal residual disease in chronic lymphocytic leukemia: should this be the goal of treatment? Curr Hematol Malig Rep. 2010;5:35–44.
29. Paiva B, Cervero J, Mateo G, Pe JJ, Montalba MA, Sureda A, Montejano L, Gutie NC, Garcı A, Mateos MV, Lo MC, Garcı R, Galende J, Herna J, Palomera L, Carrera D, Martı R, De Rubia J, Martı A, Blade J, Lahuerta JJ, Orfao A. Multiparameter flow cytometric remission is the most relevant prognostic factor for multiple myeloma patients who undergo autologous stem cell transplantation. Blood. 2008;112:4017–23.
30. Arroz M, Came N, Lin P, Chen W, Yuan C, Lagoo A, Monreal M, de Tute R, Vergilio JA, Rawstron AC, Paiva B. Consensus guidelines on plasma cell myeloma minimal residual disease analysis and reporting. Cytometry B Clin Cytom. 2016;90:31–9.
31. Fukushima PI, Nguyen PKT, O'Grady P, Stetler-Stevenson M. Flow cytometric analysis of kappa and lambda light chain expression in evaluation of specimens for B-cell neoplasia. Cytometry. 1996;26:243–52.
32. Bottcher S, Ritgen M, Buske S, Gesk S, Klapper W, Hoster E, Hiddemann W, Unterhalt M, Dreyling M, Siebert R, Kneba M, Pott C, on behalf of the EU MCL MRD Group. Minimal residual disease detection in mantle cell lymphoma: methods and significance of four-color flow cytometry compared to consensus IGH-polymerase chain reaction at initial staging and for follow-up examinations. Haematologica. 2008;93:551–9.
33. Cheminant M, Derrieux C, Touzart A, Schmit S, Grenier A, Trinquand A, Delfau-Larue MH, Lhermitte L, Thieblemont C, Ribrag V, Cheze S, Sanhes L,

Jardin F, Lefrère F, Delarue R, Hoster E, Dreyling M, Asnafi V, Hermine O, Macintyre E. Minimal residual disease monitoring by 8-color flow cytometry in mantle cell lymphoma: an EU-MCL and LYSA study. Haematologica. 2016;101:336–45.

34. Chovancová J, Bernard T, Stehlíková O, Šálek D, Janíková A, Mayer J, Doubek M. Detection of minimal residual disease in mantle cell lymphoma-establishment of novel eight-color flow cytometry approach. Cytometry B Clin Cytom. 2015;88:92–100.
35. Flores-Montero J, Flores LS, Paiva B, Puig N, García-Sánchez O, Böttcher S, van der Velden VHJ, Pérez-Morán J-J, Vidriales M-B, García-Sanz R, Jimenez C, González M, Martinez-López J, Mateos AC, Grigore G-E, Fluxá R, Pontes R, Caetano J, Sedek L, del Cañizo M-C, Bladé J, Lahuerta J-J, Aguilar C, Bárez A, García-Mateo A, Labrador J, Leoz P, Aguilera-Sanz C, San-Miguel J, Mateos M-V, Durie B, van Dongen JJM, Orfao A. Next generation flow (NGF) for highly sensitive and standardized detection of minimal residual disease in multiple myeloma. Leukemia. 2017;31(10):2094–103.
36. Costa ES, Pedreira CE, Barrena S, Lecrevisse Q, Flores J, Quijano S, Almeida J, del Carmen G, Bottcher S, van Dongen JJM, Orfao A. Automated pattern-guided principal component analysis vs expert-based immunophenotypic classification of B-cell chronic lymphoproliferative disorders: a step forward in the standardization of clinical immunophenotyping. Leukemia. 2010;24:1927–33.
37. van Dongen JJM, Lhermitte L, Bottcher S, Almeida J, van der Velden VHJ, Flores-Montero J. EuroFlow antibody panels for standardized n-dimensional flow cytometric immunophenotyping of normal, reactive and malignant leukocytes. Leukemia. 2012;26:1908–75.
38. Kalina T, Flores-Montero J, van der Velden VHJ, Martin-Ayuso M, Böttcher S, Ritgen M, Almeida J, Lhermitte L, Asnafi V, Mendonça A, de Tute R, Cullen M, Sedek L, Vidriales MB, Pérez JJ, te Marvelde JG, Mejstrikova E, Hrusak O, Szczepański T, van Dongen JJM, Orfao A. EuroFlow standardization of flow cytometer instrument settings and immunophenotyping protocols. Leukemia. 2012;26:1986–2010.
39. Theunissen P, Mejstrikova E, Sedek L, van der Sluijs-Gelling AJ, Gaipa G, Bartels M, Sobral da Costa E, Kotrová M, Novakova M, Sonneveld E, Buracchi C, Bonaccorso P, Oliveira E, te Marvelde JG, Szczepanski T, Lhermitte L, Hrusak O, Lecrevisse Q, Grigore GE, Froňková E, Trka J, Brüggemann M, Orfao A, van Dongen JJM, van der Velden VHJ. Standardized flow cytometry for highly sensitive MRD measurements in B-cell acute lymphoblastic leukemia. Blood. 2017;129:347–57.
40. Kalina T, Flores-Montero J, Lecrevisse Q, Pedreira CE, van der Velden VHJ, Novakova M, Mejstrikova E, Hrusak O, Böttcher S, Karsch D, Sedek Ł, Trinquand A, Boeckx N, Caetano J, Asnafi V, Lucio P, Lima M, Helena Santos A, Bonaccorso P, van der Sluijs-Gelling AJ, Langerak AW, Martin-Ayuso M, Szczepański T, van Dongen JJM, Orfao A. Quality assessment program for EuroFlow protocols: summary results of four-year (2010-2013) quality assurance rounds. Cytometry A. 2015;87:145–56.
41. Pott C, Brüggemann M, Ritgen M, Van Der Velden VHJ, Van Dongen JJM, Kneba M. MRD detection in B-cell non-Hodgkin lymphomas using Ig gene rearrangements and chromosomal translocations as targets for real-time quantitative PCR. Methods Mol Biol. 2013;971:175–200.
42. Weinberg OK, Ai WZ, Mariappan MR, Shum C, Levy R, Arber DA. "Minor" BCL2 breakpoints in follicular lymphoma: frequency and correlation with grade and disease presentation in 236 cases. J Mol Diagn. 2007;9:530–7.
43. Vitolo U, Ladetto M, Boccomini C, Baldini L, De Angelis F, Tucci A, Botto B, Chiappella A, Chiarenza A, Pinto A, De Renzo A, Zaja F, Castellino C, Bari A, Alvarez De Celis I, Evangelista A, Parvis G, Gamba E, Lobetti-Bodoni C, Ciccone G, Rossi G. Rituximab maintenance compared with observation after brief first-line R-FND chemoimmunotherapy with rituximab consolidation in patients age older than 60 years with advanced follicular lymphoma: a phase III randomized study by the Fondazione Italiana Lin. J Clin Oncol. 2013;31:3351–9.
44. Pott C, Hoster E, Kehden B, Unterhalt M, Herold M, van der Jagt R, Janssens A, Kneba M, Mayer M, Pocock C, Danesi N, Fingerle-Rowson G, Harbron C, Mundt K, Marcus RE, Hiddemannnn W. Minimal residual disease in patients with follicular lymphoma treated with Obinutuzumab or rituximab as first-line induction Immunochemotherapy and maintenance in the phase 3 GALLIUM study. Blood. 2016;128:abstract 623.
45. Rimokh R, Berger F, Delsol G, Digonnet I, Rouault JP, Tigaud JD, Gadoux M, Coiffier B, Bryon PA, Magaud JP. Detection of the chromosomal translocation t(11;14) by polymerase chain reaction in mantle cell lymphomas. Blood. 1994;83:1871–5.
46. Pott C, Tiemann M, Linke B, Ott MM, von Hofen M, Bolz I, Hiddemann W, Parwaresch R, Kneba M. Structure of Bcl-1 and IgH-CDR3 rearrangements as clonal markers in mantle cell lymphomas. Leukemia. 1998;12:1630–7.
47. Pott C, Hoster E, Delfau-Larue MH, Beldjord K, Bottcher S, Asnafi V, Plonquet A, Siebert R, Callet-Bauchu E, Andersen N, van Dongen JJ, Klapper W, Berger F, Ribrag V, van Hoof AL, Trneny M, Walewski J, Dreger P, Unterhalt M, Hiddemann W, Kneba M, Kluin-Nelemans HC, Hermine O, Macintyre E, Dreyling M. Molecular remission is an independent predictor of clinical outcome in patients with mantle cell lymphoma after combined immunochemotherapy: a European MCL intergroup study. Blood. 2010;115:3215–23.
48. Voena C, Malnati M, Majolino I, Faga G, Montefusco V, Farina L, Santoro A, Ladetto M, Boccadoro M, Corradini P. Detection of minimal residual disease by real-time PCR can be used as a surrogate marker to evaluate the graft-versus-myeloma effect after

allogeneic stem cell transplantation. Bone Marrow Transplant. 2003;32:791–3.
49. Donovan JW, Ladetto M, Zou G, Neuberg D, Poor C, Bowers D, Gribben JG. Immunoglobulin heavy-chain consensus probes for real-time PCR quantification of residual disease in acute lymphoblastic leukemia. Blood. 2000;95(8):2651–8.
50. Ladetto M, Sametti S, Donovan JW, Ferrero D, Astolfi M, Mitterer M, Ricca I, Drandi D, Corradini P, Coser P, Pileri A, Gribben JG, Tarella C. A validated real-time quantitative PCR approach shows a correlation between tumor burden and successful ex vivo purging in follicular lymphoma patients. Exp Hematol. 2001;29:183–93.
51. Bruggemann M, Droese J, Bolz I, Luth P, Pott C, von Neuhoff N, Scheuering U, Kneba M. Improved assessment of minimal residual disease in B cell malignancies using fluorogenic consensus probes for real-time quantitative PCR. Leukemia. 2000;14:1419–25.
52. Van Der Velden V, Cazzaniga G, Schrauder A, Hancock J, Bader P, Panzer-Grumayer E, Flohr T, Sutton R. Analysis of minimal residual disease by Ig/TCR gene rearrangements: guidelines for interpretation of real-time quantitative PCR data. Leukemia. 2007;21:604–11.
53. Logan AC, Gao H, Wang C, Sahaf B, Jones CD, Marshall EL, Buño I, Armstrong R, Fire AZ, Weinberg KI, Mindrinos M, Zehnder JL, Boyd SD, Xiao W, Davis RW, Miklos DB. High-throughput VDJ sequencing for quantification of minimal residual disease in chronic lymphocytic leukemia and immune reconstitution assessment. Proc Natl Acad Sci. 2011;108:21194–9.
54. Faham M, Zheng J, Moorhead M, Carlton VEH, Stow P, Coustan-Smith E, Pui CH, Campana D. Deep-sequencing approach for minimal residual disease detection in acute lymphoblastic leukemia. Blood. 2012;120:5173–80.
55. Martinez-Lopez J, Lahuerta JJ, Pepin F, González M, Barrio S, Ayala R, Puig N, Montalban MA, Paiva B, Weng L, Jiménez C, Sopena M, Moorhead M, Cedena T, Rapado I, Mateos MV, Rosiñol L, Oriol A, Blanchard MJ, Martínez R, Bladé J, San Miguel J, Faham M, García-Sanz R. Prognostic value of deep sequencing method for minimal residual disease detection in multiple myeloma. Blood. 2014;123:3073–9.
56. Stamatopoulos K, Kosmas C, Belessi C, Stavroyianni N, Kyriazopoulos P, Papadaki T. Molecular insights into the immunopathogenesis of follicular lymphoma. Immunol Today. 2000;21:298–305.
57. Wu D, Emerson RO, Sherwood A, Loh ML, Angiolillo A, Howie B, Vogt J, Rieder M, Kirsch I, Carlson C, Williamson D, Wood BL, Robins H. Detection of minimal residual disease in B lymphoblastic leukemia by high-throughput sequencing of IGH. Clin Cancer Res. 2014;20:4540–8.
58. Bystry V, Reigl T, Krejci A, Demko M, Hanakova B, Grioni A, Knecht H, Schlitt M, Dreger P, Sellner L, Herrmann D, Pingeon M, Boudjoghra M, Rijntjes J, Pott C, Langerak AW, Groenen PJTA, Davi F, Brüggemann M, Darzentas N. ARResT/interrogate: an interactive immunoprofiler for IG/TR NGS data. Bioinformatics. 2017;33:435–7.
59. van Dongen JJM, van der Velden VHJ, Brüggemann M, Orfao A. Minimal residual disease (MRD) diagnostics in acute lymphoblastic leukemia (ALL): need for sensitive, fast and standardized technologies. Blood. 2015;125:3996–4009.
60. van der Velden VHJ, Cazzaniga G, Schrauder A, Hancock J, Bader P, Panzer-Grumayer ER, Flohr T, Sutton R, Cave H, Madsen HO, Cayuela JM, Trka J, Eckert C, Foroni L, Zur Stadt U, Beldjord K, Raff T, van der Schoot CE, van Dongen JJM. Analysis of minimal residual disease by Ig//TCR gene rearrangements: guidelines for interpretation of real-time quantitative PCR data. Leukemia. 2007;21:604–11.
61. Sundaresan TK, Sequist LV, Heymach JV, Riely GJ, Jänne PA, Koch WH, Sullivan JP, Fox DB, Maher R, Muzikansky A, Webb A, Tran HT, Giri U, Fleisher M, Yu HA, Wei W, Johnson BE, Barber TA, Walsh JR, Engelman JA, Stott SL, Kapur R, Maheswaran S, Toner M, Haber DA. Detection of T790M, the acquired resistance EGFR mutation, by tumor biopsy versus noninvasive blood-based analyses. Clin Cancer Res. 2016;22:1103–10.
62. Brown JR, Feng Y, Gribben JG, Neuberg D, Fisher DC, Mauch P, Nadler LM, Freedman AS. Long-term survival after autologous bone marrow transplantation for follicular lymphoma in first remission. Biol Blood Marrow Transplant. 2007;13:1057–65.
63. Mandigers CMPW, Meijerink JPP, Mensink EJBM, Tonnissen ELRTM, Hebeda KM, Bogman MJJT, Raemaekers JMM. Lack of correlation between numbers of circulating t(14;18)-positive cells and response to first-line treatment in follicular lymphoma. Blood. 2001;98:940–4.
64. van Oers MHJ, Van Glabbeke M, Giurgea L, Klasa R, Marcus RE, Wolf M, Kimby E, Veer M, Vranovsky A, Holte H, Hagenbeek A. Rituximab maintenance treatment of relapsed/resistant follicular non-Hodgkin's lymphoma: long-term outcome of the EORTC 20981 phase III Randomized Intergroup Study. J Clin Oncol. 2010;28:2853–8.
65. Ladetto M, Lobetti-Bodoni C, Mantoan B, Ceccarelli M, Boccomini C, Genuardi E, Chiappella A, Baldini L, Rossi G, Pulsoni A, Di Raimondo F, Rigacci L, Pinto A, Galimberti S, Bari A, Rota-Scalabrini D, Ferrari A, Zaja F, Gallamini A, Specchia G, Musto P, Rossi FG, Gamba E, Evangelista A, Vitolo U. Persistence of minimal residual disease in bone marrow predicts outcome in follicular lymphomas treated with a rituximab-intensive program. Blood. 2013;122:3759–66.
66. Pott C, Sehn LH, Belada D, Gribben J, Hoster E, Kahl B, Kehden B, Nicolas-Virelizier E, Spielewoy N, Fingerle-Rowson G, Harbron C, Mundt K, Wassner-Fritsch E, Cheson BD. MRD response in relapsed/refractory FL after obinutuzumab plus bendamus-

tine or bendamustine alone in the GADOLIN trial. Leukemia. 2020;34:522–32.
67. Corradini P, Astolfi M, Cherasco C, Ladetto M, Voena C, Caracciolo D, Pileri A, Tarella C. Molecular monitoring of minimal residual disease in follicular and mantle cell non-Hodgkin's lymphomas treated with high-dose chemotherapy and peripheral blood progenitor cell autografting. Blood. 1997;89:724–31.
68. Andersen NS, Donovan JW, Borus JS, Poor CM, Neuberg D, Aster JC, Nadler LM, Freedman AS, Gribben JG. Failure of immunologic purging in mantle cell lymphoma assessed by polymerase chain reaction detection of minimal residual disease. Blood. 1997;90:4212–21.
69. Rambaldi A, Lazzari M, Manzoni C, Carlotti E, Arcaini L, Baccarani M, Barbui T, Bernasconi C, Dastoli G, Fuga G, Gamba E, Gargantini L, Gattei V, Lauria F, Lazzarino M, Mandelli F, Morra E, Pulsoni A, Ribersani M, Rossi-Ferrini PL, Rupolo M, Tura S, Zagonel V, Zaja F, Zinzani P, Reato G, Foa R. Monitoring of minimal residual disease after CHOP and rituximab in previously untreated patients with follicular lymphoma. Blood. 2002;99:856–62.
70. Ladetto M, De Marco F, Benedetti F, Vitolo U, Patti C, Rambaldi A, Pulsoni A, Musso M, Liberati AM, Olivieri A, Gallamini A, Pogliani E, Scalabrini DR, Callea V, Di Raimondo F, Pavone V, Tucci A, Cortelazzo S, Levis A, Boccadoro M, Majolino I, Pileri A, Gianni AM, Passera R, Corradini P, Tarella C, for G. I. T. di M. O. (GITMO). Prospective, multicenter randomized GITMO/IIL trial comparing intensive (R-HDS) versus conventional (CHOP-R) chemoimmunotherapy in high-risk follicular lymphoma at diagnosis: the superior disease control of R-HDS does not translate into an overall survival. Blood. 2008;111:4004–13.
71. Federico M, Mannina D, Versari A, Ferrero S, Marcheselli L, Boccomini C, Dondi A, Tucci A, Guerra L, Galimberti S, Cavallo F, Olivieri J, Corradini P, Arcaini L, Chauvie S, Del Giudice I, Rusconi C, Pinto A, Molinari A, Pulsoni A, Merli M, Kovalchuk S, Nassi L, Bolis S, Gattei V, Manni M, Pileri S, Brugiatelli M, Luminari S. Response oriented maintenance therapy in advanced follicular lymphoma. Results of the interim analysis of the Foll12 trial conducted by the Fondazione Italiana Linfomi. Hematol Oncol. 2019;37:abstract 104.
72. Dogliotti I, Drandi D, Genuardi E, Ferrero S. New molecular technologies for minimal residual disease evaluation in B-cell lymphoid malignancies. J Clin Med. 2018;7:288.
73. Ferrero S, Ladetto M, Beldjord K, Drandi D, Stelitano C, Bernard S, Castagnari B, Bouabdallah K, Cesaretti M, Alvarez I, Gressin R, Ponzoni M, Tripodo C, Traverse-Glehen A, Baseggio L, Liberati A, Merli M, Tessoulin B, Patti C, Cabras M, Feugier P, Pozzi S, Zucca E, Iannitto E, Thieblemont C. First application of minimal residual disease analysis in splenic marginal zone lymphoma trials: preliminary results from Brisma/Ielsg36 phase II study. Hematol Oncol. 2019;37:224–5.
74. Pott C, Schrader C, Gesk S, Harder L, Tiemann M, Raff T, Bruggemann M, Ritgen M, Gahn B, Unterhalt M, Dreyling M, Hiddemann W, Siebert R, Dreger P, Kneba M. Quantitative assessment of molecular remission after high-dose therapy with autologous stem cell transplantation predicts long-term remission in mantle cell lymphoma. Blood. 2006;107:2271–8.
75. Hermine O, Hoster E, Walewski J, Bosly A, Stilgenbauer S, Thieblemont C, Szymczyk M, Bouabdallah R, Kneba M, Hallek M, Salles G, Feugier P, Ribrag V, Birkmann J, Forstpointner R, Haioun C, Hänel M, Casasnovas RO, Finke J, Peter N, Bouabdallah K, Sebban C, Fischer T, Dührsen U, Metzner B, Maschmeyer G, Kanz L, Schmidt C, Delarue R, Brousse N, Klapper W, Macintyre E, Delfau-Larue M-H, Pott C, Hiddemann W, Unterhalt M, Dreyling M. Addition of high-dose cytarabine to immunochemotherapy before autologous stem-cell transplantation in patients aged 65 years or younger with mantle cell lymphoma (MCL Younger): a randomised, open-label, phase 3 trial of the European Mantle Cell Lymphoma Network. Lancet (London, England). 2016;388:565–75.
76. Kolstad A, Laurell A, Jerkeman M, Grønbæk K, Elonen E, Räty R, Pedersen LB, Loft A, Bogsrud TV, Kimby E, Hansen PB, Fagerli UM, Nilsson-Ehle H, Lauritzsen GF, Lehmann AK, Sundstrom C, Karjalainen-Lindsberg ML, Ralfkiaer E, Ehinger M, Delabie J, Bentzen H, Schildt J, Kostova-Aherdan K, Frederiksen H, De Nully Brown P, Geisler CH. Nordic MCL3 study: 90Y-ibritumomab-tiuxetan added to BEAM/C in non-CR patients before transplant in mantle cell lymphoma. Blood. 2014;123:2953–9.
77. Lenz G, Dreyling M, Schiegnitz E, Forstpointner R, Wandt H, Freund M, Hess G, Truemper L, Diehl V, Kropff M, Kneba M, Schmitz N, Metzner B, Pfirrmann M, Unterhalt M, Hiddemann W. Myeloablative radiochemotherapy followed by autologous stem cell transplantation in first remission prolongs progression-free survival in follicular lymphoma: results of a prospective, randomized trial of the German Low-Grade Lymphoma Study Group. Blood. 2004;104:2667–74.
78. Dreyling M, Lenz G, Hoster E, Van Hoof A, Gisselbrecht C, Schmits R, Metzner B, Truemper L, Reiser M, Steinhauer H, Boiron JM, Boogaerts MA, Aldaoud A, Silingardi V, Kluin-Nelemans HC, Hasford J, Parwaresch R, Unterhalt M, Hiddemann W. Early consolidation by myeloablative radiochemotherapy followed by autologous stem cell transplantation in first remission significantly prolongs progression-free survival in mantle-cell lymphoma: results of a prospective randomized trial of the European. Blood. 2005;105:2677–84.
79. Callanan M, Delfau MH, Macintyre E, Thieblemont C, Oberic L, Gyan E, Bouabdallah K, Gressin R, Damaj G, Casasnovas O, Ribrag V, Gimenez E, Hermine O, Le Gouill S. Predictive power of early, sequential MRD monitoring in peripheral blood and

bone marrow in patients with mantle cell lymphoma following autologous stem cell transplantation with or without rituximab maintenance ; interim results from the LyMa-MRD project. Blood. 2015;126:Abstract 338.
80. Ferrero S, Barbero S, Lo Schirico M, Evangelista A, Cifaratti A, Drandi P, Genuardi E, Grimaldi D, Monitillo L, Zaccaria JM, Benedetti S, Casaroli F, Zanni M, Castellino C, Pavone V, Petrini G, Re F, Hohaus S, Musuraca G, Cascavilla N, Congiu AG, Liberati AM, Ciccone G, Vitolo U, Cortelazzo S, Ladetto M. Comprehensive minimal residual disease (MRD) analysis of the Fondazione Italiana Linfomi (FIL) MCL0208 clinical trial for younger patients with mantle cell lymphoma: a kinetic model ensures a more refined risk stratification. Blood. 2018;132:abstract 920.
81. Rawstron AC, Kennedy B, Evans PAS, Davies FE, Richards SJ, Haynes AP, Russell NH, Hale G, Morgan GJ, Jack AS, Hillmen P. Quantitation of minimal disease levels in chronic lymphocytic leukemia using a sensitive flow cytometric assay improves the prediction of outcome and can be used to optimize therapy. Blood. 2001;98:29–35.
82. van Dongen JJM, Langerak AW, Brüggemann M, Evans PAS, Hummel M, Lavender FL, Delabesse E, Davi F, Schuuring E, García-Sanz R, van Krieken JHJM, Droese J, González D, Bastard C, White HE, Spaargaren M, González M, Parreira A, Smith JL, Morgan GJ, Kneba M, Macintyre EA. Design and standardization of PCR primers and protocols for detection of clonal immunoglobulin and T-cell receptor gene recombinations in suspect lymphoproliferations: report of the BIOMED-2 concerted action BMH4-CT98-3936. Leukemia. 2003;17:2257–317.
83. Raponi S, Della Starza I, De Propris MS, Del Giudice I, Mauro FR, Marinelli M, Di Maio V, Piciocchi A, Foa R, Guarini A. Minimal residual disease monitoring in chronic lymphocytic leukaemia patients. A comparative analysis of flow cytometry and ASO IgH RQ-PCR. Br J Haematol. 2014;166:360–8.
84. Moreno C, Villamor N, Colomer D, Esteve J, Gine E, Muntan A, Campo E, Bosch F. Clinical significance of minimal residual disease, as assessed by different techniques, after stem cell transplantation for chronic lymphocytic leukemia. Significance. 2006;107:4563–9.
85. Rawstron A, Fazi C, Agathangelidis A, Villamor N, Letestu R, Nomdedeu J, Palacio C, Stehlikova O, Kreuzer K, Liptrot S, O'brien D, De Tute R, Marinov I. A complementary role of multiparameter flow cytometry and high-throughput sequencing for minimal residual disease detection in chronic lymphocytic leukemia: an European Research Initiative on CLL study. Leukemia. 2015;30:929–36.
86. Rawstron AC, Villamor N, Ritgen M, Bö Ttcher S, Ghia P, Zehnder JL, Lozanski G, Colomer D, Moreno C, Geuna M, Evans PAS, Natkunam Y, Coutre SE, Avery ED, Rassenti LZ, Kipps TJ, Caligaris-Cappio F, Kneba M, Byrd JC, Hallek MJ, Montserrat E, Hillmen P, Böttcher S, Ghia P, Zehnder JL, Lozanski G, Colomer D, Moreno C, Geuna M, Evans PAS, Natkunam Y, Coutre SE, Avery ED, Rassenti LZ, Kipps TJ, Caligaris-Cappio F, Kneba M, Byrd JC, Hallek MJ, Montserrat E, Hillmen P. International standardized approach for flow cytometric residual disease monitoring in chronic lymphocytic leukaemia. Leukemia. 2007;21:956–64.
87. Hallek M, Cheson BD, Catovsky D, Caligaris-Cappio F, Dighiero G, Döhner H, Hillmen P, Keating M, Montserrat E, Chiorazzi N, Stilgenbauer S, Rai KR, Byrd JC, Eichhorst B, O'Brien S, Robak T, Seymour JF, Kipps TJ. iwCLL guidelines for diagnosis, indications for treatment, response assessment, and supportive management of CLL. Blood. 2018;131:2745–60.
88. Goede V, Fischer K, Busch R, Engelke A, Eichhorst B, Wendtner CM, Chagorova T, de la Serna J, Dilhuydy M-S, Illmer T, Opat S, Owen CJ, Samoylova O, Kreuzer K-A, Stilgenbauer S, Döhner H, Langerak AW, Ritgen M, Kneba M, Asikanius E, Humphrey K, Wenger M, Hallek M. Obinutuzumab plus chlorambucil in patients with CLL and coexisting conditions. N Engl J Med. 2014;370:1101–10.
89. Eichhorst B, Fink AM, Bahlo J, Busch R, Kovacs G, Maurer C, Lange E, Köppler H, Kiehl M, Sökler M, Schlag R, Vehling-Kaiser U, Köchling G, Plöger C, Gregor M, Plesner T, Trneny M, Fischer K, Döhner H, Kneba M, Wendtner CM, Klapper W, Kreuzer KA, Stilgenbauer S, Böttcher S, Hallek M. First-line chemoimmunotherapy with bendamustine and rituximab versus fludarabine, cyclophosphamide, and rituximab in patients with advanced chronic lymphocytic leukaemia (CLL10): an international, open-label, randomised, phase 3, non-inferiority trial. Lancet Oncol. 2016;17:928–42.
90. Böttcher S. Paving the road to MRD-guided treatment in CLL. Blood. 2014;123:3683–4.
91. Kwok M, Rawstron AC, Varghese A, Evans PAS, O'Connor SJM, Doughty C, Newton DJ, Moreton P, Hillmen P. Minimal residual disease is an independent predictor for 10-year progression-free and overall survival in CLL. Blood. 2016;128:2770–3.
92. Langerak AW, Ritgen M, Goede V, Robrecht S, Bahlo J, Fischer K, Steurer M, Trněný M, Mulligan SP, Mey UJM, Trunzer K, Fingerle-Rowson G, Humphrey K, Stilgenbauer S, Böttcher S, Brüggemann M, Hallek M, Kneba M, van Dongen JJM. Prognostic value of MRD in CLL patients with comorbidities receiving chlorambucil plus obinutuzumab or rituximab. Blood. 2019;133:494–7.
93. von Tresckow J, Cramer P, Bahlo J, Robrecht S, Langerbeins P, Fink A-M, Al-Sawaf O, Illmer T, Klaproth H, Estenfelder S, Ritgen M, Fischer K, Wendtner C-M, Kreuzer K-A, Stilgenbauer S, Böttcher S, Eichhorst BF, Hallek M. CLL2-BIG: sequential treatment with bendamustine, ibrutinib and obinutuzumab (GA101) in chronic lymphocytic leukemia. Leukemia. 2019;33:1161–72.
94. Trotman J, Fournier M, Lamy T, Seymour JF, Sonet A, Janikova A, Shpilberg O, Gyan E, Tilly H, Estell J,

Forsyth C, Decaudin D, Fabiani B, Gabarre J, Salles B, Van Den Neste E, Canioni D, Garin E, Fulham M, Vander Borght T, Salles G. Positron emission tomography-computed tomography (PET-CT) after induction therapy is highly predictive of patient outcome in follicular lymphoma: analysis of PET-CT in a subset of PRIMA trial participants. J Clin Oncol. 2011;29:3194–200.

95. Trotman J, Barrington SF, Belada D, Meignan M, MacEwan R, Owen C, Ptáčník V, Rosta A, Fingerle-Rowson GR, Zhu J, Nielsen T, Sahin D, Hiddemann W, Marcus RE, Davies A, Hertzberg M, Grigg A, Cannell P, Quach H, Opat S, Tam C, Marlton P, Janssens A, Offner F, Van eygen K, Sangha R, Mckay P, Wilson J, Van Der Jagt R, Roitman D, Trneny M, Mayer J, Le Du K, Solal-Celigny P, Cartron G, Foussard C, Frickhofen N, Schmidt P, Graeven U, Gaska T, Schlag R, Sökler M, Prange-Krex G, Florschütz A, Lindemann H-W, Schimmelpfennig C, Tonndorf S, Hänel M, Hess G, Schalk E, Hütten H, Doelken G, Pfreundschuh M, Keller U, Herold M, Forstpointner R, Vehling-Kaiser U, Hoffmann M, Borbenyi Z, Udvardy M, Demeter J, Rambaldi A, Morra E, Massimo F, Majolino I, Balzarotti M, Semenzato G, Canales Albendea MA, Peñalver Parraga FJ, Soler Campos A, Sancho Cia JM, Marquez Navarro JA, Grande Garcia C, Nilsson-Ehle H, Mccarthy H, Pocock C, Sadullah S, Malladi R, Radford J, Kanfer E, Kruger A, Culligan D, Dyer M, Pettengell R, Seymour J, Gribben J, Al-Ismail S, Al-Refaie F, Blesing N, Macnamara C, O'callaghan A, Haynes A, Follows G, Johnson R, Cunningham D, Bowles K, Collins G, Gallop-Evans E, Robinson S, Subash C, Bailey J, Holden V, Neidhart J, De Oliveira M, Tezcan H, Kim K, Kambhampati S, Lanier K, Mcclean J, Tobinai K, Hatake K, Ogura M, Uchida T, Ando K, Kinoshita T, Höhler T, Stauder H, Kirsch A, Koenigsmann M, Kremers S, Illmer T, Witzens-Harig M, La Roseé P, Dürig J, Kneba M, Hensel M, Fuxius S, Bergmann L, Hübel K, Buske C, Marks R, Wulf G, Lerchenmueller C, Schmits R, Reinwald M, Lengfelder E, Scott F, Chou T, Taniwaki M, Yoshida I, Ishizawa K, Uike N, Uoshima N, Kamitsuji Y, Iida S, Ohmine K, Nosaka K, Ide K, Ishikawa T, Desjardins P, Finn N, Zhu J, Li W, Yu L, Ren H, Shi YK, Wu G, Hong X, Zhang Q, Feng J, Zhan R, Lin T, Leppa S, Costello R, Tempescul A, Sanhes L, Tournilhac O, Kirchen H, Hebart H, Weide R, Jentsch-Ullrich K, Avivi I, Nagler A, Gurion R, Shpilberg O, Leoni P, Baldini L, Samoylova O, Myasnikov A, Tan T-D, Chang H, Kumagai K, Tsukamoto N, Tsukasaki K, Beatty P, Usui N, Izutsu K, Murayama T, Ichinohe T, Kubo K, Ishida F, Beck JT, Griesinger F, Osmanov D, Dakhil S, Clavert A, Maruyama D, Terui Y, Yamamoto K, Eigendorff E, Kobayashi T, Ichikawa S, Choi I, Wada K, Kikukawa Y, Matsuoka M, Yoshino T, Minami Y. Prognostic value of end-of-induction PET response after first-line immunochemotherapy for follicular lymphoma (GALLIUM): secondary analysis of a randomised, phase 3 trial. Lancet Oncol. 2018;19:1530–42.

96. Pott C, Davies A, Hiddemann W, Hoster E, Marcus R, Schmidt C, Harbron C, Mundt K, Nielsen T, Trotman J. Metabolic (PET) and MRD response confer reduced risk of progression or death in patients treated within the phase III Gallium study. Hemasphere. 2018;2:1–1113.

4 PET Imaging

Stefano Luminari and Judith Trotman

4.1 Introduction

18F-fluoro-deoxy-glucose positron emission tomography (FDG-PET) is a functional imaging technique that, combined with computed tomography (CT), adds useful detail in staging and restaging of lymphomas. Overall, FDG-PET-CT (PET) has been proven to increase the accuracy of staging compared to conventional CT scanning and has been recommended as the standard imaging modality for all FDG-avid lymphomas since 2014 [1, 2]. Most PET data has been obtained from Hodgkin and aggressive non-Hodgkin lymphomas and allowed us to define the concept of metabolic response (CMR) [3], to validate the prognostic role of achieving a CMR at different timepoints and provide a platform for the evaluation of response-adapted therapies, mainly in Hodgkin lymphoma [4]. Indolent lymphomas were excluded from PET studies for many years mainly due to the heterogeneous and generally reduced FDG avidity and clinical ambivalence about the role of PET in an "incurable" group of lymphomas. More recently, assisted by the improvement in PET technology, accumulated evidence is favoring the use of PET for staging and response assessment of low-grade lymphomas, with particularly robust data in follicular lymphoma (FL). In addition to the visual assessment of FDG-PET that is usually based on the identification of focal uptake at nodal or extranodal sites, functional imaging allows the quantification of the degree of FDG uptake. The most frequently used quantitative parameter is the standard uptake values (SUV), that is, the ratio of the image-derived radioactivity concentration and the whole-body concentration of the injected radioactivity. SUV and SUV-derived parameters (i.e., SUV_{max}, SUV_{mean}, SUV_{peak}, etc.) provide additional detail to better characterize sites with disseminated lymphoma involvement (bone marrow, spleen, extranodal sites).

Indolent lymphomas are a unique disease model to utilize PET in staging. Low-grade lymphomas are characterized by high intra-patient heterogeneity mainly in terms of the variability of organ involvement (nodal, extranodal, bone marrow) and in terms of tumor biology with heterogeneity of the clonal mechanisms and microenvironment underlying tumor spread and aggressive behavior. In this chapter the main

S. Luminari (✉)
Surgical, Medical and Dental Department of Morphological Sciences Related to Transplant, Oncology and Regenerative Medicine, University of Modena and Reggio Emilia, Reggio Emilia, Italy

Hematology, Azienda USL IRCCS Reggio Emilia, Reggio Emilia, Italy
e-mail: sluminari@unimore.it

J. Trotman
Concord Repatriation General Hospital and University of Sydney, Sydney, Australia
e-mail: Judith.Trotman@health.nsw.gov.au

M. Dreyling, M. Ladetto (eds.), *Indolent Lymphomas*, Hematologic Malignancies,
https://doi.org/10.1007/978-3-030-55989-2_4

studies describing the use of PET for staging and restaging of indolent lymphomas are outlined. Most of the data has been acquired in FL, the most frequent subtype, which commonly shows the highest FDG avidity compared to other indolent subtypes [5]. Data supporting the use of PET in the other indolent subtypes, including small lymphocytic lymphoma (SLL), marginal zone lymphomas (MZL), and lymphoplasmacytic lymphoma (LPL), is still limited due to typical leukemic presentation and the low proliferation index of these cases.

4.2 PET in Staging

The use of PET for baseline staging of lymphoma in clinical practice became standard in 2014 [1, 2]. Staging obtained with PET/CT is more accurate compared to contrast-enhanced CT scan (Ce/CT) mainly due to the greater sensitivity of PET in more frequent detection of both extranodal and nodal sites of disease. In a large cohort of 142 FL patients prospectively enrolled in the Italian FOLL05 clinical trial, PET identified more nodal areas than CT in 32% of the patients and additional extranodal sites (ENS) in 47% patients. Similarly, a central review of available PET-CT scans in the PRIMA study demonstrated extranodal involvement in 31/59 (52.5%) patients. The most frequently discovered new ENS were bone/bone marrow, spleen, skin, and gastrointestinal tract [6, 7].

With the higher sensitivity of PET, upstaging of disease occurs in a significant proportion of patients, ranging from 18 to 31% overall [8–10]. In the FOLL05 study, 62% patients with early stage (I and II) defined by CT were upstaged on PET imaging [7]. The actual effect of PET in the staging of patients with disseminated disease is mitigated by the histologic assessment of bone marrow (BM) that is frequently found positive (40–70% cases) on BM biopsy (BMB) [11]. Of particular clinical relevance is the role of PET in the identification of truly localized disease in a minority of patients, who also have no evidence of disease in BM biopsy. This concept mainly applies to FL patients, for whom published data confirms the improvement of survival of truly localized disease treated with radiotherapy [12], compared to historical series, but could also be relevant for other indolent subtypes (i.e., marginal zone lymphomas), who are eligible for potentially curative localized radiotherapy. Higher sensitivity in nodal assessment can also modify the FLIPI score although no comparison in patient outcomes has been made between CT-based FLIPI vs. PET-based FLIPI [7].

Assessment of BM involvement with FDG-PET when staging indolent lymphoma is controversial. BM involvement is the most frequently detected ENS in baseline PET staging of FL, although initial reports suggested a low sensitivity in detecting bone marrow involvement (BMI) by PET/CT. In one study BMB biopsy and PET were compared for initial staging in a cohort of 45 FL patients; PET detected 13 cases (29%) of BMI: five with a diffuse and eight with a focal pattern of FDG uptake. BMB was positive in all patients with diffuse uptake and in only three out of eight with a focal uptake [13]. In another retrospective study on 64 FL patients, the pattern of FDG uptake was suggestive of BMI in 13 out of 24 (56%) patients with BMI; nine had a diffuse uptake (all with a positive BMB) and four had focal FDG uptake (all with a negative BMB). Overall, the sensitivity of FDG-PET in detecting BMI was 54% [14]. In this study some degree of diffuse FDG uptake could be observed in patients with a false negative PET scan, suggesting that applying a more sensitive threshold to detect a diffusely abnormal FDG uptake in BM may better predict BMB-proven BMI. This concept has been investigated by Perry et al. in a retrospective study of 68 FL patients; PET assessment was consistent with BMI in 16 patients (23.5%); 13 had a positive BMB. All eight patients with focal and five of eight patients with a diffuse FDG uptake had a positive BMB. On the other hand, a diffuse "nonspecific" FDG uptake was observed in 17 patients (32.7%) with a negative BMB. A quantitative assessment of PET using SUV, an SUV_{mean} value < than 1.7 or higher than 2.7, was able to distinguish patients with a non-involved BM from those with a "true" BMI, showing sensitivity and specificity of 100% in both cases. Out of 20 scans showing an "intermediate" SUV_{mean} value between 1.7 and 2.7, only five patients had a biopsy-proven BMI [15].

A particular interest of functional imaging in the baseline staging of indolent lymphomas is the potential for early detection of transformation into a large B-cell lymphoma. Several attempts have been made to correlate the histologic FL grade and FL transformation with the intensity of FDG uptake in PET/CT. The correlation of SUV with histologic grading has not led to firm conclusions [8, 14, 16], while a correlation with proliferation index has been recently suggested [16]. In a retrospective, single-institution study by Schoder et al., in which FDG uptake was compared between 28 patients with indolent and 63 with aggressive lymphomas, 81% of indolent lymphomas had an SUV below 10, while most patients with SUV above 13 had aggressive histology. On the other hand, a low FDG uptake was not always an indicator of indolent disease: of the 63 patients with aggressive disease, 22 (35%) had lesions with an SUV < 13. For the eight patients with transformed lymphoma, SUVs ranged from 4.8 to 29.8. Three of the eight patients had an SUV < 10 [17]. According to similar studies, an SUV of 13–14 has been suggested as the cutoff to achieve the best balance between sensitivity and specificity to confirm low-grade histology [8, 18–20]. Higher SUV values of 17–21 have been reported to achieve higher specificity [19, 20]. All these early studies are small, and there has been no prospective study of the association of SUV_{max} and biopsy-proven histologic transformation in patients initially diagnosed with FL. In addition to considering absolute SUV values, the concept of $SUV_{gradient}$ has also been identified as the intra-patient difference between sites with the highest and lowest SUV_{max} values. In one study, transformed lymphomas had high $SUV_{gradients}$ between 10 and 15 that were 2.6–4.8 values higher than non-transformed cases [8, 18]. Conversely, abstract data from 522 baseline PET scans performed in the GALLIUM study suggests that there is no correlation between either baseline SUV_{max} or $SUV_{gradient}$ in the prediction of histologic transformation, which occurred in only 2.5% of patients during 5 years of follow-up [21]. Median (range) baseline SUV_{max} in patients with HT was 12.4 (8.14, 27.95) vs. 11.8 (3.05, 64.43) in those without HT. Median (range) baseline $SUV_{gradient}$, defined as the difference between $bSUV_{max}$ of the most and least FDG-avid lymphoma sites, was 6.6 (1.08, 23.91) vs. 7.14 (0.00, 59.81), respectively. In conclusion, while PET may be useful to increase the suspicion for de novo aggressive transformation of an indolent lymphoma, functional imaging cannot be considered as a sole surrogate of transformation. The diagnosis of transformation requires histologic confirmation, and in the absence of clinical features suggestive of transformation, the cost, inconvenience and risk of repeat biopsy driven by PET status need careful consideration.

The prognostic value of quantitative parameters obtained from baseline PET/CT has also been investigated in two large prospective studies. Data suggest that high SUV has no correlation with inferior patient outcome, and one study suggested an inferior 5-year progression-free survival (PFS) in patients with an SUV_{max} less than 9.4 [21, 22].

Moving from semi-quantitative metrics of FDG avidity, such as SUV_{max}, dedicated software has enabled the quantification of the metabolically active tumor volume (MTV) [23]. The latter, calculated on baseline FDG-PET scan, is demonstrated to be a strong predictor of treatment outcome in Hodgkin lymphoma [24], diffuse large B-cell lymphoma [25], primary mediastinal B-cell lymphoma [26], and peripheral T-cell lymphoma [27]. In a recent study by Meignan et al., baseline TMTV as a dichotomized variable was the strongest pretreatment predictor of outcome in a high tumor burden follicular lymphoma population treated mostly with R-CHOP immunochemotherapy. The 29% patients who had a high TMTV > 510 cm^3 had an inferior 5-year PFS, with a median PFS of <3 years and an increased risk of death. Conversely, a metabolic volume below this cutoff in the remaining 71% patients predicted a median PFS beyond 6 years. Importantly, TMTV was a strong predictor of early progression within the first 1–2 years after commencing therapy. Unlike the original FLIPI, FLIPI2 was also an independent predictor of PFS in this study and the combination of TMTV > 510 cm^3 with intermediate- to high-risk

FLIPI2 stratified the population into three risk categories based on the presence or absence of any of these two adverse factors. The 14% patients with both high TMTV and intermediate- to high-risk FLIPI2 had a very poor 46% PFS and 86% overall survival (OS) at 2 years [28]. Conversely, unpublished abstract data from the GALLIUM study has suggested no prognostic impact of baseline PET metrics (TMTV, total lesion glycolysis, or SUV_{max}) on PFS or OS in the treatment of patients with high tumor burden FL in need of therapy. In this study all patients were prescribed antibody maintenance and most patients were treated with bendamustine [29]. This raises the issue of the applicability of retrospective studies of baseline PET metrics to the modern immunochemotherapy era.

In summary, PET is now the accepted imaging modality for the staging of indolent lymphoma. With greater disease sensitivity than standard CT, a significant proportion of patients with otherwise early stage are "upstaged," and hence the outcomes, and curative potential, of local radiotherapy for patients with localized disease after PET staging are likely higher than earlier. For patients with advanced-stage FL in need of therapy, while re-biopsy may be considered for patients with a very high SUV_{max}, there is no solid prospective data in support of this. The rate of de novo histologic transformation in patients with biopsy-demonstrated indolent lymphoma in the absence of other clinical indicators is low. Furthermore, while intuitively patients with a higher SUV_{max} and higher TMTV are assumed to have poorer outcomes, the prospective data does not support this. It is possible that the FDG uptake in indolent lymphomas, specifically in FL, may relate as much to the microenvironmental cells, including T cells, as the B-cell component. Further prospective research in this area is greatly needed.

4.3 PET Response Assessment

4.3.1 Interim PET

There is little data available on the predictive power of mid-treatment PET in indolent lymphoma, with the only known publication being of PET after four cycles of R-CHOP in the LYSA PET Folliculaire study. The estimated PFS at 2 years was 86% in patients with a negative PET at cycle 4% vs. 61% in those with a positive PET ($P < 0.0046$) and 87% in patients with a negative PET at the end of treatment vs. 51% in those with a positive PET ($P < 0.001$; Fig. 4.2). Of importance, while 2-year OS also significantly differed according to final PET results, the PET status after cycle 4 did not have a significant impact on OS [30].

Evaluation by PET before four cycles of therapy, as has been evaluated in other lymphoma subtypes, has never been evaluated in patients with follicular lymphoma. This data does not support the use of interim PET in routine management of follicular lymphoma. Furthermore, it must be noted that the clinical imperative to perform interim PET in follicular lymphoma, with a median overall survival approaching two decades, is not as great as with aggressive lymphoma.

4.3.2 End-of-Induction Assessment

CT-based assessment with cumbersome measurements of the sum of the product of the diameter of up to six target lesions has been the cornerstone of response assessment for FL for decades. However, with approximately 95% of patients having a response to rituximab chemotherapy, the poor discriminatory capacity of the 1999 IWC contrast-enhanced CT-based response assessment consigns most responding patients (with an unconfirmed complete response or partial response) to an uncertain remission in which only close clinical follow-up identifies those with early relapse [1].

4.3.2.1 PET Response

An initial hypothesis-generating retrospective analysis of end-of-induction (EOI) PET scans performed in the prospective PRIMA (Primary Rituximab and Maintenance) study demonstrated that of 122 PET-CT scans performed at the end of the induction immunochemotherapy, 32 (26%) were reported as positive by the local investigator. Patients remaining PET positive had a significantly inferior PFS at 42 months of 32.9% (95% CI 17.2–49.5%, $P < 0.0001$) compared to 70.7% in those who became PET negative (95% CI 59.3–79.4%). While PET status correlated with conventional response criteria ($P = 0.0006$), it was PET status, but not conventional response [complete or unconfirmed complete response (CR/CRu) vs. partial response (PR)], 1999 IWC, that was an independent predictive factor for lymphoma progression. The risk of death was also increased in PET-positive patients (hazard ratio [HR] 7.0; $P = 0.0011$) [31]. In an independent central review of available PETs in accordance with the Deauville 5-point scale, applying a cutoff >4, there was a significantly inferior 42-month PFS in patients with a positive PET scan of 25.0% (95% CI 3.7–55.8%) vs. 61.4% (95% CI 45.4–74.1) in patients with a negative scan ($P = 0.01$; HR 3.1; 95% CI, 1.2–7.8) [6].

Another retrospective analysis of PET scans conducted in the prospective Italian FOLL05 study made similar conclusions. Again, using local investigator assessment, 49/202 (24%) patients remained PET positive after rituximab chemotherapy induction. With a median follow-up of 34 months, the 3-year PFS was 66% (95% CI 57–74%) and 35% (95% CI 18–52%; HR 2.6, 95% CI 1.6–4.2), respectively, for patients with negative and positive EOI PET ($P < 0.001$). In a multivariate analysis, postinduction PET (HR 2.6, 95% CI 1.5–4.3, $P < 0.001$) was independent of conventional response, FLIPI, and treatment arm. Also, the prognostic role of EOI PET was maintained within each FLIPI risk group [32].

The first prospective observational study of EOI PET after R-CHOP (without maintenance rituximab) was the French PET Folliculaire study [30]. Central review of PET scans was performed by three experienced nuclear medicine physicians using the Deauville 5-point scale. There was good concordance between reviewers (*K* coefficient 0.7) when using the liver as the threshold to define positivity, with lower concordance when assigning the mediastinal blood pool activity as a reference (*K* coefficient 0.57). Therefore, the liver threshold (≥4) was again used to evaluate outcomes. The estimated PFS at 2 years was 87% in patients with a negative PET at the end of treatment vs. 51% in those with a positive PET ($P < 0.001$). Two-year OS also significantly differed according to final PET results: 100% vs. 88% ($P < 0.0128$). This was the first prospective study to confirm the importance of applying the deauville score (DS) and 2014 Lugano criteria for EOI PET assessment after treatment of FL.

The better reporter concordance with the cutoff of ≥4, and the better separation of the PFS curves applying this cutoff, were the basis for applying these criteria in a pooled analysis of 246 centrally reviewed scans, by three PET physicians, from the aforementioned PET Folliculaire, PRIMA, and FOLL05 studies [33]. Forty-one (16.7%) scans were positive with a cutoff ≥4 (i.e., lymphoma FDG uptake moderately > liver uptake), with substantial reporter concordance. With a median follow-up of 55 months, the HR for PFS and OS of EOI PET-positive vs. PET-negative patients was 3.9 (95% CI 2.5–5.9, $P < 0.0001$) and 6.7 (95% CI 2.4–18.5, $P = 0.0002$), respectively. For patients remaining PET positive, 4-year PFS was 23.2% (95% CI 11·1–37.9%) vs. 63.4% (95% CI 55.9–70.0%) in those who became PET negative ($P < 0.0001$) (see Fig. 4.1a). Four-year OS was 87.2% (95% CI 71.9–94.5%) vs. 97.1% (95% CI 93.2–98.8%) ($P < 0.0001$), providing the first large body of evidence of the impact of postinduction PET status on OS (Figs. 4.1 and 4.2). Conversely, conventional CT-based response (complete response/unconfirmed complete remission vs. partial response) was weakly predictive of PFS (HR 1.7, $P = 0.02$) but not OS. These results suggest that performed on its own, conventional response assessment may be misleading, creating false optimism for a few PET-positive patients in CRu, but more importantly unwarranted pessimism for many PET-negative patients achieving only a PR on the conventional CT-based assessment.

More recently, data from the GALLIUM study confirmed the highly predictive power of postinduction PET status after either rituximab or obinutuzumab chemotherapy (bendamustine, CHOP, or CVP) for FL [34]. Of 595 patients included in the PET intention-to-treat population, 508 and 519 were included in an OS and PFS

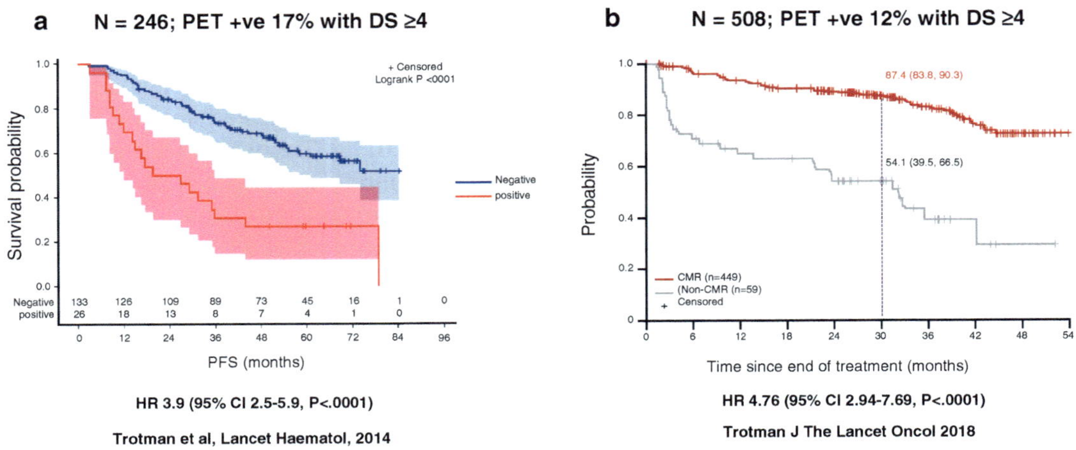

Fig. 4.1 Postinduction PET in follicular lymphomas, progression-free survival (PFS) data from a pooled analysis of three retrospective studies (**a**) and from the GALLIUM trial (**b**). *DS* Deauville score, *HR* hazard ratio, *CI* confidence interval. (Reprinted with permission)

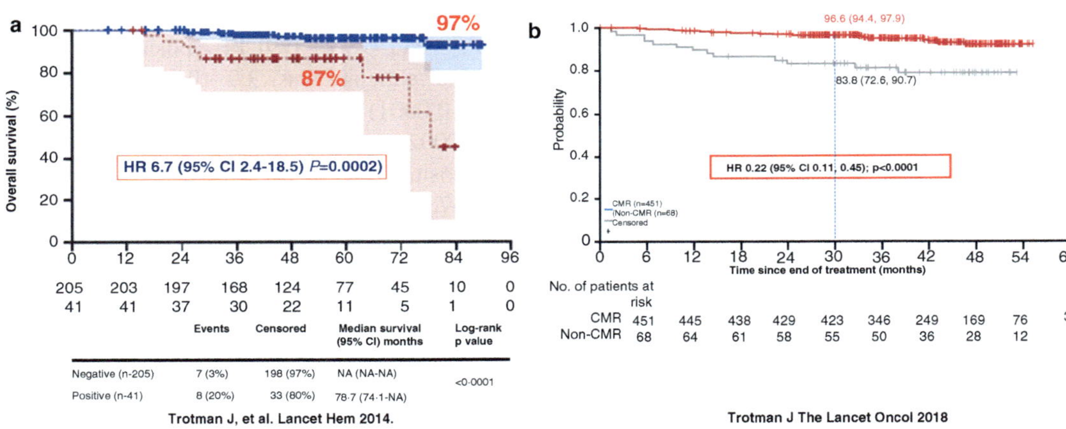

Fig. 4.2 Postinduction PET in follicular lymphomas, overall survival (OS) data from a pooled analysis of three retrospective studies (**a**) and from the GALLIUM trial (**b**). *CMR* complete metabolic response, *HR* hazard ratio, *CI* confidence interval. (Reprinted with permission)

landmark analysis, respectively, applying the Lugano 2014 response criteria, which incorporates the 5 point scale (5PS). Following induction therapy, 454/595 (76.3%) obtained complete metabolic response (CMR). With median 43.3 months' follow-up, postinduction PET-CT was highly prognostic for PFS and OS (CMR vs. non-CMR: HR 0.2, 95% CI 0.1–0.3, $P < 0.0001$ and HR 0.2, 95% CI 0·.1–0.5, $P < 0.0001$, respectively). Two-and-a-half-year PFS from EOI was 87.4% (95% CI 83.8–90.2) for CMR patients vs. 54.9% (95% CI 40.5–67.3) for non-CMR patients; 2.5-year OS was 96.6% (95% CI 94.4–97.9) vs. 84.0% (95% CI 72.9–90.8) (Fig. 4.1b). Having a CT-based CR at EOI as assessed by an independent review committee (IRC) was significantly prognostic for PFS only (CR vs. non-CR: HR 0.5; 95% CI 0.3–0.7; $P = 0.001$); OS (CR vs. non-CR: HR 0.5; 95% CI 0.3–1.2; $P = 0.124$). With a fivefold increased rate of early progression and death in patients who failed to obtain CMR, this data validates the prognostic impact of PET, confirming that PET rather than contrast-enhanced CT scanning should be considered the new gold standard for response assessment in clinical practice and a platform for the study of response-adapted therapy. Two large studies are under way (the Italian FOLL12 trial and British-led PETReA study), which individualize postinduction treatment based on risk according to metabolic response. Both trials include treatment-naïve patients with advanced-stage FL in need of systemic therapy meeting GELF criteria. The Italian FOLL12 study was designed to establish noninferiority in terms of PFS of a standard approach consisting of immunochemotherapy followed by rituximab maintenance for all patients regardless of metabolic and molecular response, compared with a response-adapted approach that used postinduction metabolic and molecular response; in the experimental arm, patients achieving complete metabolic response were not treated with rituximab maintenance but were treated with only 4 weekly rituximab doses in the case of molecular residual; patients without complete metabolic response (i.e., DS 4–5 at the end-of-induction PET) had to receive one dose of radioimmunotherapy with ibritumomab tiuxetan before starting rituximab maintenance. The trial has completed recruitment of 810 patients, and preliminary results were recently disclosed (REF FEDERICO ICML 2019). The study was not able to show the noninferiority of the response-adapted approach compared to standard therapy in terms of PFS. In the currently recruiting PETReA (PET response-adapted therapy) trial (EUDRACT 2016-004010-10), patients who obtain complete metabolic response are randomized to rituximab maintenance compared with observation. This will quantify the PFS benefit of maintenance rituximab and assess the trade-off with toxicity in this good-risk population. Similarly, a trial of therapeutic escalation, comparing the addition of lenalidomide to maintenance rituximab with rituximab alone, is appropriate in the 12% of patients who fail to obtain a complete metabolic response, in whom the GALLIUM study demonstrated a 45% risk of progression within only 30 months after induction and a 16% risk of early death. Final study results of the FOLL12 and PETReA trials integrating efficacy and safety data will allow more definitive assessment of the risk/benefit ratio of response-adapted therapy in FL.

With a median overall survival now extending to 20 years, progression-free survival is the widely accepted clinical endpoint after the first-line treatment of follicular lymphoma. Several studies have shown that the time to next treatment usually closely follows progression. Determining whether these published studies of postinduction PET can be utilized for a formal by-trial surrogacy analysis, for either PFS or OS, is a current task of the Mayo-clinic-led follicular lymphoma analysis of surrogacy hypothesis (FLASH) consortium.

4.4 PET in Other Indolent B-Cell Lymphomas

Indolent non-follicular lymphomas (INFL) include marginal zone lymphoma (MZL), lymphoplasmacytic lymphoma (LPL), and small lymphocytic lymphomas (SLL). Data regarding the avidity of FDG and its prognostic significance in INFL are scarce and conflicting [1, 2], and the standard use of PET in the staging and response assessment is not yet recommended (REF Cheson 2014, Barrington). Nonetheless, FDG avidity has been documented mainly for MZL and has been correlated with histologic characteristics. A recent study of 69 patients with gastric mucosal associate lymphoid tissue (MALT) lymphoma demonstrated FDG avidity in 52%, which correlated with morphological characteristics, tumor stage, and Ki-67 proliferative index [35]. In another study of 72 patients with extragastric MALT lymphoma, 75% were FDG avid, and FDG avidity was significantly correlated with Ki-67 proliferative index [36]. PET at baseline was also retrospectively assessed on a series of 110 patients with MZL, showing FDG avidity in 70%, 62.5% for MALT, 76.4% for nodal marginal zone lymphoma (nMZL), and 76.4% for splenic marginal zone lymphoma (SMZL).

Overall, FDG-avid INFL are characterized by a low median SUV_{max} ranging from 5 to 7 [37, 38]. PET interpretation in INFL is further complicated by the frequent bone marrow involvement that is often not detected on PET and does not obviate the need for a bone marrow biopsy (BMB) in the initial patient assessment.

Regarding the prognostic role of EOI PET/CT in MZL, a retrospective study of 32 patients showed that CMR was associated with better PFS [38].

4.5 Conclusion

There is sufficient robust data from several prospective trials [30–34] to utilize the 2014 Lugano staging and response criteria for the assessment of FL [1, 2], and EOI PET status is an appropriate platform for prognostication and study of response-adapted approaches. Further study of baseline quantitative measures, such as SUV_{max} and TMTV, is required to determine the appropriateness of using such measures in this indolent lymphoma. The role of PET in other indolent lymphomas requires additional prospective study.

References

1. Cheson BD, Fisher RI, Barrington SF, Cavalli F, Schwartz LH, Zucca E, et al. Recommendations for initial evaluation, staging, and response assessment of Hodgkin and non-Hodgkin lymphoma: the Lugano classification. J Clin Oncol. 2014;32:3059–67.
2. Barrington SF, Mikhaeel NG, Kostakoglu L, Meignan M, Hutchings M, Müeller SP, et al. Role of imaging in the staging and response assessment of lymphoma: consensus of the international conference on Malignant Lymphomas Imaging Working Group. J Clin Oncol. 2014;32(27):3048–58.
3. Meignan M, Gallamini A, Haioun C. Report on the first international workshop on interim-PET scan in lymphoma. Leuk Lymphoma. 2009;50(8):1257–60.
4. Johnson P, Federico M, Kirkwood A, Fosså A, Berkahn L, Carella A, et al. Adapted treatment guided by interim PET-CT scan in advanced Hodgkin's lymphoma. N Engl J Med. 2016;374(25):2419–29.
5. Weiler-Sagie M, Bushelev O, Epelbaum R, Dann EJ, Haim N, Avivi I, et al. 18F-FDG avidity in lymphoma readdressed: a study of 766 patients. J Nucl Med. 2010;51(1):25–30.
6. Tychyj-Pinel C, Ricard F, Fulham M, Fournier M, Meignan M, Lamy T, et al. PET/CT assessment in follicular lymphoma using standardized criteria: central review in the PRIMA study. Eur J Nucl Med Mol Imaging. 2014;41(3):408–15.
7. Luminari S, Biasoli I, Arcaini L, Versari A, Rusconi C, Merli F, et al. The use of FDG-PET in the initial staging of 142 patients with follicular lymphoma: a retrospective study from the FOLL05 randomized trial of the Fondazione Italiana Linfomi. Ann Oncol. 2013;24(8):2108–12.
8. Karam M, Novak L, Cyriac J, Ali A, Nazeer T, Nugent F. Role of fluorine-18 fluoro-deoxyglucose positron emission tomography scan in the evaluation and follow-up of patients with low-grade lymphomas. Cancer. 2006;107(1):175–83.
9. Wirth A, Foo M, Seymour JF, MacManus MP, Hicks RJ. Impact of [18F] fluorodeoxyglucose positron emission tomography on staging and management of early-stage follicular non-Hodgkin lymphoma. Int J Radiat Oncol Biol Phys. 2008;71(1):213–9.
10. Janikova A, Bolcak K, Pavlik T, Mayer J, Kral Z. Value of [18F]fluorodeoxyglucose positron emission tomography in the management of follicular lymphoma: the end of a dilemma? Clin Lymphoma Myeloma. 2008;8(5):287–93.
11. Armitage JO. A clinical evaluation of the International Lymphoma Study Group classification of non-Hodgkin's lymphoma. Blood. 1997;89(11):3909–18.
12. Brady JL, Binkley MS, Hajj C, Chelius M, Chau K, Balogh A, et al. Definitive radiotherapy for localized follicular lymphoma staged by 18 F-FDG PET-CT: a collaborative study by ILROG. Blood. 2019;133(3):237–45.
13. Le Dortz L, De Guibert S, Bayat S, Devillers A, Houot R, Rolland Y, et al. Diagnostic and prognostic impact of 18F-FDG PET/CT in follicular lymphoma. Eur J Nucl Med Mol Imaging. 2010;7(12):2307–14.
14. Wöhrer S, Jaeger U, Kletter K, Becherer A, Hauswirth A, Turetschek K, et al. 18F-fluoro-deoxy-glucose positron emission tomography (18F-FDG-PET) visualizes follicular lymphoma irrespective of grading. Ann Oncol. 2006;17(5):780–4.
15. Perry C, Lerman H, Joffe E, Sarid N, Amit O, Avivi I, et al. The value of PET/CT in detecting bone marrow involvement in patients with follicular lymphoma. Medicine (United States). 2016;95(9):e2910.
16. Novelli S, Briones J, Flotats A, et al. PET/CT assessment of follicular lymphoma and high grade B cell lymphoma - good correlation with clinical and histological features at diagnosis. Adv Clin Exp Med. 2015;24(2):325–30.
17. Schöder H, Noy A, Gönen M, Weng L, Green D, Erdi YE, et al. Intensity of 18fluorodeoxyglucose uptake in positron emission tomography distinguishes between indolent and aggressive non-Hodgkin's lymphoma. J Clin Oncol. 2005;23(21):4643–51.
18. Noy A, Schöder H, Gönen M, Weissler M, Ertelt K, Cohler C, et al. The majority of transformed lymphomas have high standardized uptake values (SUVs) on positron emission tomography (PET) scanning similar to diffuse large B-cell lymphoma (DLBCL). Ann Oncol. 2009;20(3):508–12.
19. Bodet-Milin C, Kraeber-Bodéré F, Moreau P, Campion L, Dupas B, Le Gouill S. Investigation of

FDG-PET/CT imaging to guide biopsies in the detection of histological transformation of indolent lymphoma. Haematologica. 2008;93(3):471–2.
20. Wondergem MJ, Rizvi SNF, Jauw Y, Hoekstra OS, Hoetjes N, Van De Ven PM, et al. 18F-FDG or 3′-deoxy-3′-18F-fluorothymidine to detect transformation of follicular lymphoma. J Nucl Med. 2015;56(2):216–21.
21. Mir F, Barrington SF, Meignan M, Brown H, Nielsen T, Sahin D, et al. Baseline Suvmax did not predict histological transformation from follicular lymphoma to aggressive lymphoma in the phase III GALLIUM study. Blood. 2018;132(Suppl 1):4160. https://doi.org/10.1182/blood-2018-99-116686.
22. Cottereau AS, Versari A, Chartier L, Dupuis J, Tarantino V, Casasnovas R-O, et al. Low Suvmax measured on baseline FDG-PET/CT and elevated β2 microglobulin are negative predictors of outcome in high tumor burden follicular lymphoma treated by immunochemotherapy: a pooled analysis of three prospective studies. Blood. 2016;128(22):1101. https://doi.org/10.1182/blood.V128.22.1101.1101.
23. Bai B, Bading J, Conti PS. Tumor quantification in clinical positron emission tomography. Theranostics. 2013;3(10):787–801.
24. Song MK, Chung JS, Lee JJ, Jeong SY, Lee SM, Hong JS, et al. Metabolic tumor volume by positron emission tomography/computed tomography as a clinical parameter to determine therapeutic modality for early stage Hodgkin's lymphoma. Cancer Sci. 2013;104(12):1656–61.
25. Mikhaeel NG, Smith D, Dunn JT, Phillips M, Møller H, Fields PA, et al. Combination of baseline metabolic tumour volume and early response on PET/CT improves progression-free survival prediction in DLBCL. Eur J Nucl Med Mol Imaging. 2016;43(7):1209–19.
26. Ceriani L, Martelli M, Zinzani PL, Ferreri AJM, Botto B, Stelitano C, et al. Utility of baseline 18FDG-PET/CT functional parameters in defining prognosis of primary mediastinal (thymic) large B-cell lymphoma. Blood. 2015;126(8):950–6.
27. Cottereau AS, Hapdey S, Chartier L, Modzelewski R, Casasnovas O, Itti E, et al. Baseline total metabolic tumor volume measured with fixed or different adaptive thresholding methods equally predicts outcome in peripheral T cell lymphoma. J Nucl Med. 2017;58(2):276–81.
28. Meignan M, Cottereau ASAS, Versari A, Chartier L, Dupuis J, Boussetta S, et al. Baseline metabolic tumor volume predicts outcome in high-tumor-burden follicular lymphoma: a pooled analysis of three multicenter studies. J Clin Oncol. 2016;34:3618–26.
29. Barrington SF, Trotman J, Sahin D, Belada D, Davies A, MacEwan R, et al. Baseline PET-derived metabolic tumor volume metrics did not predict outcomes in follicular lymphoma patients treated with first-line immunochemotherapy and antibody maintenance in the phase III GALLIUM study. Blood. 2018;132(Suppl 1):2882. https://doi.org/10.1182/blood-2018-99-117235.
30. Dupuis J, Berriolo-Riedinger A, Julian A, Brice P, Tychyj-Pinel C, Tilly H, et al. Impact of [18F]fluorodeoxyglucose positron emission tomography response evaluation in patients with high-tumor burden follicular lymphoma treated with immunochemotherapy: a prospective study from the Groupe d'Etudes des Lymphomes de l'Adulte and GOELAMS. J Clin Oncol. 2012;30(35):4317–22.
31. Trotman J, Fournier M, Lamy T, Seymour JF, Sonet A, Janikova A, et al. Positron emission tomography-computed tomography (PET-CT) after induction therapy is highly predictive of patient outcome in follicular lymphoma: analysis of PET-CT in a subset of PRIMA trial participants. J Clin Oncol. 2011;29(23):3194–200.
32. Luminari S, Biasoli I, Versari A, Rattotti S, Bottelli C, Rusconi C, et al. The prognostic role of post-induction FDG-PET in patients with follicular lymphoma: a subset analysis from the FOLL05 trial of the Fondazione Italiana Linfomi (FIL). Ann Oncol. 2014;25(2):442–7.
33. Trotman J, Luminari S, Boussetta S, Versari A, Dupuis J, Tychyj C, et al. Prognostic value of PET-CT after first-line therapy in patients with follicular lymphoma: a pooled analysis of central scan review in three multicentre studies. Lancet Haematol. 2014;1(1):e17–27.
34. Trotman J, Barrington SF, Belada D, Meignan M, MacEwan R, Owen C, et al. Prognostic value of end-of-induction PET response after first-line immunochemotherapy for follicular lymphoma (GALLIUM): secondary analysis of a randomised, phase 3 trial. Lancet Oncol. 2018;19(11):1530–42.
35. Albano D, Bertoli M, Ferro P, Fallanca F, Gianolli L, Picchio M, et al. 18F-FDG PET/CT in gastric MALT lymphoma: a bicentric experience. Eur J Nucl Med Mol Imaging. 2017;44(4):589–97.
36. Albano D, Bosio G, Giubbini R, Bertagna F. 18F-FDG PET/CT and extragastric MALT lymphoma: role of Ki-67 score and plasmacytic differentiation. Leuk Lymphoma. 2017;58(10):2328–34.
37. Vaxman I, Bernstine H, Kleinstern G, Hendin N, Shimony S, Domachevsky L, et al. FDG PET/CT as a diagnostic and prognostic tool for the evaluation of marginal zone lymphoma. Hematol Oncol. 2019;37(2):168–75.
38. Park JH, Kim S, Ryu JS, Lee SW, Park CS, Huh J, et al. Complete metabolic response (CMR) in positron emission tomography–computed tomography (PET-CT) scans may have prognostic significance in patients with marginal zone lymphomas (MZL). Hematol Oncol. 2018;36(1):56–61.

5 Role of Radiotherapy

Lena Specht, Mario Levis, and Umberto Ricardi

5.1 Introduction

Indolent lymphomas are highly radiosensitive, and some of the first patients to receive radiation therapy (RT) were patients with indolent lymphomas [1]. Reports of durable remissions and even cures with RT were published already in the 1930s [2–4]. With advances in technology, extended treatment fields could be irradiated [1]. In the first reports, extended-field RT (EFRT) yielded superior relapse-free survival compared with more limited involved-field RT (IFRT), but there was no difference in overall survival (OS) [5].

Modern imaging with computed tomography (CT), magnetic resonance (MR), and in particular positron emission tomography (PET) scanning has enabled much more accurate staging of patients. Most importantly, it is now possible to select patients with a truly localized disease for whom RT may be curative and to define accurately areas affected by the disease, enabling better targeting and use of smaller radiation treatment volumes [6]. Modern advanced treatment planning and delivery techniques have made it possible to irradiate the involved tissue volume with great accuracy while minimizing radiation doses to the normal tissues [7–11].

5.2 Evolution of Modern Lymphoma Radiotherapy

Modern RT has led to substantial reductions of radiation fields, moving from the old concept of EFRT and IFRT to the modern, state-of-the-art involved-site radiotherapy (ISRT). In the following, we briefly describe the historical processes that led to the introduction of ISRT.

1. EFRT was created at a time when RT was the only curative treatment modality. Radiation was delivered to large volumes of tissue, including prophylactic RT to lymph nodes with no evidence of lymphoma involvement, but which were suspected of harboring microscopic disease. In the most extreme form of EFRT, all major lymph node regions in the body were irradiated, so-called total nodal irradiation (TNI). Excellent remission rates (100%) and progression-free survival rates (80%) were achieved, particularly in patients with Hodgkin lymphoma, which is characterized by predictable, contiguous spread of the disease [12]. However, many patients developed long-term complications, the most

L. Specht
Department of Oncology, Rigshospitalet, Copenhagen, Denmark
e-mail: lena.specht@regionh.dk

M. Levis (✉) · U. Ricardi
Department of Oncology, University of Torino, Torino, Italy
e-mail: mario.levis@unito.it; umberto.ricardi@unito.it

M. Dreyling, M. Ladetto (eds.), *Indolent Lymphomas*, Hematologic Malignancies,
https://doi.org/10.1007/978-3-030-55989-2_5

serious ones being second cancers and cardiovascular disease, from the inevitable, unintended, and extensive irradiation of healthy organs.

2. When effective chemotherapy for many lymphoma types was introduced, it was gradually realized that the very extensive EFRT was no longer needed in patients receiving combined modality treatment. Also, it was realized that many lymphoma types do not spread contiguously and that, therefore, the prophylactic radiotherapy to neighboring lymph node regions was not useful, even in patients treated with RT as the primary treatment modality. Treatment fields were therefore reduced to IFRT, including only the regions containing lymph nodes with known involvement. Both EFRT and IFRT are based on lymph node regions, and the definition of these regions was usually the one that was used in the Ann Arbor staging system [13], despite the fact that these regions were never meant to be used in RT planning. EFRT and IFRT stem from a time when two-dimensional RT planning was used and only X-rays were available, so the knowledge of the precise location and extent of disease was not available. Hence, the definition of RT fields was based on anatomic landmarks, usually bony structures, leading to the inclusion of large volumes of normal tissues in the RT fields.
3. Technological developments in imaging, treatment planning, and treatment machines have revolutionized RT during the recent couple of decades, and these very significant improvements are now also applied in the treatment of lymphomas [14, 15]. This has led to a veritable paradigm shift in lymphoma RT. In fact, the combination of three-dimensional planning, modern imaging and advanced techniques, such as three-dimensional conformal RT, intensity-modulated RT (IMRT), volumetric arc therapy (VMAT) and proton therapy, allowed to irradiate exclusively and with high precision the volume that needs RT, and no more than that, using advanced techniques such as three-dimensional conformal RT, intensity-modulated RT (IMRT), volumetric arc therapy (VMAT), and proton therapy. The modern concept used in lymphoma RT is ISRT. The target for ISRT is defined according to the internationally recognized guidelines developed by the International Commission on Radiation Units and Measurements (ICRU) [16], which have been used for solid tumors for many years. The clinical target volume in the ICRU system is the volume of tissue that contains macroscopic malignant disease and/or subclinical malignant disease with a certain probability of occurrence considered relevant for therapy. For lymphomas treated primarily with combined modality therapy, including effective systemic therapy, the target is only the initially macroscopically involved lymphoma volume, as the systemic treatment is able to deal with the initial microscopic disease. In indolent lymphomas, however, when using RT as the primary curative treatment without any effective systemic therapy, the target is the macroscopically involved lymphoma volume and the lymph nodes in the vicinity, which although of normal size, might contain microscopic disease. This means that the target volume is somewhat more generous when RT is the sole treatment modality, including also adjacent lymph nodes to the involved site, with a generous margin dictated by the clinical situation [8]. In primary extranodal disease, there is often multifocal disease within the affected organ, so here the target volume includes in many cases the entire organ [11]. Even with these somewhat more generous target volumes, the irradiated volume is significantly smaller with ISRT than with IFRT, because it does not target whole anatomic regions.

5.3 Radiotherapy in Indolent Lymphomas

5.3.1 Early-Stage Nodal Indolent Lymphomas

5.3.1.1 Follicular Lymphoma

Follicular lymphomas (FL) grades 1, 2, and 3A are considered indolent, whereas grade 3B is biologically closer to diffuse large B-cell lymphoma. Most patients have widespread disease at diagnosis, but around 20% are in stage I or II. Localized disease, that is, stage I or stage II in contiguous areas, is curable with local RT. A large series of patients treated with RT in the past have been published, documenting long-term relapse-free survival of around 40% [17–24]. Although treatment with extended-field RT yielded higher relapse-free survival than more limited treatment fields, there was no difference in overall survival [25]. The addition of chemotherapy or rituximab improves relapse-free survival but has no impact on overall survival [26–28].

Analyses of large patient databases indicate that the use of RT improves overall survival in early-stage FL [23, 24]. Despite this, the use of RT seems to be decreasing [23, 24]. Due to this inappropriate management, RT is an increasingly underused treatment approach in the modern therapy for patients with early-stage FL.

Modern imaging with PET scanning has increased the accuracy of the staging, thereby improving the proper identification of patients with early-stage FL who may benefit from RT alone [29]. This has led to an improvement in the outcome for patients with early-stage FL treated with RT alone, with a 5-year progression-free survival (PFS) ranging from 70 to 75% in two large retrospective cohorts [30, 31]. Some prognostic factors may still compromise the outcome. As an example, in the series from ILROG [30], stage II disease and BCL2 expression were associated with a lower PFS at 5 years (49.5% and 62.5%, respectively), and these patients might, therefore, be candidates for additional treatment.

In the past, radiation doses of 30–40 Gy have been used for the curative treatment of follicular lymphomas. However, a large randomized British study showed no advantage of 40 Gy compared with 24 Gy [32], and this is now the recommended dose [8].

Modern RT for localized follicular lymphoma is limited to the macroscopic lymphoma volume and the adjacent lymph nodes in that site with a generous margin to encompass suspected subclinical disease, as no curative systemic treatment is administered. Despite the fact that no randomized trial has been conducted to date to compare large fields with small fields, Campbell et al. [33] showed that there is no significant difference in PFS (48% vs 50%, $p = 0.5$) between IFRT and RT to a volume that is close to ISRT. Both the volumes and the doses are reduced very significantly compared with the past, and side effects from the treatment are minor in most cases [8]. Figure 5.1 shows a RT plan for a follicular lymphoma located in the right groin.

A recent UK prospective randomized trial (FORT) [34] compared very low-dose RT (LDRT,

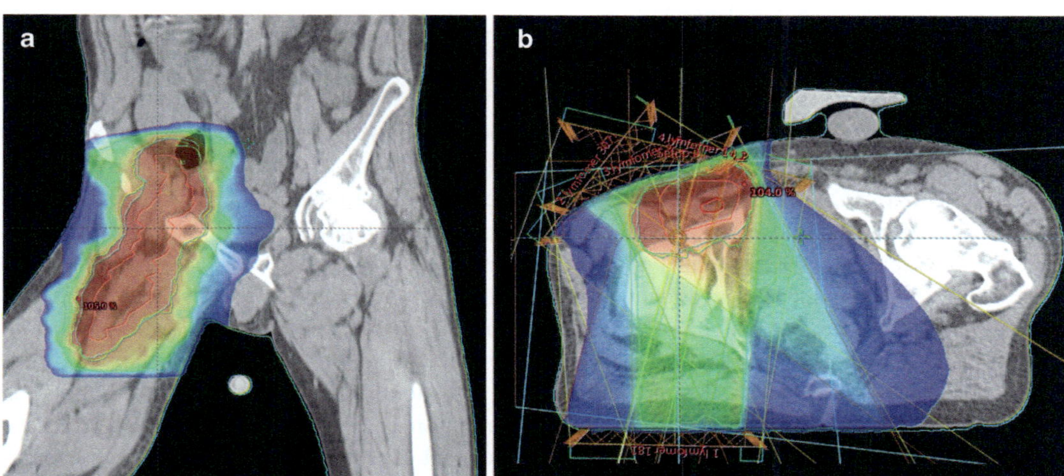

Fig. 5.1 Radiotherapy plan (intensity-modulated radiation therapy (IMRT)) for a localized follicular lymphoma in the left inguinofemoral region. (**a**) Coronal view, (**b**) axial view

4 Gy in two fractions) with the modern standard regimen of 24 Gy in 12 fractions in patients with FL or marginal zone lymphomas: higher response rates were shown with 24 Gy (ORR: 91% vs. 81%; CRR 67% vs. 49%). Moreover, patients treated with 4 Gy had a shorter time to progression (HR 3.42), while there were no differences in terms of overall survival. Given these results, 24 Gy remains the standard of treatment for FL patients, with LDRT representing a valuable alternative for frail patients or palliative treatment.

5.3.1.2 Mantle Cell Lymphoma

Mantle cell lymphomas are most commonly widely disseminated at diagnosis. However, 10–15% of patients present with early-stage disease. Despite the poor response to systemic treatments of mantle cell lymphomas, they are exquisitely radiosensitive and potentially curable with RT if truly localized. In a large series from ILROG, 10-year survival was over 70% for patients treated with RT with or without systemic treatment [35]. It was evident that localized mantle cell lymphoma represents a subgroup with special characteristics and a better prognosis than the usual disseminated mantle cell lymphoma regardless of treatment. These patients, who are often older, seem to be suitable for less-intensive treatment with abbreviated chemotherapy and rituximab and RT to achieve disease control with limited toxicity.

5.3.1.3 Nodal Marginal Zone Lymphoma, Lymphoplasmacytic Lymphoma, Small Lymphocytic Lymphoma

Localized cases of these indolent lymphoma types are rare, and few reports of treatment results are available. They seem to be highly radiosensitive, and radiation seems to improve the outcome in this particular setting. In fact, a recent analysis of the National Cancer Database [36] shows that the omission of RT is detrimental in early-stage marginal zone lymphomas, with a 5- and 10-year OS of 86.7 and 68.8% for radiation group compared to 78 and 54.3% for patients not treated ($p < 0.001$). Therefore, these patients should be treated with local irradiation according to the principles outlined for FL.

5.3.2 Early-Stage Extranodal Indolent Lymphomas

Lymphomas that present primarily with lesions wholly or predominantly confined outside lymph node areas, with or without the involvement of adjacent or draining lymph nodes, are defined as primary extranodal lymphomas [37]. They must be distinguished from disseminated lymphomas with extranodal spread, which are not considered primary extranodal lymphomas and often have a different clinical behavior. The term *primary extranodal* lymphoma is therefore only relevant for early-stage disease. The treatment of lymphomas in general is determined on the basis of the histopathologic type and the anatomic extent of the disease. However, for extranodal lymphomas, the specific organ involvement must also be taken into account.

5.3.2.1 Mucosa-Associated Lymphoid Tissue (MALT) Lymphoma

MALT lymphomas are extranodal marginal zone lymphomas. They occur most commonly in the stomach, less commonly in other parts of the gastrointestinal tract, second-most commonly in the ocular adnexae, and then in a descending order in the lungs, skin, salivary glands, female breast, soft tissues, thyroid, and infrequently in many other organs (Fig. 5.2) [38]. These lymphomas are virtually always localized to the organ in question, sometimes with the involvement of regional lymph nodes. In some localizations, the lymphoma is associated with an infection, notably *Helicobacter pylori* in the stomach and in some geographical areas *Chlamydia psittaci* in the orbit. Sometimes antibiotics active against the infectious organism may bring the lymphoma in remission [39]. Otherwise, primary RT is the treatment of choice in most situations. It is curative in the majority of patients. A recent retrospective analysis from Memorial Sloan Kettering Cancer Center [40] showed high PFS

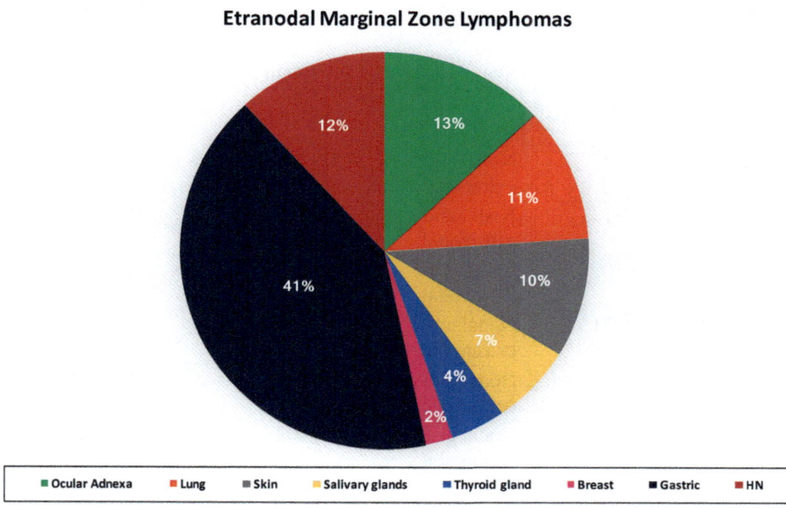

Fig. 5.2 Frequency rates of extranodal marginal zone lymphomas according to site of involvement

and OS rates at 5 years (60% and 89%, respectively) in a large group of 244 early-stage MALT lymphoma patients receiving RT alone with curative intent. Moreover, the cumulative incidence of disease-specific death at 5 years was only 1.3%. Although indolent lymphomas are highly responsive to systemic therapy, the curative potential of standard-dose systemic therapy has not been demonstrated [41].

Modern RT for extranodal marginal zone lymphomas follows in principle the guidelines for the involved-site radiation therapy for nodal indolent lymphomas [8, 11]. However, in many organs, for example, the stomach, orbit, salivary glands, thyroid gland, and breasts, lymphoma tends to be multifocal. Therefore, the involved organ is often treated in its entirety. If adjacent structures have been involved, some or all of the invaded structures may be included in the irradiated area. Uninvolved lymph nodes are not routinely included in the irradiated volume. However, first echelon nodes of uncertain status close to the primary organ may be included, for example, the perigastric lymph nodes in the lymphoma of the stomach. With regard to radiation dose, the aforementioned randomized British study also included patients with MALT lymphomas and demonstrated that a dose of 24 Gy in 12 fractions was as effective as doses of 40–45 Gy [30]. Hence, the recommended dose is 24 Gy. LDRT with 4 Gy is a feasible option in MALT lymphomas, as demonstrated by the already cited FORT trial [34], with response rates and duration almost as good as with 24 Gy. In fact, with a closer look at the study results, patients with MALT lymphomas had better response rates to LDRT compared to other indolent histologic types, as shown by a similar overall response rates (ORR) for 24 Gy and 4 Gy (92% vs 87%, respectively). Some retrospective reports have confirmed the high ORR of LDRT for MALT lymphomas (Table 5.1), which is now investigated in some prospective studies led by the MD Anderson Cancer Center (trial numbers NCT02494700 and NCT03680586).

The techniques used for RT of MALT lymphomas vary with the different involved organs [11]. RT techniques and doses for different locations are shown in Table 5.2. Results of treatment with RT are excellent, although they vary slightly depending on which extranodal organ is involved. PFS for MALT lymphomas in different organs is shown in Fig. 5.3 [42]. For the stomach, treating in deep inspiration breath hold (DIBH) may have an advantage in reducing the radiation dose to the heart, which is located right above the stomach (Fig. 5.4). Moreover, the combination of DIBH with highly conformal techniques, such as intensity-modulated RT (IMRT), allows a further reduction of the dose received by the kidneys, which are frequently located in close proximity of the target of treat-

Table 5.1 Studies investigating the role of low-dose radiotherapy (LDRT) in marginal zone lymphomas

First author, year	No. of patients	Site of disease	Treatment	Results
	MALT/ total			
Ganem, 1994 [69]	7/27	Nodal and extranodal	2 Gy × 2 in 3 days	37% CR
Sawyer, 1997 [66]	5/11	Nodal and extranodal	2 Gy × 2 in 3 days	38% CR, 56% PR
Haas, 2003 [60]	9/109	Nodal and extranodal	2 Gy × 2/4 Gy × 1	61% CR, 31% PR, 8% nonresponders
Haas, 2005 [61]	25/71	Nodal and extranodal	2 Gy × 2/4 Gy × 1	Median OS 67 months
Ng, 2006 [65]	2/10	Nodal and extranodal	2 Gy × 2	90% CR
Luthy, 2008 [63]	2/23	Nodal and extranodal	2 Gy × 2	88% CR, 12% PR
Rossier, 2011 [70]	13/43	Nodal and extranodal	2 Gy × 2	28% CR, 15% PR, 26% SD, 11% PD; median OS 41 months
Chan, 2011 [71]	5/54	Nodal and extranodal	2 Gy × 2	71% CR, 17% PR, 8% SD, 2% PD, median TTLP 1.62 years
Girinsky, 2012 [50]	10/10	Lung	2 Gy × 2	5-years OS 100%, 5-years PFS 87.5%
Russo, 2013 [72]	18/187	Nodal and extranodal	2 Gy × 2	TTFT-L 2.82 HR
Fasola, 2013 [47]	20/20	Orbit	2 Gy × 2	85% CR, 11% PR; 2-years FFLR 100%
Hoskin, 2014 [34]	72/548	Nodal and extranodal	2 Gy × 2 vs. 24 Gy × 12	55% CR
Pinnix, 2017 [48]	14/22	Ocular adnexa	2 Gy × 2	86% CR, 14% PR; ORR 100%
Konig, 2018 [73]	20/47	Nodal and extranodal	2 Gy × 2	90% CR, 3% PR; ORR 93%
Goyal, 2018 [74]	34/54	Skin	2 Gy × 2/4 Gy × 2	94% CR, 1-year failure rate: 6.7%
Ludmir, 2019 [75]	11/11	Breast	2 Gy × 2 vs 30 Gy × 15	Time from initial treatment to progression: 45.6 months; 5-years PFS 100%
Total	267/1247			

CR complete response, *PR* partial response, *SD* stable disease, *PD* progressive disease, *OS* overall survival, *PFS* progression-free survival, *TTLP* time to local progression, *TTFT-L* time to further treatment to local failure, *FFLR* freedom from local recurrence, *HR* hazard ratio, *ORR* overall response rate

ment [43, 44], without compromising target coverage. The orbital-adnexa location accounts for roughly 13% of all MALT lymphomas. Standard-dose RT (24–30 Gy) leads to excellent control rates (85–100%) [45, 46], which are partially counterbalanced by treatment-related toxicities and by a substantial risk of distant recurrence (10–25%) at 10 years after treatment. For the conjunctiva, treating with an anterior electron field while shielding the lens with a lead cylinder mounted on a haptic lens yields high lymphoma control with minimal side effects. Lower doses (2 Gy × 2) are a valuable strategy to reduce RT-related side effects, particularly cataract,

Table 5.2 Radiotherapy techniques and doses for marginal zone lymphomas in different locations

	%	Imaging	Setup	GTV	CTV	Doses	Technique	Other TP
Lymph nodes	2	CT	Depending on the site	Pre-biopsy lesion	GTV + adjacent involved lymph nodes	24 Gy/12 fx	3DCRT/ IMRT	
Stomach/ duodenum	38	CT + EGDS	Supine; Arms above head; 4DCT; Oral contrast medium	Pre-biopsy lesion + involved nodes	Whole organ	24 Gy/12 fx	IMRT	HP eradication
Ocular adnexa/ orbital cavity	14	CT/ MRI	Supine; Head mask	Pre-biopsy lesion	Entire orbit	24 Gy/12 fx OR 4 Gy/2 fx	3DCRT	*C. psittaci* eradication
Salivary glands	9	CT/ MRI	Supine; Head mask	Pre-biopsy lesion	Whole salivary gland	24 Gy/12 fx OR 4 Gy/2 fx	3DCRT	
Lung	10	CT/ HRCT	Supine; Arms above head; 4DCT	Pre-biopsy lesion	GTV + margin due to breath variations	24 Gy/12 fx OR 4 Gy/2 fx	IMRT	
H&N	12	CT/ MRI	Supine; Head mask; (bite)	Pre-biopsy lesion	Entire involved structure	24 Gy/12 fx OR 4 Gy/2 fx	IMRT	

GTV gross tumor volume, *CTV* clinical target volume, *TP* treatment possibility, *H&N* head and neck, *CT* computed tomography, *EGDS* esophagogastroduodenoscopy, *MRI* magnetic resonance imaging, *HRCT* high-resolution computed tomography, *4DCT* 4-dimensional computed tomography, *Gy* Gray, *Fx* fractions, *3DCRT* three-dimensional conformal radiation therapy, *IMRT* intensity-modulated radiation therapy. *HP Helicobacter pylori*

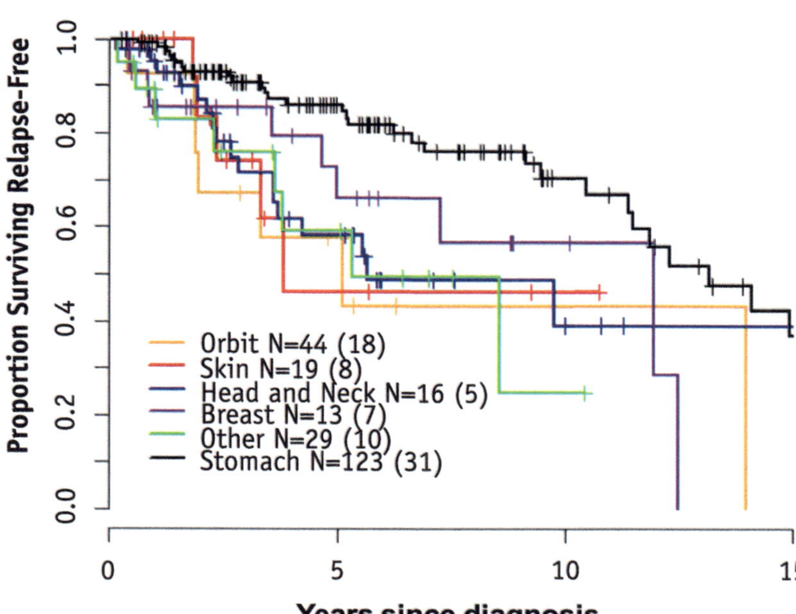

Fig. 5.3 Relapse-free survival in 244 patients from Memorial Sloan Kettering Cancer Center [42] with MALT lymphoma in different organs, treated with local radiation therapy. (Reprinted with permission)

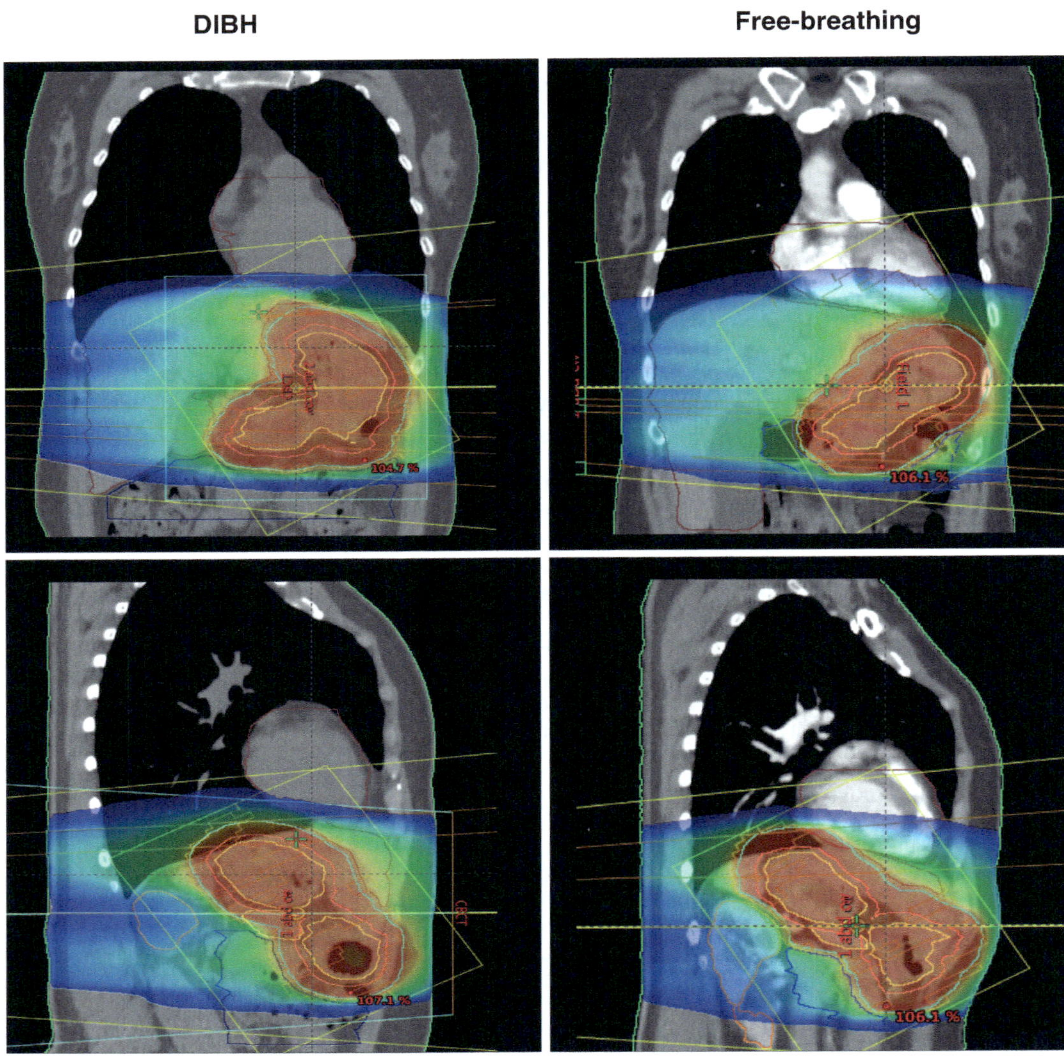

Fig. 5.4 Radiotherapy plan for a gastric MALT lymphoma; to the left side, dose distribution in deep inspiration breath hold (DIBH); to the right side, dose distribution in free breathing. Notice the sparing of the heart in the deep inspiration plan. (Coronal views in the upper row and sagittal views in the lower row)

while maintaining excellent and durable ORR, ranging from 90 to 95% [47, 48] (Fig. 5.5). Salivary gland involvement is less common (7% of MALT lymphomas) and is frequently related to autoimmune disorders (e.g., Sjogren syndrome). The prognosis is usually very good, with 5-year overall survival of at least 90% [49] for patients receiving a 3D conformal RT course with curative intent on the whole gland (Fig. 5.6). For the lung, only the lymphoma lesions with margins for microscopic extension and respiratory movement are irradiated, and treatment in DIBH may reduce the amount of normal lung tissue irradiated by inflating the lungs (Fig. 5.7). The efficacy of LDRT was also demonstrated in a small cohort of patients with lung localization, with 5-year PFS and OS of 87.5% and 100%, respectively [50].

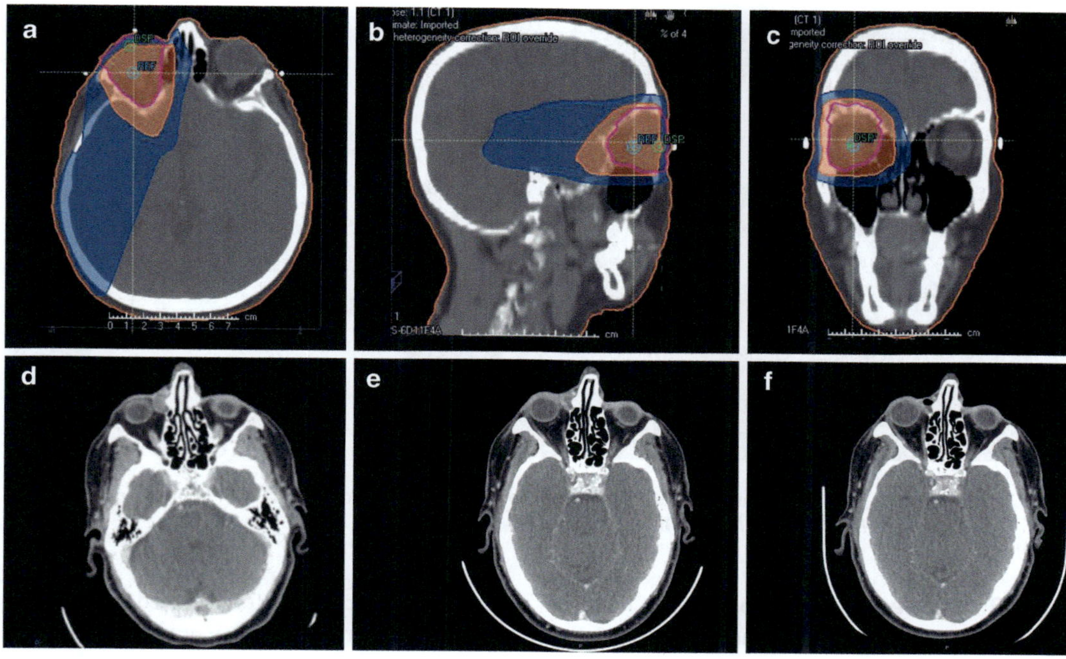

Fig. 5.5 A 68-year-old woman with right orbital-stage MALT lymphoma treated with LDRT (4 Gy in two fractions) with a curative intent. In the first row, dose distribution on an axial view (**a**), a sagittal view (**b**), and a coronal view (**c**). In the second row, disease presentation at baseline (**d**) and its evolution after LDRT at 3 months (**e**) and at 6 months (**f**) with the achievement and maintenance of a complete response at the CT scan

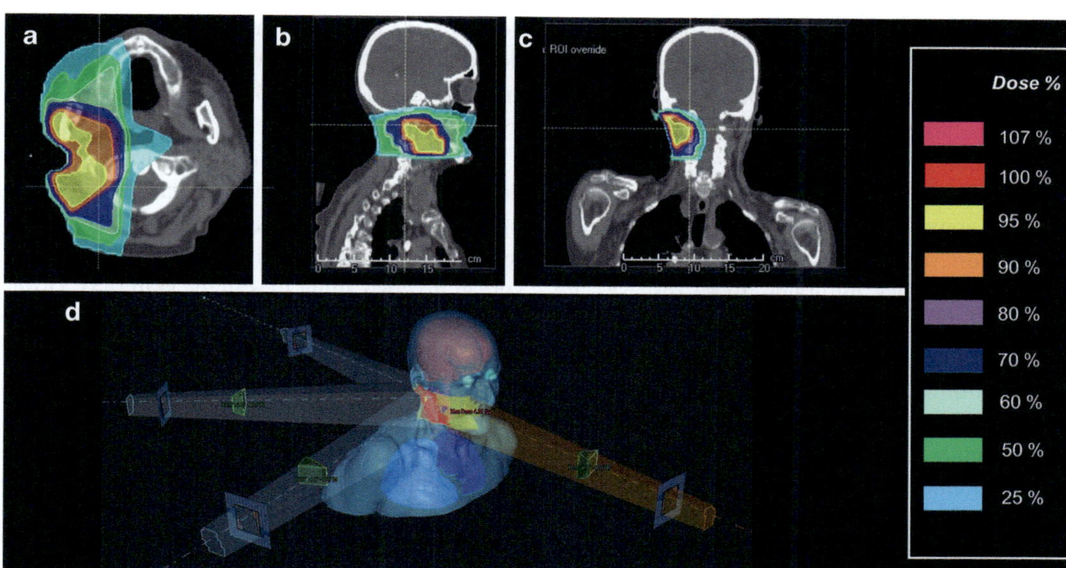

Fig. 5.6 A 75-year-old woman with stage IE MALT lymphoma of the parotid gland, treated with radiotherapy alone with curative intent (24 Gy in 12 fractions). In the upper row, dose distribution in the axial (**a**), coronal (**b**), and sagittal (**c**) views. In the lower row, beam orientation of the 3DCRT plan generated for this patient (**d**)

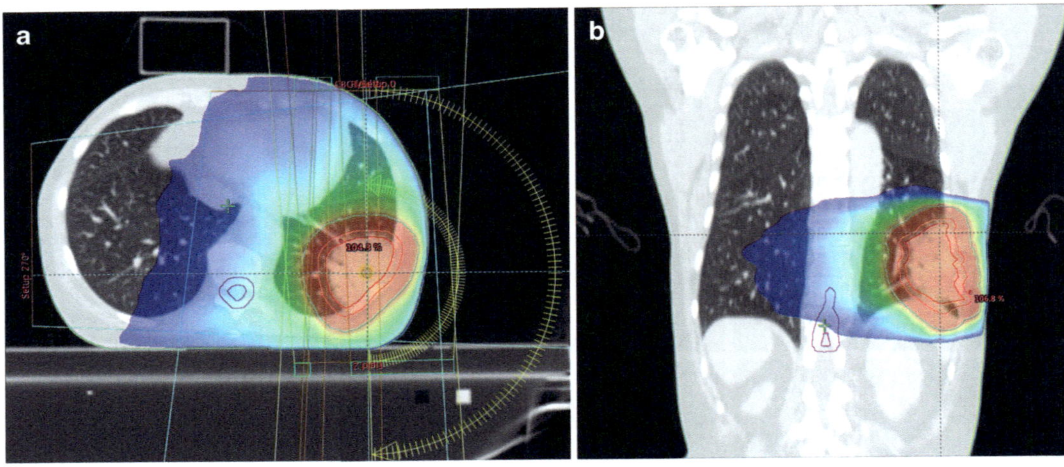

Fig. 5.7 Pulmonary MALT lymphoma treated with deep inspiration breath hold (DIBH) with highly *conformal volumetric arc therapy (VMAT)*. (**a**) *axial view;* (**b**) *coronal view*

5.3.2.2 Cutaneous Lymphoma

Approximately, one third of non-Hodgkin lymphomas present as extranodal lymphomas [51]. The most common site is the gastrointestinal tract, and the second-most common is the skin. Primary cutaneous lymphomas tend to remain localized to the skin for a long time, and they have a much more indolent course and a much better prognosis than that of lymphomas of a similar histologic subtype in other locations [52]. In recent lymphoma classifications, primary cutaneous lymphomas are therefore classified as separate entities [53].

Mycosis fungoides and Sézary syndrome are the most common primary cutaneous lymphomas in the Western world. Except for very localized mycosis fungoides infiltrates, these diseases are incurable, but they often have a very indolent course over many years. They are treated primarily with skin-directed therapies, and when infiltrates become thicker, RT is the most effective treatment for palliation. Local x-ray therapy remains a very effective treatment for primary cutaneous lymphomas. However, if it is administered over large areas, the dose to the underlying internal organs exceeds their tolerance. Electrons, by contrast, have a limited range of penetration and deposit their total energy within that range. The effect of electrons is therefore limited to superficial tissues, with the depth depending on the energy of the electrons. They can therefore be used for the treatment of larger areas, and they are today preferred for the treatment of cutaneous lymphomas because of the sparing of deeper-lying tissues [54, 55]. In mycosis fungoides, RT can be curative in patients with early localized disease, and the recommended dose is 20–24 Gy. For local palliation in patients with more widespread disease, the recommended dose is 8–12 Gy; 8 Gy may be given in one fraction, but often patients will require reirradiation, and smaller fractions of 3–5 Gy may be preferred [54, 55].

Techniques for yielding a uniform electron dose to the entire skin surface have been developed, and total skin electron beam therapy remains a highly effective treatment for widespread mycosis fungoides in the skin [54]. Doses for total skin electron beam therapy used to be 30–36 Gy. However, total skin electron beam therapy is a palliative treatment and recurrences invariably occur. Lower doses of 10–12 Gy are now more popular, as they offer advantages of briefer duration, fewer side effects, and the opportunity for retreatment, which may ultimately offer the patient better and longer overall palliation [56, 57]. Figure 5.8 shows mycosis fungoides infiltrates in the skin before and after total skin electron beam therapy.

Primary cutaneous anaplastic large-cell lymphoma, primary cutaneous follicle center lym-

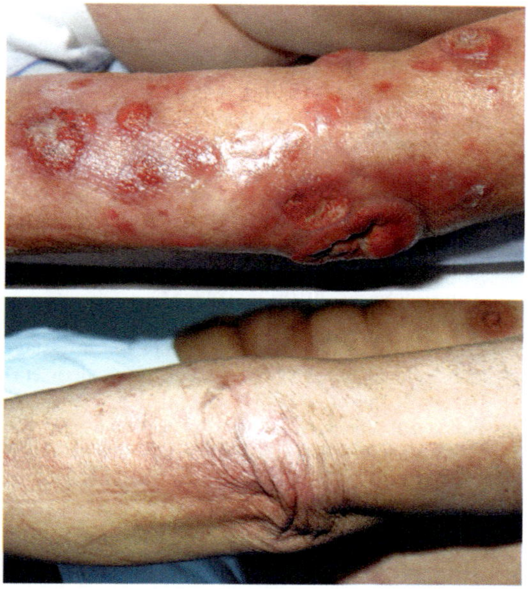

Fig. 5.8 Mycosis fungoides infiltrates in the skin before (upper panel) and 6 months after total skin electron beam therapy (lower panel)

phoma, and primary cutaneous marginal zone lymphoma are indolent lymphomas. For localized disease in the skin, local RT is the preferred treatment, usually with electrons. For multifocal disease, local RT is an excellent palliative treatment. For primary cutaneous anaplastic large-cell lymphoma, a dose of 24–30 Gy has been recommended, but recent data indicate that a dose of 20 Gy or even lower may be effective. For the very indolent primary marginal zone and follicle center lymphomas, the recommended curative radiation dose is 24–30 Gy. However, indolent B-cell lymphomas are exquisitely radiosensitive, and in the palliative setting, 2 Gy × 2 is effective and very convenient [52, 54, 55].

5.3.3 Nodal Indolent Lymphoma, Advanced Disease

Indolent lymphomas are exquisitely radiosensitive, and localized radiotherapy to LDRT can achieve excellent palliation in patients with advanced disease [58–66] (Table 5.1). A total dose of just 4 Gy given in two fractions achieves response rates around 90%, most of them complete remissions, with a response duration of over 2 years. Importantly, this treatment has very few side effects, even in situations where relatively large treatment fields are necessary, for example, whole-abdominal irradiation, and can be repeated as necessary. The biologic basis for this extreme radiosensitivity seems to be p53 induction and apoptosis [67, 68].

5.4 Conclusion

Indolent lymphomas are highly radiosensitive. In early-stage disease, both nodal and extranodal, primary involved-site RT to moderate doses (24-30 Gy) has the potential to cure many patients. In advanced disease, local palliation with a very low risk of side effects can be achieved with very low doses (4 Gy) of RT.

References

1. Specht L. The history of radiation therapy of lymphomas and description of early trials. In: Armitage JO, Coiffier B, Dalla-Favera R, Harris N, Mauch PM, editors. Non-Hodgkin's lymphomas. 2nd ed. Baltimore: Lippincott Williams & Wilkins; 2009. p. 12–24.
2. Berven E. Le traitement radiologique des tumeurs malignes de la cavité buccale. Acta Radiol. 1932;13:213–31.
3. Finzi NS. The Roentgen treatment of lymphadenoma. Am J Roentgenol. 1938;39:261–2.
4. Hynes JF, Frelick RW. Roentgen therapy of malignant lymphoma with special reference to segmental radiation therapy. Results 1935-1945. Am J Roentgenol. 1953;70:247–57.
5. Paryani SB, Hoppe RT, Cox RS, Colby TV, Rosenberg SA, Kaplan HS. Analysis of non-Hodgkin's lymphomas with nodular and favorable histologies, stages I and II. Cancer. 1983;52:2300–7.
6. Mikhaeel NG, Milgrom SA, Terezakis S, Berthelsen AK, Hodgson D, Eich HT, et al. The optimal use of imaging in radiation therapy for lymphoma—guidelines from the International Lymphoma Radiation Oncology Group (ILROG). Int J Radiat Oncol Biol Phys. 2019;104(3):501–12.
7. Aznar MC, Maraldo MV, Schut DA, Lundemann M, Brodin NP, Vogelius IR, et al. Minimizing late effects for patients with mediastinal Hodgkin lymphoma: deep inspiration breath-hold, IMRT, or both? Int J Radiat Oncol Biol Phys. 2015;92:169–74.

8. Illidge T, Specht L, Yahalom J, Aleman B, Berthelsen AK, Constine L, et al. Modern radiation therapy for nodal non-Hodgkin lymphoma—target definition and dose guidelines from the International Lymphoma Radiation Oncology Group (ILROG). Int J Radiat Oncol Biol Phys. 2014;89:49–58.
9. Maraldo MV, Brodin NP, Aznar MC, Vogelius IR, Munck Af RP, Petersen PM, Specht L. Estimated risk of cardiovascular disease and secondary cancers with modern highly conformal radiotherapy for early-stage mediastinal Hodgkin lymphoma. Ann Oncol. 2013;24:2113–8.
10. Rechner LA, Maraldo MV, Vogelius IR, Zhu XR, Dabaja BS, Brodin NP, et al. Life years lost attributable to late effects after radiotherapy for early stage Hodgkin lymphoma: the impact of proton therapy and/or deep inspiration breath hold. Radiother Oncol. 2017;125:41–7.
11. Yahalom J, Illidge T, Specht L, Hoppe RT, Li YX, Tsang R, Wirth A. Modern radiation therapy for extranodal lymphomas: field and dose guidelines from the International Lymphoma Radiation Oncology Group. Int J Radiat Oncol Biol Phys. 2015;92:11–31.
12. Crnkovich MJ, Leopold K, Hoppe RT, Mauch PM. Stage I to IIB Hodgkin's disease: the combined experience at Stanford University and the Joint Center for Radiation Therapy. J Clin Oncol. 1987;5(7):1041–9.
13. Kaplan HS, Rosenberg SA. The treatment of Hodgkin's disease. Med Clin North Am. 1966;50:1591–610.
14. Specht L, Yahalom J. The concept and evolution of involved site radiation therapy for lymphoma. Int J Clin Oncol. 2015;20:849–54.
15. Specht L. Radiotherapy for Hodgkin lymphoma, reducing toxicity while maintaining efficacy. Cancer J. 2018;24:237–43.
16. DeLuca P, Jones D, Gahbauer R, Whitmore G, Wambersie A. Prescribing, recording, and reporting photon-beam intensity-modulated radiation therapy (IMRT). J ICRU. 2010;10:1–106.
17. Ahmed N, Owen TE, Rubinger M, Williams G, Nugent Z, Ahmed S, Cooke A. Early stage W.H.O. grade I and II follicular lymphoma treated with radiation therapy alone. PLoS One. 2013;8:e65156.
18. Barzenje DA, Cvancarova SM, Liestol K, Fossa A, Delabie J, Kolstad A, Holte H. Radiotherapy compared to other strategies in the treatment of stage I/II follicular lymphoma: a study of 404 patients with a median follow-up of 15 years. PLoS One. 2015;10:e0131158.
19. Choi SH, Cho J, Kim JS, Cheong JW, Suh CO. Radiotherapy as an effective treatment modality for follicular lymphoma: a single institution experience. Radiat Oncol J. 2015;33:310–9.
20. Guadagnolo BA, Li S, Neuberg D, Ng A, Hua L, Silver B, et al. Long-term outcome and mortality trends in early-stage, Grade 1-2 follicular lymphoma treated with radiation therapy. Int J Radiat Oncol Biol Phys. 2006;64:928–34.
21. Heinzelmann F, Engelhard M, Ottinger H, Bamberg M, Weinmann M. Nodal follicular lymphoma: the role of radiotherapy for stages I and II. Strahlenther Onkol. 2010;186:191–6.
22. Mac Manus MP, Hoppe RT. Is radiotherapy curative for stage I and II low-grade follicular lymphoma? Results of a long-term follow-up study of patients treated at Stanford University. J Clin Oncol. 1996;14:1282–90.
23. Pugh TJ, Ballonoff A, Newman F, Rabinovitch R. Improved survival in patients with early stage low-grade follicular lymphoma treated with radiation: a surveillance, epidemiology, and end results database analysis. Cancer. 2010;116:3843–51.
24. Vargo JA, Gill BS, Balasubramani GK, Beriwal S. What is the optimal management of early-stage low-grade follicular lymphoma in the modern era? Cancer. 2015;121:3325–34.
25. Wilder RB, Jones D, Tucker SL, Fuller LM, Ha CS, McLaughlin P, et al. Long-term results with radiotherapy for stage I-II follicular lymphomas. Int J Radiat Oncol Biol Phys. 2001;51:1219–27.
26. Janikova A, Bortlicek Z, Campr V, Kopalova N, Benesova K, Belada D, et al. Radiotherapy with rituximab may be better than radiotherapy alone in first-line treatment of early-stage follicular lymphoma: is it time to change the standard strategy? Leuk Lymphoma. 2015;56:2350–6.
27. MacManus M, Fisher R, Roos D, O'Brien P, Macann A, Davis S, et al. Randomized trial of systemic therapy after involved-field radiotherapy in patients with early-stage follicular lymphoma: TROG 99.03. J Clin Oncol. 2018;36:2918–25.
28. Sancho JM, Ribera JM, Vaquero M, Oriol A, Hernandez-Rivas JA, Feliu E. Non-gastrointestinal malt lymphomas: a study of 10 cases and comparison with 27 patients with gastrointestinal MALT lymphoma. Haematologica. 2000;85:557–9.
29. Wirth A, Foo M, Seymour JF, MacManus MP, Hicks RJ. Impact of [18f] fluorodeoxyglucose positron emission tomography on staging and management of early-stage follicular non-Hodgkin lymphoma. Int J Radiat Oncol Biol Phys. 2008;71:213–9.
30. Brady JL, Binkley MS, Hajj C, Chelius M, Chau K, Balogh A, et al. Definitive radiotherapy for localized follicular lymphoma staged by (18)F-FDG PET-CT: a collaborative study by ILROG. Blood. 2019;133:237–45.
31. Ng SP, Khor R, Bressel M, MacManus M, Seymour JF, Hicks RJ, Wirth A. Outcome of patients with early-stage follicular lymphoma staged with (18) F-Fluorodeoxyglucose (FDG) positron emission tomography (PET) and treated with radiotherapy alone. Eur J Nucl Med Mol Imaging. 2019;46:80–6.
32. Lowry L, Smith P, Qian W, Falk S, Benstead K, Illidge T, et al. Reduced dose radiotherapy for local control in non-Hodgkin lymphoma: a randomised phase III trial. Radiother Oncol. 2011;100:86–92.
33. Campbell BA, Voss N, Woods R, Gascoyne RD, Morris J, Pickles T, et al. Long-term outcomes for patients with limited stage follicular lymphoma: involved regional radiotherapy versus involved node radiotherapy. Cancer. 2010;116(16):3797–806.

34. Hoskin PJ, Kirkwood AA, Popova B, Smith P, Robinson M, Gallop-Evans E, et al. 4 Gy versus 24 Gy radiotherapy for patients with indolent lymphoma (FORT): a randomised phase 3 non-inferiority trial. Lancet Oncol. 2014;15:457–63.
35. Dabaja BS, Zelenetz AD, Ng AK, Tsang RW, Qi S, Allen PK, et al. Early-stage mantle cell lymphoma: a retrospective analysis from the International Lymphoma Radiation Oncology Group (ILROG). Ann Oncol. 2017;28:2185–90.
36. Ling DC, Vargo JA, Balasubramani GK, Beriwal S. Underutilization of radiation therapy in early-stage marginal zone lymphoma negatively impacts overall survival. Pract Radiat Oncol. 2015;6:97–105.
37. Specht L. Radiotherapy studies and extra-nodal non-Hodgkin lymphomas, progress and challenges. Clin Oncol (R Coll Radiol). 2012;24:313–8.
38. Khalil MO, Morton LM, Devesa SS, Check DP, Curtis RE, Weisenburger DD, Dores GM. Incidence of marginal zone lymphoma in the United States, 2001-2009 with a focus on primary anatomic site. Br J Haematol. 2014;165:67–77.
39. Ferreri AJ, Ponzoni M, Guidoboni M, Resti AG, Politi LS, Cortelazzo S, et al. Bacteria-eradicating therapy with doxycycline in ocular adnexal MALT lymphoma: a multicenter prospective trial. J Natl Cancer Inst. 2006;98:1375–82.
40. Teckie S, Qi S, Chelius M, Lovie S, Hsu M, Noy A, et al. Long-term outcome of 487 patients with early-stage extra-nodal marginal zone lymphoma. J Ann Oncol. 2017;28(5):1064–9.
41. Zelenetz AD, Gordon LI, Wierda WG, Abramson JS, Advani RH, Andreadis CB, et al. Non-Hodgkin's lymphomas, version 4.2014. J Natl Compr Cancer Netw. 2014;12:1282–303.
42. Teckie S, Qi S, Lovie S, Navarrett S, Hsu M, Noy A, et al. Long-term outcomes and patterns of relapse of early-stage extranodal marginal zone lymphoma treated with radiation therapy with curative intent. Int J Radiat Oncol Biol Phys. 2015;92:130–7.
43. Van der Geld YG, Senan S, van Sornsen de Koste JR, Verbakel WF, Slotman BJ, Lagerwaard FJ. A four-dimensional CT-based evaluation of techniques for gastric irradiation. Int J Radiat Oncol Biol Phys. 2007;69:903–9.
44. Watanabe M, Isobe K, Takisima H, Uno T, Ueno N, Kawakami H, et al. Intrafractional gastric motion and interfractional stomach deformity during radiation therapy. Radiother Oncol. 2008;87:425–31.
45. Stefanovic A, Lossos IS. Extranodal marginal zone lymphoma of the ocular adnexa. Blood. 2009;114:501–10.
46. Goda JS, Le LW, Lapperrier NJ, Millar BA, Payne D, Gospodarowicz MK, et al. Localized orbital mucosa associated lymphoma tissue lymphoma managed with primary radiation therapy: efficacy and toxicity. Int J Radiat Oncol Biol Phys. 2011;81:e659–66.
47. Fasola CE, Jones JC, Huang DD, Le QT, Hoppe RT, Donaldson SS. Low dose radiation therapy (2 Gy x 2) in the treatment of orbital lymphoma. Int J Radiat Oncol Biol Phys. 2013;86:930–5.
48. Pinnix CC, Dabaja BS, Milgrom SA, Smith GL, Abou Z, Nastoupil L, et al. Ultra-low-dose radiotherapy for definitive management of ocular adnexal B-cell lymphoma. Head Neck. 2017;39:1095–100.
49. Shum JW, Emmerling M, Lubek JE, Ord RA. Parotid lymphoma: a review of clinical presentation and management. Oral Surg Oral Med Oral Pathol Oral Radiol. 2014;118(1):e1–5. https://doi.org/10.1016/j.oooo.2013.10.013.
50. Girinsky T, Paumier A, Ferme C, Hanna C, Ribrag V, Leroy-Ladurie F, Ghalibafian M. Low-dose radiation treatment in pulmonary mucosa-associated lymphoid tissue lymphoma: a plausible approach? A single-institution experience in 10 patients. Int J Radiat Oncol Biol Phys. 2012;83:e385–9.
51. Newton R, Ferlay J, Beral V, Devesa SS. The epidemiology of non-Hodgkin's lymphoma: comparison of nodal and extra-nodal sites. Int J Cancer. 1997;72:923–30.
52. Willemze R, Hodak E, Zinzani PL, Specht L, Ladetto M. Primary cutaneous lymphomas: ESMO clinical practice guidelines for diagnosis, treatment and follow-up. Ann Oncol. 2018;29:iv30–40.
53. Swerdlow SH, Campo E, Harris NL, Jaffe ES, Pileri SA, Stein H, et al. WHO classification of tumours of haematopoietic and lymphoid tissues (revised 4th ed.). Lyon: IARC; 2017.
54. Specht L, Dabaja B, Illidge T, Wilson LD, Hoppe RT. Modern radiation therapy for primary cutaneous lymphomas: field and dose guidelines from the International Lymphoma Radiation Oncology Group. Int J Radiat Oncol Biol Phys. 2015;92:32–9.
55. Specht L, Skov L. Cutaneous lymphomas. Clin Oncol. 2019;31(11):797–807.
56. Hoppe RT, Harrison C, Tavallaee M, Bashey S, Sundram U, Li S, et al. Low-dose total skin electron beam therapy as an effective modality to reduce disease burden in patients with mycosis fungoides: results of a pooled analysis from 3 phase-II clinical trials. J Am Acad Dermatol. 2015;72:286–92.
57. Kamstrup MR, Lindahl LM, Gniadecki R, Iversen L, Skov L, Petersen PM, et al. Low-dose total skin electron beam therapy as a debulking agent for cutaneous T-cell lymphoma: an open-label prospective phase II study. Br J Dermatol. 2012;166(2):399–404.
58. Ganem G, Cartron G, Girinsky T, Haas RL, Cosset JM, Solal-Celigny P. Localized low-dose radiotherapy for follicular lymphoma: history, clinical results, mechanisms of action, and future outlooks. Int J Radiat Oncol Biol Phys. 2010;78:975–82.
59. Girinsky T, Guillot-Vals D, Koscielny S, Cosset JM, Ganem G, Carde P, et al. A high and sustained response rate in refractory or relapsing low-grade lymphoma masses after low-dose radiation: analysis of predictive parameters of response to treatment. Int J Radiat Oncol Biol Phys. 2001;51:148–55.
60. Haas RL, Poortmans P, de Jong D, Aleman BM, Dewit LG, Verheij M, et al. High response rates and lasting remissions after low-dose involved field

radiotherapy in indolent lymphomas. J Clin Oncol. 2003;21:2474–80.
61. Haas RL, Poortmans P, de Jong D, Verheij M, van der Hulst M, de Boer JP, Bartelink H. Effective palliation by low dose local radiotherapy for recurrent and/or chemotherapy refractory non-follicular lymphoma patients. Eur J Cancer. 2005;41:1724–30.
62. Johannsson J, Specht L, Mejer J, Jensen BA. Phase II study of palliative low-dose local radiotherapy in disseminated indolent non-Hodgkin's lymphoma and chronic lymphocytic leukemia. Int J Radiat Oncol Biol Phys. 2002;54:1466–70.
63. Luthy SK, Ng AK, Silver B, Degnan KO, Fisher DC, Freedman AS, Mauch PM. Response to low-dose involved-field radiotherapy in patients with non-Hodgkin's lymphoma. Ann Oncol. 2008;19:2043–7.
64. Murthy V, Thomas K, Foo K, Cunningham D, Johnson B, Norman A, Horwich A. Efficacy of palliative low-dose involved-field radiation therapy in advanced lymphoma: a phase II study. Clin Lymphoma Myeloma. 2008;8:241–5.
65. Ng M, Wirth A, Ryan G, MacManus M, Davis S. Value of low-dose 2 x 2 Gy palliative radiotherapy in advanced low-grade non-Hodgkin's lymphoma. Australas Radiol. 2006;50:222–7.
66. Sawyer EJ, Timothy AR. Low dose palliative radiotherapy in low grade non-Hodgkin's lymphoma. Radiother Oncol. 1997;42:49–51.
67. Haas RL, de Jong D, Valdes Olmos RA, Hoefnagel CA, van den Heuvel I, Zerp SF, et al. In vivo imaging of radiation-induced apoptosis in follicular lymphoma patients. Int J Radiat Oncol Biol Phys. 2004;59:782–7.
68. Knoops L, Haas R, de Kemp S, Majoor D, Broeks A, Eldering E, et al. In vivo p53 response and immune reaction underlie highly effective low-dose radiotherapy in follicular lymphoma. Blood. 2007;110:1116–22.
69. Ganem G, Lambin P, Socié G, Girinsky T, Bosq J, Pico JL, et al. Potential role for low dose limited-field radiation therapy (2 x 2 Grays) in advanced low-grade non-Hodgkin's lymphomas. Hematol Oncol. 1994;12:1–8.
70. Rossier C, Schick U, Miralbell R, MIrimanoff RO, Weber DC, Qzsahin M. Low-dose radiotherapy in indolent lymphoma. Int J Radiat Oncol Biol Phys. 2011;81(3):e1–6.
71. Chan EK, Fung S, Gospodarowicz M, Hodgson D, Wells W, Sun A, et al. Palliation by low-dose local radiation therapy for indolent non-Hodgkin lymphoma. Int J Radiat Oncol Biol Phys. 2011;81:781–6.
72. Russo AL, Chen YH, Martin NE, Vinjamoori A, Luthy SK, Freedman A, et al. Low-dose involved-field radiation in the treatment of non-Hodgkin lymphoma: predictors of response and treatment failure. Int J Radiat Oncol Biol Phys. 2013;86(1):121–7.
73. König L, Hörner-Rieber J, Bernhardt D, Hommertgen A, Rieken S, Debus J, Herfarth K. Response rates and recurrence patterns after low-dose radiotherapy with 4 Gy in patients with low-grade lymphomas. Strahlenther Onkol. 2018;194(5):454–61.
74. Goyal A, Carter JB, Pashtan I, Gallotto S, Wang I, Isom S, et al. Very low-dose versus standard dose radiation therapy for indolent primary cutaneous B-cell lymphomas: a retrospective study. J Am Acad Dermatol. 2018;78(2):408–10.
75. Ludmir EB, Milgrom SA, Pinnix CC, Gunther JR, Westin J, Fayad LE, et al. Emerging treatment strategies for primary breast extranodal marginal zone lymphoma of mucosa-associated lymphoid tissue. Clin Lymphoma Myeloma Leuk. 2019;19(4):244–50.

Part I

B-Cell Lymphoma

Follicular Lymphoma

6

Alden A. Moccia, Martin Dreyling,
and Michele Ghielmini

Follicular lymphoma (FL)

Clinical outline
FL typically affects adult patient as a widespread disease involving the lymph nodes, but it can affect extranodal sites. linical features (i.e. pediatric age or anatomic primary site) may define FL subsets with proper biology and behavior.

Cytology	Centrocytes and centroblasts in variable relation; spindle cell morphology rare. In histology, number of centroblast per high power field defines the grading.	Follicular lymphoma, cytology 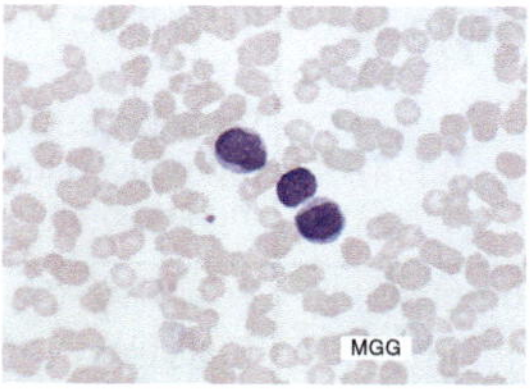
Histology	FL recapitulates the cyto-architectural and phenotypic features of germinal centers (GC) but lacking compartmentalization. Diffuse growth possible. Extrafollicular growth of cells with GC-phenotype commonly found. Accompanying sclerosis may be observed. In the bone marrow, infiltrates closely attached to bone trabeculae.	Follicular lymphoma, hystology 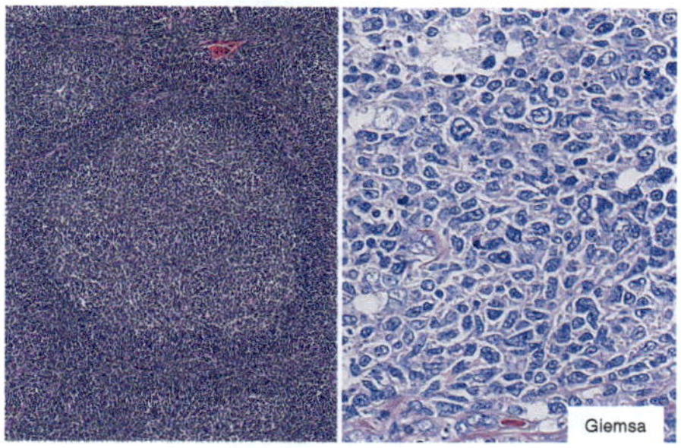

	CD20	CD5	CD23[1]	CD10[2]	BCL6[3]	cyclin D1	CD103	FMC7	IgM	light chains
notes	[1]detects typical dendritic cells too, [2]less frequent in higher grades, [3]less expressed in extrafollicular cells									
other marker	Ki67 variable. BCL2 is typically overexpressed (can undetectable due to mutations or absent in higher grade FL) Other markers of germinal center origin: LMO2, HGAL, GCET. MUM1 positivity in a minority of cases, often with high grade cytology									

■ = majority of cases positive ▒ = variable fraction of cases positive □ = negative

Main differential diagnosis	Benign follicular hyperplasia, Diffuse large B-cell lymphoma (should have lost follicular pattern and show sheets of blasts)

M. Dreyling, M. Ladetto (eds.), *Indolent Lymphomas*, Hematologic Malignancies,
https://doi.org/10.1007/978-3-030-55989-2_6

Key molecular features
IGH genes rearranged, ongoing somatic hypermutation. Frequent overexpression of BCL2 and alteration of TNFRSF14. Frequent translocations: t(14;18)(q32;q21) in approx 85% (less frequent in higher grades), *BCL6* translocation (5-10%). Lymphomas with rearrangements if *IRF4* are separated from FL as a distinct entity despite follicular growth. Frequent copy number alterations: loss of 1p (*TNFRSF14*), 6q, 10q, 17p, gains 1, 6p, 7, 8, 12q, X, 18q. Frequent mutations: *BCL2, KMT2D, TNFRSF14, EZH2, EPHA7, CREBBP, BCL6, MEF2B, EP200, TNFAIP2.*
Precursor lesions
Benign t(14;18)-positive cells in healthy donors, Follicular Neoplasia in situ
Progression
Transformation to diffuse large B-cell lymphoma; less commonly, to high grade B-cell lymphoma or B-lymphoblastic lymphoma / leukemia. Most frequent are relapses of FL not showing histological progression/transformation.

Clinically relevant pathologic features	**Relevance**	**Evidence**
Histologic grading	Prognostic: FL grades I-IIIa harbor no different prognosis.	**A**
	Prognostic: Grade as a prognostic marker only observed in older but not reproduced in more recent studies. Nevertheless, FL IIIb is commonly managed as an aggressive lymphoma.	**B**
Clinico-pathological subtypes of FL (defined by combination of localization, histology and genetics)	Prognostic (favourable): Testicular FL (Confined to testis, frequently younger patients, no t(14;18)(q32;q21) Duodenal-type FL (t(14;18)(q32;q21) positive, confined to duodenum or GI tract, low or no tendency to disseminate or transform) in situ follicular neoplasia (Incidental finding of few t(14;18)(q32;q21) positive cells in GC or lymph nodes enlarged due to other reasons).	
Related diseases	Prognostic (favourable): Primary cutaneous follicle center lymphoma (confined to skin, mostly negative for BCL2 translocation, rarely CD10 expression) Pediatric type follicular lymphoma (nodal, localized stage, cervical region, children, adolescents and young adults, no *BCL2* and *BCL6* translocations)	
***BCL2* rearrangement**	Translocation as a sole bio-marker not prognostic or predictive. Prognostic value of translocation in the context of clinico-pathological subtypes (see above)	**B**
Mutations (*EZH2, ARID1A, MEF2B, EP300, FOXO1, CREBBP, CARD11*)	Prognostic: integration of targeted sequencing for gene panels improves clinical stratification(m7-FLIPI)	**B**
Legend: A = verified in multiple studies, randomized trials and/or integrated in guidelines; B = variable between studies/needs definitive validation; C = preliminary/discrepant results.		

A. A. Moccia (✉) · M. Ghielmini
Oncology Institute of Southern Switzerland, Bellinzona, Switzerland
e-mail: Alden.Moccia@eoc.ch; Michele.Ghielmini@eoc.ch

M. Dreyling
Department of Medicine III, LMU Hospital, München, Bayern, Germany
e-mail: Martin.Dreyling@med.uni-muenchen.de

6.1 Introduction

Follicular lymphoma (FL) represents the most common indolent lymphoma in the Western world. Diagnosis is based on the peculiar histologic nodular pattern and histogenetically it arises from germinal center B-cells. The presence in the same lymph node of a diffuse pattern composed of centroblasts is considered to be in keeping with a progression to a diffuse large B-cell lymphoma.

FL is typically characterized by a relapsing and remitting course of the disease and by the risk of a transformation to a more aggressive disease. The behavior of FL is characterized by a wide heterogeneity. In some cases, the disease can be controlled for many years while in others it follows an aggressive and sometimes chemorefractory course. To date, advanced-stage FL continues to be a treatable but not curable condition. Despite an improvement in the management of patients with FL in recent years, there are still open questions that remain unsolved. In the past 30 years, new treatment approaches have partially modified the management of patients with FL, resulting in more favorable clinical outcomes. Chemotherapy in combination with a monoclonal anti-CD20 antibody is currently the standard of care for patients with advanced-stage FL in need of treatment. The median overall survival (OS) has dramatically improved, in particular, since the advent of rituximab in the treatment armamentarium. Chemotherapy-free approaches based on anti-CD20 antibodies (in particular, rituximab) also represent an option for many patients. Fortunately, for patients relapsing after first-line therapy, there is a wide variety of strategies ranging from targeted therapies up to stem cell transplantation. In this chapter, we review the current knowledge of FL pathology and epidemiology and the critical issues encountered in the clinical practice when treating patients with FL.

6.2 Epidemiology

FL is the second most common lymphoma in the Western world, accounting for approximately 20% of all NHL and up to 70% of indolent lymphomas. The median age at diagnosis is in the mid-1960s. The incidence in Europe is 2.18 cases per 100,000 persons per year [1] and has been stable over time. There is a large variability in terms of incidence, depending in particular on ethnicity: it tends to be higher in Whites than in Black and Asian populations [2]. Numerous potential risk factors have been associated with NHL, even though there is a lack of consensus regarding specific risk factors for the development of FL. Factors traditionally associated with NHL are in particular specific chemical agents (agricultural pesticides, hair dyes), infections (HIV, human T lymphotropic virus type 1 (HTLV-1), Epstein-Barr virus, hepatitis C, *Borrelia burgdorferi*), autoimmune diseases (Lupus erythematosus, rheumatoid arthritis, Sjögren syndrome, Hashimoto's thyroiditis), multicentric Castleman disease, and inflammatory gastrointestinal diseases. Of note, the risk of FL tends to be slightly increased among relatives of a person with FL [3].

6.3 Pathology

FL is diagnosed according to the criteria of the fourth World Health Organization (WHO) classification updated in 2017 [4]. FL is a neoplasm composed of germinal center B-cells exhibiting most frequently a partially follicular growth pattern, which tends to reproduce the architecture of normal germinal centers of secondary follicles. Neoplastic follicles are often poorly defined and usually have attenuated mantle zones. FL is composed of a mixture of centrocytes (cleaved follicle center cells) and centroblasts (large, noncleaved follicle center cells) surrounded by nonmalignant cells including macrophages, T-cells, and follicular dendritic cells. Centroblasts are generally the minority. The presence of diffuse areas composed predominantly of centroblasts is considered to be equivalent to diffuse large B cell lymphoma (DLBCL). Grading of FL is primarily based on the count of centroblasts per high-power field (HPF): grade 1 (0–5 centroblasts per HPF) and grade 2 (6–15 centroblasts per HPF) tend to share similar clinical characteristics and are considered to be of low-grade. FL of grade 3 are considered to be high-grade and they are further divided into 3A and 3B neoplasms, both exhibiting >15 centroblasts per HPF, with confluent sheets of centroblasts defining grade 3B [5]. Grade 3B cases tend to have a more aggressive clinical course and are biologically distinct from other FL, resembling DLBCL in their clinical behavior and response to therapy. Table 6.1 summarizes the main characteristics distinguishing grades 1–3A from grade 3B.

Histology at the time of transformation is generally in keeping with DLBCL (80%); rarely patients may present with a composite lymphoma (14%) or a lymphoma morphologically similar to a high-grade B-cell lymphoma (6%) [6].

6.4 Immunophenotype and molecular markers

The immunophenotype of FL is usually confirmed by immunohistochemistry or using flow cytometry. Immunophenotyping studies have demonstrated that FL cells are derived from normal germinal B cells. Tumor cells typically express monoclonal surface immunoglobulin and pan-B cell antigens (CD19, CD20, CD79a), complement receptor (CD21 and CD35), and CD10 (60%) and nuclear BCL-6. CD10 expression is often stronger in the follicle than in the interfollicular cells; some cases, in particular grade 3B, tend to lack CD10 but retain BCL6 expression. Unlike small lymphocytic and mantle cell lymphoma, FL lacks expression of CD5 and CD43 (most cases) and there is no staining for MUM1. Cytoplasmic staining for BCL-2 protein is strongly positive in almost all grade 1/2 tumors [7].

FL is characterized by the reciprocal translocation t(14;18)(q32;q21), which is present in 85–90% of cases [8]. This translocation leads to the placement of the B cell lymphoma 2 (BCL2) gene under the inductive influence of transcriptional enhancers associated with IGH, resulting in overexpression of the anti-apoptotic BCL2 protein, in turn leading to increased cell survival. This somatic rearrangement is thought to constitute the first step of lymphomagenesis. Nevertheless, the t(14;18) translocation alone is considered insufficient for the development of FL [9]. The development of FL requires further acquired aberrations in genes controlling the normal germinal center B-cells development. The complexity of the disease is also related to the importance of its interactions with the microenvironment that substantially influence disease development. Moreover, the relevance of normal tumor-infiltrating immune and stromal cells have been recognized to play a crucial role. In a model proposed by Scott et al., FL's neoplastic cells tend to "colonize" reactive germinal center that supports their proliferation and survival, and they "reeducate" the tumor microenvironment to their advantage, escaping immune surveillance [10]. This is well illustrated by the TNFRSF14 and STAT6 mutations which induce this interaction with the microenvironment [11]. In the early stages of development, the neoplastic cells, through the deregulation of a set of genes (KMT2D, MLL2, CREBBP, TNFRSF14, EZH2, RRAGC), acquire specific aberrations that inhibit apoptosis and increase BCR signaling. The acquisition of additional aberrations that enable proliferation (i.e., MYC p53 pathway, FOXO1) changes the nature of the tumor, frequently leading to histologic transformation.

Table 6.1 Grading of follicular lymphoma

Grade 1–2	*0–15 centroblasts per HPF*
1	0–5 centroblasts per HPF
2	6–15 centroblasts per HPF
Grade 3	*>15 centroblasts per HPF*
3A	Centrocytes present
3B	Solid sheets of centroblasts

HPF high-power (40× objective, 0.159 mm^2) microscopic field

6.5 Pathological Variants

In the revised 2017 WHO classification, several variants of FL have been described.

In situ follicular neoplasia (ISFN) is a pathologic diagnosis used to describe the identification of follicles that have a high content of BCL2-rearrangement-positive B cells within a lymph node that otherwise lacks the diagnostic features of FL. ISFN may be associated with progression to overt FL even though the risk is typically considered to be low [12].

Pediatric-type FL is rare, diagnosed mainly in children, and has distinctive clinical and pathological features. It tends to be more frequently localized, and patients typically do not experience a relapse after excision. Pathologically it is characterized by large follicles, with a large number of centroblasts often resembling FL grade 2/3 but lack the t(14;18). The prognosis of pediatric FL appears to be good.

Duodenal-type FL is a distinct subtype from other gastrointestinal FL. It typically presents as solitary or multiple polypoid lesions, which are confined to the mucosa and submucosa of the second part of the duodenum. This subtype of FL tends to have an indolent course and rarely progress into overt FL. Typically is associated with an excellent outcome and may even spontaneously regress [4, 13].

Even though the majority of FL cases harbor the t(14;18) translocation, there is a small subset of cases who do not present this genetic alteration. This entity is described as t(14;18)-negative FL. These patients have similar outcomes as patients with an FL that harbors the translocation, but this entity is associated with a distinct molecular feature that includes the absence of CD10 expression and the presence of BCL6 alterations, IRF4 expression, and proliferation signatures [14].

6.6 Staging

A careful history and physical examination are crucial in evaluating a new patient with FL to define the extent of disease. Treatment decisions depend upon the distinction between early-stage and advanced disease. The majority of patients with FL present with painless lymph nodes enlargement. The most frequently involved sites included cervical, inguinal, and axillary regions. It is also crucial to determine the presence of systemic symptoms (also called "B symptoms") including fever (temperature >38°), night sweats, and unexplained weight loss (>10% of body weight over the past 6 months). B symptoms represent an adverse prognostic factor and their resolution is frequently related to treatment response. Retroperitoneal adenopathies are usually asymptomatic, even though they may lead to abdominal discomfort and obstructive uropathy. Mesenteric or pelvic adenopathy may induce bowel obstruction or perforation.

FL is diagnosed by bioptic lymph node examination; fine-needle aspiration does not provide adequate material for an accurate diagnosis and tumor grading.

Laboratory studies should include a complete blood count, with the examination of the peripheral smear processed to search for circulating lymphoma cells. Lactate dehydrogenase (LDH) and beta2-microglobulin are indirect parameters of tumor load that have independent prognostic value. Serum creatinine and uric acid are essential in identifying risk for tumor lysis syndrome. Impaired renal function may also be related to ureteral obstruction. An isolated elevation in alkaline phosphatase should prompt an evaluation of the skeletal system. A serum protein electrophoresis may reveal a monoclonal gammopathy. It is also recommended to determine several viral serologies, in particular for HIV, hepatitis B (HBV), and hepatitis C (HCV). Although HBV is not crucially related to any NHL, reactivation of chronic hepatitis in patients receiving cytotoxic chemotherapy or immunotherapy is a well-recognized complication. When the hepatitis B surface antigen and hepatitis B core antibody are positive, viral load assessment by measuring HBV DNA should be performed and a specific antiviral treatment initiated, particularly when rituximab is part of the treatment.

Imaging studies represent a key component of the staging evaluation. Moreover, they may help in the selection of the site of biopsy. The preferred imaging modality for staging patients with NHL depends on the 18F-fluorodeoxyglucose (FDG) avidity of the histologic subtype. Indolent lymphomas are generally characterized by variable FDG avidity. Increasing evidence supports the role of FDG-PET in FDG-avid indolent non-Hodgkin lymphoma, in particular in FL [15]. More recently, formal guidelines for the use of FDG-PET in FL recommend its use for initial staging, evaluation, and response assessment after first-line therapy [16, 17].

FDG-PET may offer several advantages over conventional CT-scan, in particular the potential evaluation of large-cell transformation and the identification of patients at high risk of relapse at the end of therapy. Nevertheless, the exact impact of FDG-PET on outcome in FL remains to be defined and implementation of this tool into clinical management is based primarily on retrospective observations.

FL frequently presents with a bone marrow involvement. Bone marrow assessment should include both an aspirate and biopsy. The aspirate is useful for morphologic analysis, flow cytometry, and cytogenetics.

6.7 Clinical Presentation

The majority of patients with FL present with painless lymphadenopathy in the cervical, axillary, inguinal, and femoral regions [18], while large mediastinal masses are rare. The adenopathy sometimes waxes and wanes spontaneously, but rarely disappears completely. Only a minority of patients (accounting for approximately 15–20%) present with limited-stage disease, namely stage I or II. Despite the presence of widespread disease at diagnosis, the majority of patients are asymptomatic at the time of diagnosis. In contrast to aggressive lymphomas, constitutional symptoms (B symptoms) are rare and are present in approximately 20% of all cases. Only a minority of patients present with an increased LDH or cytopenias in the peripheral blood and no specific laboratory abnormalities have been associated with FL. Central nervous system involvement is rare, even though peripheral nerve compression and epidural tumor masses causing cord compression may be observed.

6.8 Risk Stratification and Prognosis

FL prognosis has evolved over the past decades and the outcome of patients with FL has improved considerably when comparing earlier treatment eras (1960s–1990s, the median survival being in the range of 10 years) to more recent eras, with a median survival in the range of 18 years [19]. This substantial improvement in survival can mainly be attributed to advances in frontline management, namely the use of monoclonal antibodies, superiority in diagnostic measures and supportive treatment and the availability of more active treatments for patients with transformed follicular lymphoma [20].

Several clinical prognostic factors have been identified as indicators of survival in patients with FL at the time of diagnosis.

Histologic grade has historically been an important factor in the determination of patient risk at the time of diagnosis. Low-grade histologies, namely grades 1, 2, and 3A, tend to have a very similar outcome with indolent behavior. However, patients with FL grade 3B tend to have more aggressive disease and they can be potentially cured with anthracycline-based chemotherapy [21].

The Follicular Lymphoma International Prognostic Index (FLIPI) is among the most well-validated prognostic tools in FL [18]. The FLIPI was developed before the rituximab era and it includes five main prognostic factors: number of involved nodal areas >4, LDH (normal vs. elevated), age (≤or >60 years), stage (I, II vs. III, IV), and the hemoglobin level (normal vs. <120 g/l). Patients are classified into the following prognostic groups based on the predicted outcome: low risk (0–1 factors), 90% 5-year OS; intermediate risk (two factors, 78% 5-year OS); high risk (three or more factors, 52% 5-year OS). The FLIPI has subsequently been validated in the rituximab era by the German Low-Grade Study Group in a cohort of 362 patients treated with rituximab, cyclophosphamide, doxorubicin, vincristine, and prednisone (R-CHOP) [22].

The FLIPI-2 score was derived from a large multicenter study including more than 1000 patients with FL, in need of treatment and receiving rituximab. The FLIPI-2 identified five parameters, some of which overlap with the original FLIPI: age >60 years, serum beta-2 microglobulin level higher than the upper limit of normal, hemoglobin level <120 g/l, bone marrow involvement and greatest diameter of the largest involved node more than 6 cm as independent risk factor for progression-free survival (PFS). Three-year PFS rates of patients with low (0 factors), intermediate (1–2 factors), or high (3–5 factors) FLIPI-2 scores were 91, 69%, and 51%, respectively, whereas 3-year survival rates were 99%, 96%, and 84%, respectively [23]. Prognostic scoring systems are summarized in Table 6.2. A simplified version of the FLIPI-2 based on serum beta-2 microglobulin level and an assessment of bone marrow involvement was proposed using data from the PRIMA study and validated in a separate cohort [24].

The recently proposed m7-FLIPI index combines the mutation status of seven clinically relevant genes (i.e., EZH2, ARID1A, MEF2B, EP300, FOXO1, CREBBP, and CARD11) with the FLIPI and the Eastern Cooperative Oncology Group (ECOG) Performance Status [25]. This model was created using the clinical and genetic data from two studies including patients with previously untreated symptomatic, advanced stage FL treated with either R-CHOP or R-CVP (rituximab, cyclophosphamide, vincristine, and prednisolone). This index was then validated in an independent cohort of 107 patients with symptomatic FL treated with R-CVP.

The French group has investigated the prognostic role of gene expression pattern and identified a 23 gene set identifying a high-risk patient cohort. Again, these results were confirmed in an independent validation set [26].

Both molecular scores represent a first step towards the incorporation of genetic findings in the determination of outcome in patients with FL, but it remains primarily a research tool not applicable to routine clinical practice.

Approximately 20% of patients with FL will experience an early progression of disease (POD) after chemo-immunotherapy, usually defined as progression or relapse within the first 2 years of diagnosis/treatment (POD24). The clinical impact of POD24 was investigated in a pivotal analysis conducted from the National LymphoCare Study (NLCS) including patients with FL treated over 200 locations across the United States. Patients with POD24 had a poorer outcome compared to the reference group (patients without early progression), with 5-year overall survival (OS) at 50% versus 90%, respectively. This finding was maintained even after adjusting for the FLIPI score and was validated in an independent cohort of patients from the

Table 6.2 Prognostic scoring systems in follicular lymphoma

Variables	Risk groups	Number of factors	5-year OS, %
FLIPI [18]			
Age >60	Low	0–1	90
Ann Arbor stage III/IV	Intermediate	2	78
Hemoglobin <12 g/dl	High	3 or more	52
Elevated LDH			
>4 nodal sites			
FLIPI-2 [23]			
Age >60	Low	0	79
Elevated B2M	Intermediate	1–2	51
Lymph node mass >6 cm	High	3 or more	18
BM involvement			
Hemoglobin <12 g/dl			

B2M beta 2 microglobulin, *BM* bone marrow

University of Iowa and the Mayo Clinic [27]. These results highlighted an important and previously under-appreciated population of patients with poor survival.

The prognostic role of POD24 was also separately studied in patients treated with the so-called chemotherapy-free approaches. The Nordic Lymphoma Group recently published the results of two prospective trials including 321 patients with indolent lymphoma (84% with FL) treated with single-agent rituximab (148 randomly allocated to the addition of interferon alfa-2a) with more than 10 years of follow-up. Patients with POD24 appeared to have a significantly worse outcome in comparison to the reference group (10-year survival rate of 59% vs. 81% for those with more prolonged remission) [28]. These results were validated in an independent cohort of patients treated in three Swiss Groups of Clinical Cancer Research (SAKK) trials [29].

In conclusion, at present, the optimal way in which to implement prognostic indexes in FL remains largely unknown and none of these scoring indexes serves as a guide for treatment initiation. In the future, the identification of predictive biomarkers will possibly help to establish the role of individual therapies.

6.9 First-Line Treatment

FL is characterized by a heterogeneous clinical presentation and it is generally considered to be incurable when it presents in an advanced stage. The variability of presentation at the time of diagnosis and the fact that most patients are completely asymptomatic result in differences in strategies for the initial management. Most patients present with slow-growing adenopathies and they do not necessarily need an active treatment at the time of diagnosis. Treatment of FL typically depends on the stage at presentation. Patients with limited-stage (stage I–II) are candidates for radiation therapy, which may be curative in a significant proportion of patients. In contrast, patients with advanced-stage disease (stage III–IV) are considered not to be curable with conventional therapies. For this reason, a pretreatment evaluation is needed to determine the extent of the disease. Moreover, it should provide information concerning the fitness of the patient, in particular, performance status and the presence of comorbidities.

6.10 Initial Treatment of Limited-Stage FL

Approximately 10–20% of FLs are diagnosed at an early stage (stage I or II) [30]. Radiation therapy (RT) has been traditionally the treatment of choice for this group of patients, with the potential induction of sustained remissions [31]. The definition of this particular group of patients is currently more accurate with the use of FDG-PET, which allows the identification of a truly localized disease [32]. Despite the reduced number of randomized clinical trials (Table 6.3.), radiation therapy alone is usually the preferred modality, resulting in 10-year overall survival rates of 60–80% [38]. Alternatively, an initial watchful waiting policy has also been proposed for selected patients, with few retrospective clinical trials reporting similar survival outcomes [30]. Nonetheless, a recent analysis based on the Surveillance, Epidemiology, and End Results (SEER) Program registry suggested a survival benefit in patients with early-stage FL treated with RT in comparison to observation [31]. Systemic therapy with immunotherapy alone (i.e., rituximab) or chemo-immunotherapy has rarely been studied in patients with early-stage FL. McManus et al. conducted a multicenter phase III trial including 150 FL patients with stage I and II. Patients were randomly assigned to RT alone or RT followed by six cycles of chemotherapy. The majority of patients had stage I disease and chemotherapy regimen consisted of CVP with rituximab added after a protocol amendment. With a median follow-up of 9.6 years, the additional chemotherapy appeared to improve PFS (59 vs. 41% at 10 years; HR 0.57, 95% CI 0.34–0.95), even though this was not translated into superior OS [41]. In another prospective phase II study, the combination of involved field radiation and rituximab achieved

Table 6.3 Selected trials including patients with early-stage follicular lymphoma

Author (year)	Stage	*n*	Median RT dose	Survival (%)
Herfarth et al. (2018) [33]	I (56%) II (44%)	85	30–40 Gy	5-year PFS 78 5-year OS 96
Tsang et al. (2005) [34]	I (64%) II (36%)	573	35 Gy	10-year FFTF 48 10-year OS >60
Brady et al. (2019) [35]	I (80%) II (20%)	512	>24 Gy	5-year FFTF 69 5-year OS 96
Vaughan Hudson et al. (1994) [36]	I (100%)	208	35 Gy	10-year FFTF 47 10-year OS 64
Mac Manus et al. (1996) [37]	I (41%) II (59%)	177	35–50 Gy	10-year FFTF 44 10-year OS 64
Wilder et al. (2001) [38]	I (41%) II (59%)	80	40 Gy	10-year FFTF 41 15-year OS 43
Soubeyran et al. (1988) [39]	I (44%) II (56%)	103	35–40 Gy	10-year FFTF 49 10-year OS 56
Guckenberger et al. (2012) [40]	I (47%) II (34%) III (19%)	107	25–45 Gy	10-year FFTF 58 10-year OS 64

PFS progression-free survival, *FFTF* freedom from treatment failure, *OS* overall survival, *Gy* gray

comparable rates of long-term remissions (78% at 5 years) [33]. Similar results have been obtained by adding rituximab to RT therapy: results of a multicenter study conducted in Italy showed that 10-year PFS was significantly longer ($p < 0.05$) in the rituximab RT group (four rituximab courses (375 mg/m^2, days 1, 8, 15, 22) before RT) (64.6%) compared to RT alone (50.7%), whereas the 10-year OS projections were not significantly different [42].

The dose and field of RT varied largely among studies. The radiation field has been gradually narrowed based on nonrandomized evidence, but rather following the publication of trials showing similar outcomes [40]. The standard dose for involved-field radiotherapy (IF-RT) is 24 Gy, which is significantly lower than the doses delivered in the past (30–40 Gy), and this has been demonstrated in a randomized trial to be as effective as higher doses [43]. Moreover, the first report from patients treated with low-dose RT of 2 × 2 Gy, mostly for palliation of advanced-stage disease, showed very promising results in terms of disease control [44]. This lead to the launch of a prospective randomized trial, which aimed to compare 2 × 2 Gy with the standard dose of 24 Gy in patients with limited-stage FL. The preliminary results demonstrated a significantly higher rate of progression in the low-dose group and this lead to the recommendation to not adopt low-dose RT for the treatment of patients with limited stage with a potential curative intent [45].

It should also be considered that most of the relapses in patients with early-stage FL occurred outside the irradiation fields [46]. This highlights the fact that all patients with early-stage FL need to be rigorously staged before treatment start.

6.11 Initial Treatment of Advanced-Stage FL

For patients with advanced-stage disease (stage III, IV or stage II not suitable for radiotherapy) treatment decisions must be individualized according to disease and patient's specific factors. As said, advanced-stage FL is still considered to be an incurable condition, even if the disease is responsive to various treatment modalities such as chemotherapy, immunotherapy, radiotherapy, and target-therapies. Once the diagnosis of advanced-stage FL is established, the next step is to determine if the patient needs therapy, as not all patients with FL require treatment at the time of diagnosis. The crucial decision is when to treat and how to treat. Given the fact that most patients with FL will not die of disease, maintaining an optimal quality of life represents one of the principal goals of therapy. Importantly, the range of therapeutic options should be discussed together with the patient, and the treatment modality is usually selected based on characteristics of the disease, goals of treatment and perceptions of the preferences of the patient.

6.11.1 Advanced-Stage FL with Low Tumor Burden

There is a wide variety of treatment options for FL. These options include watchful waiting (observation), single-agent anti-CD20 antibody (in particular, rituximab), chemotherapy associated with an anti-CD20 antibody (rituximab or obinutuzumab). Several prospective randomized trials [47–50] demonstrated that deferring therapy until the appearance of symptoms was not detrimental in terms of OS, and a prolonged treatment-free period may decrease cost, complications, and potential drug resistance. Moreover, histologic transformation to DLBCL appeared to occur at a rate of approximately 2%/year, regardless of whether FL is treated aggressively or conservatively [51, 52].

A landmark prospective randomized trial validating the role of watchful waiting as an initial management strategy in advanced-stage FL with low tumor burden was conducted by Ardeshna in 2003. More than 300 patients with advanced-stage asymptomatic FL were randomized to active treatment with an alkylating agent (oral chlorambucil) versus delayed therapy until the time of progression or symptomatic disease. With a median follow-up of 16 years, no difference in terms of OS was observed between the two treatment arms. Of note, nearly 20% of patients did not require any active treatment [48]. Even though other randomized trials have addressed the same question and have obtained similar results [47, 53], the fact that these studies were conducted in an era where rituximab (which has been shown to lead to an improvement in OS in patients with FL in need of therapy) was not available should be underlined. Therefore, we do not know how the impact on survival of rituximab in combination with chemotherapy could have affected the natural history of the disease in this population.

A relevant follow-up study was published in 2014 using rituximab as first-line treatment [54]. In this British trial, patients with low tumor burden FL were randomly assigned to receive either (1) rituximab induction given weekly for 4 weeks, (2) rituximab induction followed by maintenance rituximab every 2 months for 2 years, or (3) watchful waiting. The rituximab induction alone arm was closed prematurely due to slow accrual, and the study was subsequently amended to a two-arms study. With a median follow-up of 4 years, there was no difference in time to next treatment between the induction alone versus induction followed by maintenance group (HR = 0.75, $p = 0.33$), even though the amended trial was underpowered for the comparison of the two groups. Rates of histologic transformation and OS were similar between the two approaches. Nevertheless, there was a significant difference in the time to start of new therapy, with 46% (95% CI 39–53) of patients in the watchful waiting group not needing treatment at 3 years compared with 88% [55–64] in the maintenance rituximab group (hazard ratio [HR] 0.21, 95% CI 0.14–0.31; $p < 0.0001$). Rituximab therapy was associated with improved quality of life measures, reflecting a decrease in anxiety in patients receiving active treatment. This study provided the rationale for single-agent rituximab as an option for patients with newly diagnosed asymptomatic FL with low tumor burden, although the lack of an OS benefit indicates that "watchful waiting" remains an appropriate approach in this population.

If single-agent rituximab should be the first line treatment choice, then the next question is, which is the optimal schedule and how to administer it. In the RESORT trial, 289 patients with FL and low tumor burden were randomized after induction with four doses of weekly rituximab to receive maintenance rituximab (one dose every 13 weeks until progression) or retreatment with rituximab only at the time of progression. With a median follow-up of 4.5 years, time to treatment failure (approximately 4 years) and quality of life were similar in the two arms, and a reduced number of rituximab doses were used in the group without maintenance (median 4 vs. 18 doses) [65].

6.11.2 Advanced-Stage FL with High Tumor Burden

In evaluating the best time for treatment initiation, the best approach is to consider the presence or absence of symptoms along with the estimation of tumor burden. The *Groupe d'Etude des Lymphomes Folliculaires* (GELF) criteria have been proposed to identify those patients who would benefit from therapy rather than observation [47]. The GELF criteria are clinical parameters, which represent a surrogate of tumor burden: patients with high tumor burden, according to these criteria, are generally treated upfront with active systemic treatment. In the original GELF study patients considered to have a low tumor burden, were randomly assigned to one of three arms: arm 1, watchful waiting (n = 66); arm 2, prednimustine 200 mg/m^2/day for 5 days per month for 18 months (n = 64); or arm 3, interferon alfa 5 MU/day for 3 months, then 5 MU three times per week for 15 months (n = 63). Watchful waiting approach did not appear to be detrimental in comparison to early treatment. Since then, the subsequent clinical trials conducted by the same group evaluating different regimens of chemo-immunotherapy included patients with high tumor burden based on these criteria. The British National Lymphoma Investigation (BNLI) criteria have also been validated, and they are frequently used to assess the tumor burden and the optimal timing of initial treatment [54]. In the BNLI criteria, osseous lesions and bone marrow infiltration are also considered as a trigger for initiating treatment. Table 6.4. summarizes the main criteria for starting therapy in FL.

The current standard approach for patients with advanced-stage FL with high tumor burden consists of immuno-chemotherapy with an anti-CD20 monoclonal antibody in combination with a chemotherapy component (Table 6.5). Systemic treatment with rituximab alone was also shown to be useful as well as other chemo-free combinations, for example, rituximab and lenalidomide. Chemotherapy regimens frequently used are primarily based on alkylating agents (such as CVP, CHOP), based on a purine analog (i.e., fludarabine) alone or in combination with mitoxantrone (FM) or more recently including bendamustine.

The combination of rituximab with chemotherapy represents one of the standard of care for front-line treatment. Four prospective trials comparing different regimens with or without R have shown a significant benefit in PFS and OS in patients treated with rituximab [72–75]. No significant side effects were associated with the addition of rituximab. The question concerning the chemotherapy backbone should be considered has not being put to rest. The FOLL05 trial compared in 534 patients with advanced-stage FL, three most popular regimens, namely R-CVP, R-CHOP, and R-FM. R-CHOP and R-FM exhibited a superior PFS in comparison to R-CVP with a 3-year PFS of 52.68% and 63% (p = 0.011), respectively. Nevertheless, no differences were observed in terms of OS [69, 76].

Table 6.4 Comparison of criteria for starting treatment

Groupe d'Etude des Lymphome Folliculaires (GELF) [47]	Largest nodal (or extranodal) size >7 cm At least three nodal sites of >3 cm Presence of systemic symptoms Presence of serous effusion Substantial enlargement of the spleen Risk of vital organ compression Presence of leukemia or blood cytopenias
British National Lymphoma Investigation (BNLI) [54]	Presence of pruritus or B symptoms Rapid disease progression during the past 3 months Life-threatening organ involvement Significant bone marrow infiltration resulting in bone marrow depression (defined as hemoglobin level <100 g/l, white cell count <3.0 × 10^9 l^{-1} or platelets count <100 × 10^9 l^{-1} in the absence of other causes) Localized bone lesion Renal infiltration Macroscopic liver involvement

Table 6.5 Selected trials including patients with high-tumor-burden follicular lymphoma at diagnosis

Author (year)	Phase	*n*	Treatment	Maintenance	Survival
Rummel et a. (2013) [66]	III	549	R-CHOP R-B	NO	Median PFS 31.2 Median PFS 69.5 m
Flinn et al. (2019) [67]	III	447	R-CHOP, R-CVP R-B	NO	5-y PFS 55.8%, 5-y OS 81.7% 5-y PFS 65.5%, 5-y OS 85.0%
Salles et al. (2011) [68]	III	1217	R-CVP, R-CHOP, R-FCM	NO YES	3-y PFS 74·9% 3-y PFS 57·6%
Luminari et al. (2018) [69]	III	534	R-CVP R-CHOP R-FM	NO	8-y PFS 42%, 8-y OS 85% 8-y PFS 49%, 8-y OS 83% 8-y PFS 52%, 8-y OS 79%
Marcus et al. (2017) [70]	III	1202	R-CHOP, R-B, R-CVP G-CHOP, G-R, G-CVP	YES	3-y PFS 73%, 3-y OS 92.1% 3-y PFS 80%, 3-y OS 94.0%
Morschhauser et al. (2018) [71]	III	1030	R-CHOP, R-B, R CVP R^2	YES	3-y PFS 78%, 3-y OS 94% 3-y PFS 77%, 3-y OS 94%

PFS progression-free survival, *OS* overall survival, *R-CHOP* rituximab, cyclophosphamide, doxorubicin, vincristine, and prednisone, *R-CVP* rituximab, cyclophosphamide, vincristine, and prednisolone, *R-B* rituximab and rituximab, *G* obinutuzumab, R^2 rituximab and lenalidomide, *m* months, *y* years, *w* weeks

For patients without evidence of histologic transformation, bendamustine has become an important agent. Rummel et al. conducted a randomized prospective clinical trial, including patients with advanced-stage untreated indolent and mantle cell lymphoma treated with bendamustine and rituximab (B-R) or R-CHOP. The B-R combination appeared to improve PFS in this population and induced less alopecia, cytopenia, and infections in comparison to R-CHOP [66]. There was no difference in OS (70% vs. 66% at 10 years), and the number of second malignancies was similar between the two treatment arms (39 vs. 47 cases).

A similar study was conducted in the United States (the BRIGHT trial) and evaluated the B-R combination in comparison to R-CHOP and R-CVP as an upfront treatment for 447 patients with indolent and mantle cell lymphoma. B-R appeared not to be inferior to the other two regimens in terms of complete response (CR) rate (31 vs. 25%, respectively; $p = 0.0225$) and overall response (97–91%, respectively; $p = 0.0102$) [77]. In the updated 5-year follow-up analysis, PFS for patients treated with B-R was 65% (95% CI, 58.5–71.6) compared to 55.8% (95% CI, 48.4–62.5; HR = 0.61 95% CI, 0.45–0.85; $p = 0.0025$) for the entire group. There was no significant difference in OS between the groups. Of note, patients with grade 3A FL were excluded from this trial. In terms of toxicity profiles, B-R was associated with higher rates of nausea/vomiting, secondary malignancies, and lower rates of peripheral neuropathy/paresthesia and alopecia. Patients treated with R-CHOP/R-CVP had more hematological toxicity than B-R, even though the infection rate appeared to be higher in the latter group [67].

In conclusion, B-R appeared to be a valid option for those patients who want to avoid alopecia or severe neutropenia. Moreover, the schedule of B-R given for two consecutive days but less frequently (every 4 weeks), might be interesting to some patients for logistical reasons. Obinutuzumab is a type II anti-CD20 monoclonal antibody, which has been recently approved in combination with chemotherapy for first-line patients with FL. The approval followed the results published of the prospective randomized GALLIUM trial, including 1202 patients with untreated follicular lymphoma in need of therapy. Patients were randomized to an obinutuzumab-based induction and maintenance strategy versus a rituximab-based induction and maintenance. Participating centers were free to select one of the following chemotherapy regimens associated with the anti-CD20 antibody for induction: bendamustine (57%), CHOP (33%), or CVP

(10%). Responding patients were then allocated to receive up to 2 years of maintenance with the same antibody they received during induction. Results from the preplanned interim analysis showed that the experimental arm was associated with an improved PFS (3-year PFS 83 vs. 79; HR 0.68, 95% CI 0.54–0.87). After a median follow-up of 34.5 months (range, 0–54.5 months) similar results were seen concerning ORR, CR, OS, and rates of histologic transformation. Nevertheless, the obinutuzumab-based strategy was also associated with a higher rate of grade 3/4 adverse events (75 vs. 68%), in particular, infusion-related reactions (59 vs. 49%), febrile neutropenia (6.9% vs. 4.9%) and grade 3/4 infections (20% vs. 15.6%). Unexpectedly, several fatal events were observed in both arms (4% and 4.3% for patients receiving obinutuzumab and rituximab, respectively). Moreover, a higher incidence of grade 3/4 toxicity was observed in patients treated with bendamustine in both arms, in particular infections and secondary malignancies [70, 78]. In conclusion, although these results suggest an improvement in PFS with the use of obinutuzumab, it is currently not clear whether this will translate into a survival benefit after a longer follow-up. For the time being the use of either anti-CD20 antibody appears to be reasonable.

Besides the combination with cytotoxic agents, several patients may also be treated successfully with "chemotherapy-free" approaches. Single-agent rituximab appears to be an adequate initial treatment, in particular for those patients with comorbidities and/or with disease progressing slowly over a long time. Rituximab has low toxicity profiles, and in general, it induced reasonable response rates. The SAKK investigated the role of rituximab monotherapy in newly diagnosed patients and pretreated patients with FL. Rituximab monotherapy given at the dose of 375 mg/m^2/week for a total of four doses followed by four additional doses administered every 2 months, induced an overall response rate ranging from 46% to 67% for patients at relapse or treatment-naïve, respectively [79]. With the long-term follow-up of 9.5 years, it appears that 35% of patients with previously untreated FL who responded to rituximab induction and were treated with four doses of rituximab maintenance did not progress after 8 years [80]. To better define the optimal duration of rituximab maintenance, the same group compared a long-term approach (maximum of 5 years or until disease progression or unacceptable toxicity) versus a short-term schedule (four administrations administered every 2 months). Long-term rituximab maintenance did not appear to improve event-free survival (EFS), which was the primary endpoint of the trial [81].

Another chemotherapy-free approach using rituximab (*R*) as a backbone is the combination with lenalidomide, also known as the R^2 regimen. Three prospective phase II trials conducted in the United States and Europe demonstrated that the R^2 regimen induces a high rate of CR in treatment-naive patients with FL with 3-year PFS with 2-year PFS 86% [82–84]. These promising results led to the launch of an international open-label phase III trial (the RELEVANCE trial), which accrued 1030 patients with advanced-stage FL in need of treatment. Patients were randomly allocated to receive R^2 (lenalidomide given at a dose of 20 mg/day on days 2 through 22 of each 28-day cycle for six cycles, followed by lenalidomide at a dose of 10/20 mg/day for 12 cycles) or chemotherapy with rituximab, which consisted of either CVP, CHOP, or B, depending on the investigator's choice. In each treatment arm, patients were treated for a total of 30 months. With a median follow-up of 38 months, no significant differences were observed in terms of CR rates (48% (95% CI, 44–53) vs. 53% (95% CI, 49–57), $p\,0 = 0.13$), PFS at 3 years (77% vs. 78%; HR 1.1, 95% CI 0.85–1.43), and OS at 3 years (94% vs. 94%; HR 1.16, 95% CI 0.72–1.86). In terms of toxicity, a higher percentage of patients in the rituximab chemotherapy arm presented with grade III/IV neutropenia (32% vs. 50%) and febrile neutropenia of any grade (2% vs. 7%). Patients treated with R^2 presented more rash (43% vs. 24%), diarrhea (37% vs. 19%), and tumor flare reaction (6% vs. <1%) [71]. In conclusion, based on these results, the R^2 regimen represents a new treatment option for previously untreated patients with FL, but has been not yet registered in the first-line indication.

6.11.3 The Role of Maintenance Therapy

Disease relapse represents a matter of concern of patients with FL, and the identification of further ways to extend the period of remission continues to be an essential goal for clinicians and investigators. A possible strategy to achieve this objective is with the implementation of the so-called maintenance therapy, to be proposed after successful induction therapy. Anti-CD20 monoclonal antibodies appear to be an attractive option for maintenance therapy because they are associated with only limited acute toxicity and no significant long-term or cumulative toxicity. Moreover, the long half-life of these compounds allows for spaced treatments while maintaining long-term drug exposure. The role of maintenance therapy has been investigated in patients with either low and high tumor burden, after first-line treatment and in the relapse setting. The RESORT trial included only patients with low tumor burden treated with an induction therapy of 4 weekly doses of rituximab. Patients were then randomized to receive either maintenance rituximab every 3 months indefinitely or rituximab re-treatment upon progression. At a median follow-up of 4.5 years, PFS in both study arms were comparable but patients receiving maintenance therapy were less likely to require cytotoxic chemotherapy even though the estimated OS at 5 years was similar in both groups (94%) and no difference in terms of rate of histologic transformation was observed [85]. Nevertheless, the benefit in terms of disease control must be weighed against the higher amount of rituximab used in the maintenance arm.

Other clinical trials have assessed the role of maintenance rituximab after an induction based on single-agent rituximab. The SAKK 35/98 trial included newly diagnosed and previously treated FL. Patients were treated with a rituximab induction (4 weekly doses) and then randomized to receive either maintenance rituximab given every 2 months for four infusions or no further treatment. With a median follow-up of 10 years, the median EFS was significantly longer in the rituximab maintenance arm in comparison to the observation arm (24 months vs. 13 months, $p < 0.001$) [80]. In a subsequent trial conducted by the same group (the SAKK 35/03 trial) 270 patients with untreated, relapsed, stable, or chemoresistant FL were treated with an induction therapy which was identical to the previously described study and were then randomly assigned to receive a short-term maintenance (rituximab every 2 months for four additional doses) or a long-term maintenance (rituximab every 2 months until progression or unacceptable toxicity for a maximum of 5 years). No differences were seen in terms of the primary endpoint (EFS), and slightly more adverse events were observed in the long-term schedule [81].

In patients responding to an induction therapy based on immune-chemotherapy (i.e., R-CHOP, R-CVP, and rituximab fludarabine cyclophosphamide), the role of maintenance rituximab was primarily addressed in the PRIMA trial. In this trial, 1019 patients with previously untreated FL, demonstrating an initial response to induction, were randomly assigned to maintenance rituximab (375 mg/m2 administered every 2 months for 24 months) or placebo. Improvement in PFS was observed in the maintenance arm at a median follow-up of 36 months (74.9% vs. 57.6%), but no difference could be demonstrated in terms of OS. Rituximab maintenance was also associated with a higher percentage of patients in CR or unconfirmed CR at 24 months (72% vs. 52%), but was associated with a higher overall rate of severe (grade III/IV) adverse events (24% vs. 17%) and a higher percentage of infection (39% vs. 24%) [68]. With a longer follow-up of 73 months the PFS benefit in the maintenance arm was maintained (42.7% vs. 59.2%; HR 0.58, 95% CI 0.48–0.69; $p < 0.0001$) and no unexpected toxicity were observed. Nevertheless, the use of maintenance rituximab did not translate into an improvement in OS even with a longer follow-up [86].

In a large meta-analysis including seven trials evaluating rituximab maintenance after chemotherapy or chemo-immunotherapy (a total of 2315 patients with FL), maintenance rituximab appeared to improve the PFS (HR 0.57; 95% CI 0.51–0.64) and OS (HR 0.79; 95% CI 0.66–0.96) even though it was associated with a greater risk of adverse events (34% vs. 24%) [87].

It continues to be a matter of debate if these results should also be applied for patients treated with B-R as induction therapy. Several trials reported a higher rate of mortality not related to lymphoma, in particular in patients receiving maintenance after bendamustine-based combinations [70, 88], and the main cause of mortality in these patients was *Pneumocystis jirovecii* pneumonia. Nonetheless, it should be underlined that in this trial, the chemotherapy backbone was not randomly assigned. Moreover, the optimal duration of maintenance therapy is mostly unknown and continues to remain a matter of discussion. Many clinicians decide to administer maintenance with a schedule established in a specific phase III trial, such as that used in the PRIMA study (rituximab every 2 months for a total of 2 years). As previously described, trials that have investigated longer duration of maintenance have observed increased toxicity towards the end of the planned treatment. From a practical point of view, it is recommended to administer long-term prophylaxis for *Pneumocystis jirovecii* if giving rituximab maintenance after B-R induction.

6.12 The Role of High-Dose Chemotherapy and Autologous Stem-Cells Transplant

High-dose chemotherapy (HDT) followed by autologous stem cell transplant (ASCT) represents a treatment strategy that has been extensively investigated in patients with FL. Nonetheless, given the toxicity of this approach and the overall favorable outcome generally observed in patients with FL, the identification of the right timing for this procedure has always been a challenge.

Several randomized clinical trials have investigated the role of HDT, followed by ASCT in patients with FL. Three randomized trials conducted in the pre-rituximab era and one in the rituximab era have evaluated the role of upfront ASCT consolidation versus observation alone in patients with advanced-stage FL, in remission after first-line therapy. All these trials demonstrated a benefit in terms of PFS in comparison to observation alone, indeed suggesting that this approach induced improved disease control, but none showed an OS benefit [89–91]. Based on these results, HDT and ASCT are currently not recommended as consolidation in patients with FL in the first remission.

For patients with FL at relapse, the results of a single prospective trial conducted in the pre-rituximab era showed that ASCT might be superior to conventional-dose therapy. In this trial, 140 patients with refractory FL were randomized to receive chemotherapy alone versus chemotherapy, followed by ASCT using unpurged or purged stem cells. With a 69-month median follow-up, the authors could demonstrate a 2-year PFS (26% vs. 55–58%, $p = 0.0037$) benefit and 4-year OS benefit for patients who underwent ASCT (46% vs. 71–77%, $p = 0.079$) [92]. Despite these positive results, ASCT was not widely adopted as a standard of care for patients with relapsed FL, due to concern regarding early and late toxicity. Moreover, this study was performed before the advent of rituximab, when the median survival of patients with FL was shorter in comparison to the present time.

Several retrospective studies have compared the outcome of patients treated with ASCT or chemo-immunotherapy in a more recent era. Sebban et al. published a retrospective analysis including 254 patients with relapsed FL treated in two successive randomized studies with the same treatment: patients treated with HDT and ASCT presented with a higher rate of 5-year EFS (51% vs. 24%) and OS (70% vs. 42%), in comparison to patients treated with conventional therapy [93]. Similar results supporting the use of ASCT regardless of front-line rituximab exposure have been found by Le Gouill et al. in an analysis including 175 FL patients from the FL2000 [94]. A retrospective analysis using data from the National LymphoCare Study and the Center for International Blood and Marrow Transplant Research reported on the outcomes of 349 patients who progressed within 2 years or did not respond to initial rituximab-based therapy. In a planned subset analysis, the patients receiving ASCT within 1 year of treatment failure had superior OS at 5 years (73% vs. 60%) [95]. Similarly, the follow-up analysis of two prospective first-line trials confirmed the overall survival benefit in young patients who had relapsed within 24 months after a CHOP-like induction [96]. The European Group for Blood and Marrow Transplantation (EBMT) published a project which aimed to define indications for HDT and ASCT in patients with FL in the rituximab era in Europe following a RAND-modified Delphi consensus method. In patients with first chemosensitive relapse, the consensus was that HDT with ASCT represents an appropriate option to consolidate remission, especially in patients with a short response after immuno-chemotherapy or with high-risk FLIPI [97].

Even though HDT and ASCT may provide a sustained remission and possibly a cure for many patients, it is also essential to recognize the fact that this procedure is associated with significant acute and late toxicity. A primary concern is related to the risk of developing secondary malignancies, in particular, myelodysplasia (MDS) or acute myeloid leukemia (AML). A population-based cohort study including more than 7000 patients treated with ASCT, the risk of secondary malignancies appear to be moderately increased (standardized incidence ratios (SIR) 1.4) compared with the general population but was significantly elevated for MDS/AML (SIR = 20.6) [55]. For this reason, patients should be counseled regarding this risk and other related potential late effects.

6.13 The Role of Allogeneic Stem Cell Transplantation

Allogeneic stem cell transplantation with myeloablative conditioning was associated with a lower relapse rate but higher transplant-related mortality and finally, a similar OS [56]. This observation suggested the presence of graft versus lymphoma effect. To decrease the toxicity of allo-SCT reduced-intensity conditioned (RIC-alloSCT) has been developed. Several clinical trials demonstrated the feasibility of this approach also in patients who were early pretreated [57, 58]. The outcomes following a RIC-alloSCT showed a 5-year PFS rate ranging from 50% to 85%. No prospective trials have compared the efficacy of RIC-alloSCT and myeloablative conditioning alloSCT in patients with FL. RIC-alloSCT is currently the most frequently employed approach for patients over the age of 50 and with comorbidities [97].

The decision to consider either ASCT or alloSCT in patients with refractory/relapsed FL remains to be defined. There is only one prospective randomized trial addressing this issue and unfortunately, it was closed prematurely due to poor accrual [54]. Thus, based on the beforementioned European consensus, alloSCT is being recommended to be preferably discussed for patients that have relapsed after ASCT [97].

6.14 Radioimmunotherapy (RIT)

Radioimmunotherapy (RIT) is based on the use of monoclonal antibodies linked to radioisotopes. Ibritumomab tiuxetan is a murine anti-CD20 monoclonal antibody conjugated to the radioisotope yttrium-90 that is approved by the US Food and Drug Administration (FDA) for the treatment of patients with relapsed/refractory FL. Several prospective trials of RIT (mostly phase II trials) demonstrated response rates ranging from 60% to 80%, with a median PFS less than 1 year. The majority of patients who achieve a CR following RIT remained in remission for more than 3 years [59, 60]. No randomized trials have compared RIT to immuno-chemotherapy. Ibritumomab tiuxetan appeared to be safe; the most common side effects are related to the potentially prolonged hematological toxicity.

The high response rate achieved with this approach makes RIT an attractive treatment option, even though it is currently not commonly employed due to the complexity of administration.

Alternatively a consolidation approach resulted in an improved PFS in an international first-line trial [61]. However, this approach seems to be inferior to a prolonged rituximab maintenance for 2 years [62].

6.15 Management of Relapsed FL

Although the median OS for FL has improved substantially in comparison to the past decades, most patients will eventually relapse, and they will require successive treatments. The optimal approach to patients with relapsed FL remains undefined. It is crucial to recognize high-risk patients, in particular, patients presenting with a histologic transformation or those presenting with early treatment failure. The latter group is classically composed of patients with FL progressing within 24 months of initial immunochemotherapy [27]. These patients are classically treated with more aggressive approaches because they tend to have a worse outcome. For young patients without significant comorbidity, the best plan may include HDT followed by ASCT especially in early relapses. On the other hand, patients with asymptomatic relapsed FL do not necessarily require immediate treatment. The indications for treatment initiation are generally similar as used for first-line therapy. A repeated biopsy is whenever possible recommended at the time of relapse, to rule out histologic transformation to diffuse large B-cell lymphoma. Bone marrow biopsy is in general reserved for patients with significant cytopenia. The clinical feature that may be associated with histological transformation are in particular rapid discordant growth of a single nodal site, the presence of B symptoms, hypercalcemia, and increased LDH. The choice of subsequent lines of therapy largely depends on several factors, including the type of previous treatment, age, the presence of comorbidities, the duration of remission, and the patient preference. The different options available are a re-challenge with the initial treatment regimen (in particular for patients presenting with long remission), the use of non-cross resistant chemotherapy regimens or the administration of new targeted agents. The goal, in young and fit patients, is to induce a long-lasting remission. In elderly patients presenting with comorbidities, treatment for patients with relapsed FL aims to obtain a better quality of life and to reduce lymphoma-associated symptoms. As said, for patients presenting with early relapse, the use of a non-cross resistant treatment is generally recommended. Patients relapsing after a long period of remission and presenting with comorbidities may benefit from single-agent rituximab [63]. For relapsing patients having received regimens with alkylating agents, a combination including bendamustine may be considered. Several regimens have demonstrated clinical activity in this setting, but there is a limited number of randomized trials. At first relapse after immunochemotherapy, treatment option includes an anti-CD20 monoclonal antibody in association with CHOP, CVP, bendamustine, or lenalidomide, depending on the patient's history and prior therapy. In particular, the combination of bendamustine plus obinutuzumab may be preferred in patients previously treated with R-CVP or R-CHOP, if the relapse occurs less than 6–12 months from the last rituximab administration. The other way round, CHOP may be preferred for patients with previously treated with a bendamustine-based regimen.

Two phase II trials have assessed the activity and safety of combinations with bendamustine in patients with relapsed/refractory NHL (14% with FL): median PFS was in the range of 2 years and the most common side effect was hematological toxicity (in particular, leukopenia and thrombocytopenia) [64, 98]. In a randomized, noninferiority, phase III trial including 230 patients with relapsed indolent NHL and mantle cell lymphoma, fludarabine-based chemotherapy with rituximab was compared to B-R. Patients treated with the latter regimen exhibited a higher response rate and an improved PFS and OS, suggesting that this combination may be one of the preferred treatment options for patients with relapsed indolent lymphoma [99].

The decision to use rituximab maintenance at the time of relapse should be based on whether the patients are refractory to this compound. For patients considered to be rituximab refractory, rituximab maintenance is in general not proposed. In this regard, the GADOLIN trial included patients with rituximab refractory indolent NHL and randomized patients to receive either obinutuzumab (G) and bendamustine in induction followed by G maintenance or single-agent bendamustine without maintenance. The updated results of this trial showed that the G-B induction plus G maintenance significantly improves PFS and OS in comparison to bendamustine alone [100].

6.16 Novel Agents in the Management of FL

6.16.1 Lenalidomide

New compounds are frequently reserved for patients presenting with multiple relapses, but there are compounds that are now being investigated in the first-line (Table 6.6). One example is lenalidomide, which was assessed as a single agent in patients with relapsed/refractory indolent lymphoma (mostly FL) in the NHL-001 including 43 patients and showing a promising ORR of 23% (CR 7%) with a median PFS of 4.4 months [109]. The combination of lenalidomide and rituximab (also known as the R^2 combination) was tested in several phase II trials [82, 84] and subsequently in a large randomized international phase III trial (the AUGMENT trial) showing a significant clinical activity in comparison to rituximab alone [101]. In the first-line setting, the RELEVANCE trial demonstrated that the R^2 combination was comparable in term of efficacy to standard immuno-chemotherapy (R-CHOP, B-R, R-CVP) [71]. The role of lenalidomide in maintenance is currently investigated in the MAGNIFY study, a phase IIIB multicenter open-label study, where responding patients are randomized to receive either maintenance

Table 6.6 Selected trials including patients treated with "chemotherapy-free" regimens

Author (year)	Phase	*n*	Setting	Treatment	ORR	ORR, survival
Ghielmini et al. (2004) [79]	II	202	First-line FL Relapsed FL	R	46–67%	Median EFS 12–23 m
Taverna et al. (2016) [81]	II	165	First-line FM	R		
			Relapsed FL	Short-term maintenance R Long-term maintenance R	62%	Median EFS 3.4 y Median EFS 5.3 y
Zucca et al. (2019) [84]	II	154	First-line FL	R R^2	57% 78%	Median PFS 2.3 y Median PFS 5.0 y
Leonard et al. (2019) [101]	III	358	Relapsed FL	R R^2	53% 78%	2-year PFS 36% 2-year PFS 58%
Gopal et al. (2014) [102]	II	125	Relapsed indolent NHL	Idelalisib	57%	NA
Dreyling et al. (2017) [103]	II	142	Relapsed indolent NHL	Copanlisib	59%	Median EFS 11.2 m
Schmidt et al. (2018) [104]	II	98	First-line FL	Ibrutinib + obinutuzumab	90%	1-y PFS 80%,
Ogura et al. (2014) [105]	II	39	Relapsed FL	Vorinostat	49%	PFS 20 m
Morschhauser et al. (2019) [106]	II	95	Relapsed FL	Tazemetostat	74%[a]	PFS 60 w[a]
Palanca-Wessels et al. (2015) [107]	I	34	Relapsed indolent NHL	Polatuzumab vedotin	55%	Median PFS 5.7 m
Davids et al. (2017) [108]	I	106	Relapsed indolent NHL	Venetoclax	38%	Median PFS 11 m

FL follicular lymphoma, *NHL* non-Hodgkin lymphoma, *PFS* progression-free survival, *EFS* event-free survival, *R* rituximab, R^2 rituximab and lenalidomide, *m* months, *y* years, *w* weeks
[a]Mutant *EZH2* tumors

lenalidomide plus rituximab or rituximab alone (ClinicalTrials.gov Identifier: NCT01996865).

6.16.2 Phosphatidylinositol 3-Kinases (PI3K) Inhibitors

PI3K inhibitors are heterodimeric enzymes that have regulatory and catalytic subunits. Idelalisib is a selective P110δ PI3K inhibitor. In the phase I study, including heavily pretreated patients with indolent NHL, idelalisib showed an encouraging activity with an ORR of 48% [110]. Based on these promising results a subsequent phase II trial including 125 patients with indolent NHL considered to be refractory to rituximab and alkylating agents were treated with 150 mg twice daily of idelalisib until progression or unacceptable toxicity. The ORR among FL patients was 57% (95% CI 0.42–0.66) with 7% CR, and after a median follow-up of 9.7 months, the median PFS was 11.0 months, substantially longer in comparison to the PFS achieved after the previous therapies [102]. Despite the promising activity, toxicity associated with this agent has frequently been problematic. Idelalisib has been associated with immune-mediated toxicity such as transaminitis, diarrhea, and pneumonitis related to the infiltration of CD8 positive lymphocytes. Moreover, in a subsequent phase III clinical trial, an excess of mortality attributed to an increase in opportunistic infection (in particular *Pneumocystis jirovecii* pneumonia and cytomegalovirus reactivation) was observed in the idelalisib containing arm. Therefore, when treatment with idelalisib is considered, adequate pneumocystis prophylaxis and cytomegalovirus monitoring are highly recommended.

Copanlisib is another pan-class PI3K inhibitor with potent activity against PI3K-alpha and PI3K-delta isoforms which was recently approved by the FDA for the treatment of patients with relapsed FL. In a phase II study, 104 patients with FL treated with copanlisib exhibited an ORR of 59% with 12% CR and a PFS of 11.2 months [103].

6.16.3 Bruton's Tyrosine Kinase Inhibitors

Ibrutinib is an irreversible inhibitor of Bruton's tyrosine kinase (BTK), and it has a pro-apoptotic effect, disrupting cellular adhesion and migration. Two phases II studies were performed enrolling subjects with relapsed/refractory FL. Forty patients received 560 mg daily of ibrutinib until progression or unacceptable toxicity. With a median follow-up of 6.5 months, ORR was 30% (CR 2.5%), and the median PFS was 9.9 months [111]. In the second trial, 110 patients were treated with the same therapy, and after a median follow-up of 27.7 months, the median PFS was 4.6 months [112]. In a first-line trial the combination of obinutuzumab and ibrutinib was well tolerated, but rate of ongoing remissions at 1 year were inferior to conventional treatment approaches [104].

6.16.4 Epigenetic Therapies

Histone deacetylases (HDAC) represent a class of enzymes that remove acetyl groups from an ε-N-acetyl lysine amino acid on a histone, and consequently, they regulate gene transcription. HDAC inhibitors induce hyperacetylation of histones and hence the activation of the mechanism of tumor suppression and apoptosis. One of the agents which was tested in patients with FL is vorinostat. In two phase II trials, which included 17 and 39 patients, respectively, with relapsed/refractory FL, vorinostat appeared to induce an ORR of 47–49% with a median PFS of 15.6 and 20 months [105, 113].

Another compound is tazemetostat, a first-in-class oral enhancer of zeste homolog 2 (EZH2) inhibitor, which was tested as a single-agent treatment for relapsed or refractory patients with FL or DLBCL grouped by EZH2 mutational status, and demonstrated an objective response rate of 92% in FL with EZH2 mutation and 26% in FL with wild-type EZH2 [106].This may represent an example of personalized medicine in FL which may be applied more frequently in the future.

6.16.5 Antibody–Drug Conjugates

Polatuzumab vedotin is an anti-CD79B monoclonal antibody conjugated to monomethyl auristatin E (MMAE). The recommended dose, which was defined in a phase I trial, is 2.4 mg/kg. The results showed promising activity with ORR of 55% with a median PFS of 5.7 months. The most common grade 3–4 toxicities were hematologic and peripheral neuropathy [107].

6.16.6 Bcl-2 Inhibitors

Bcl-2 family proteins play as regulators of apoptosis in cancer cells. BH3-only proteins have interaction with Bax and Bak, and they induce cellular apoptosis. Venetoclax (ABT-199) is a small molecule BH3-mimetic. Venetoclax was investigating in 106 patients with relapsed/refractory B NHL treated in a phase I study, and ORR was 38% (11/29) and for CR (14%) in patients with follicular lymphoma [108]. Other studies using this compound in combination with other targeted agents are currently ongoing.

6.17 Conclusions

The optimal treatment approach for patients with FL remains undefined. In this chapter, we reviewed the current spectrum of treatment options for patients with newly diagnosed and relapsed FL. The trend observed over the last years is characterized by a shift towards more biological and targeted treatments. A plethora of new targeted agents are currently under investigation and there is a high expectation that these agents will be part of the treatment armamentarium against FL.

The management of patients with relapsed FL largely depends on patient and disease characteristics. In the next 10 years, FL will likely remain an incurable condition. Nevertheless, new approaches with less toxicity will probably further improve the outcome of those patients. The unmet medical need remains the patient not responding or rapidly progressing to immunochemotherapy. In particular for those patients, it will be crucial to investigate the efficacy of novel agents and new combinations.

References

1. Sant M, Allemani C, Tereanu C, De Angelis R, Capocaccia R, Visser O, et al. Incidence of hematologic malignancies in Europe by morphologic subtype: results of the HAEMACARE project. Blood. 2010;116(19):3724–34.
2. Morton LM, Wang SS, Devesa SS, Hartge P, Weisenburger DD, Linet MS. Lymphoma incidence patterns by WHO subtype in the United States, 1992–2001. Blood. 2006;107(1):265–76.
3. Goldin LR, Bjorkholm M, Kristinsson SY, Turesson I, Landgren O. Highly increased familial risks for specific lymphoma subtypes. Br J Haematol. 2009;146(1):91–4.
4. Swerdlow SH, Campo E, Pileri SA, Harris NL, Stein H, Siebert R, et al. The 2016 revision of the World Health Organization classification of lymphoid neoplasms. Blood. 2016;127(20):2375–90.
5. Vaidyanathan G, Czuczman MS. Follicular lymphoma grade 3: review and updates. Clin Lymphoma Myeloma Leuk. 2014;14(6):431–5.
6. Lossos IS, Gascoyne RD. Transformation of follicular lymphoma. Best Pract Res Clin Haematol. 2011;24(2):147–63.
7. Swerdlow SHCE, Harris NL, Jaffe ES, Pileri SA, Stein H, Thiele J. World Health Organization classification of tumours of haematopoietic and lymphoid tissues. Geneva: WHO; 2017.
8. Tsujimoto Y, Cossman J, Jaffe E, Croce CM. Involvement of the bcl-2 gene in human follicular lymphoma. Science. 1985;228(4706):1440–3.
9. McDonnell TJ, Korsmeyer SJ. Progression from lymphoid hyperplasia to high-grade malignant lymphoma in mice transgenic for the t(14; 18). Nature. 1991;349(6306):254–6.
10. Scott DW, Gascoyne RD. The tumour microenvironment in B cell lymphomas. Nat Rev Cancer. 2014;14(8):517–34.
11. Yildiz M, Li H, Bernard D, Amin NA, Ouillette P, Jones S, et al. Activating STAT6 mutations in follicular lymphoma. Blood. 2015;125(4):668–79.
12. Jegalian AG, Eberle FC, Pack SD, Mirvis M, Raffeld M, Pittaluga S, et al. Follicular lymphoma in situ: clinical implications and comparisons with partial involvement by follicular lymphoma. Blood. 2011;118(11):2976–84.
13. Schmatz AI, Streubel B, Kretschmer-Chott E, Puspok A, Jager U, Mannhalter C, et al. Primary follicular lymphoma of the duodenum is a distinct mucosal/submucosal variant of follicular lymphoma: a retrospective study of 63 cases. J Clin Oncol. 2011;29(11):1445–51.

14. Horsman DE, Okamoto I, Ludkovski O, Le N, Harder L, Gesk S, et al. Follicular lymphoma lacking the t(14;18)(q32;q21): identification of two disease subtypes. Br J Haematol. 2003;120(3):424–33.
15. Wohrer S, Jaeger U, Kletter K, Becherer A, Hauswirth A, Turetschek K, et al. 18F-fluoro-deoxy-glucose positron emission tomography (18F-FDG-PET) visualizes follicular lymphoma irrespective of grading. Ann Oncol. 2006;17(5):780–4.
16. Cheson BD, Fisher RI, Barrington SF, Cavalli F, Schwartz LH, Zucca E, et al. Recommendations for initial evaluation, staging, and response assessment of Hodgkin and non-Hodgkin lymphoma: the Lugano classification. J Clin Oncol. 2014;32(27):3059–68.
17. Barrington SF, Mikhaeel NG, Kostakoglu L, Meignan M, Hutchings M, Mueller SP, et al. Role of imaging in the staging and response assessment of lymphoma: consensus of the international conference on malignant lymphomas imaging working group. J Clin Oncol. 2014;32(27):3048–58.
18. Solal-Celigny P, Roy P, Colombat P, White J, Armitage JO, Arranz-Saez R, et al. Follicular lymphoma international prognostic index. Blood. 2004;104(5):1258–65.
19. Conconi A, Motta M, Bertoni F, Piona C, Stathis A, Wannesson L, et al. Patterns of survival of follicular lymphomas at a single institution through three decades. Leuk Lymphoma. 2010;51(6):1028–34.
20. Tan D, Horning SJ, Hoppe RT, Levy R, Rosenberg SA, Sigal BM, et al. Improvements in observed and relative survival in follicular grade 1–2 lymphoma during 4 decades: the Stanford University experience. Blood. 2013;122(6):981–7.
21. Wahlin BE, Yri OE, Kimby E, Holte H, Delabie J, Smeland EB, et al. Clinical significance of the WHO grades of follicular lymphoma in a population-based cohort of 505 patients with long follow-up times. Br J Haematol. 2012;156(2):225–33.
22. Buske C, Hoster E, Dreyling M, Hasford J, Unterhalt M, Hiddemann W. The follicular lymphoma international prognostic index (FLIPI) separates high-risk from intermediate- or low-risk patients with advanced-stage follicular lymphoma treated front-line with rituximab and the combination of cyclophosphamide, doxorubicin, vincristine, and prednisone (R-CHOP) with respect to treatment outcome. Blood. 2006;108(5):1504–8.
23. Federico M, Bellei M, Marcheselli L, Luminari S, Lopez-Guillermo A, Vitolo U, et al. Follicular lymphoma international prognostic index 2: a new prognostic index for follicular lymphoma developed by the international follicular lymphoma prognostic factor project. J Clin Oncol. 2009;27(27):4555–62.
24. Bachy E, Maurer MJ, Habermann TM, Gelas-Dore B, Maucort-Boulch D, Estell JA, et al. A simplified scoring system in de novo follicular lymphoma treated initially with immunochemotherapy. Blood. 2018;132(1):49–58.
25. Pastore A, Jurinovic V, Kridel R, Hoster E, Staiger AM, Szczepanowski M, et al. Integration of gene mutations in risk prognostication for patients receiving first-line immunochemotherapy for follicular lymphoma: a retrospective analysis of a prospective clinical trial and validation in a population-based registry. Lancet Oncol. 2015;16(9):1111–22.
26. Huet S, Tesson B, Jais JP, Feldman AL, Magnano L, Thomas E, et al. A gene-expression profiling score for prediction of outcome in patients with follicular lymphoma: a retrospective training and validation analysis in three international cohorts. Lancet Oncol. 2018;19(4):549–61.
27. Casulo C, Byrtek M, Dawson KL, Zhou X, Farber CM, Flowers CR, et al. Early relapse of follicular lymphoma after rituximab plus cyclophosphamide, doxorubicin, vincristine, and prednisone defines patients at high risk for death: an analysis from the national LymphoCare study. J Clin Oncol. 2015;33(23):2516–22.
28. Lockmer S, Ostenstad B, Hagberg H, Holte H, Johansson AS, Wahlin BE, et al. Chemotherapy-free initial treatment of advanced indolent lymphoma has durable effect with low toxicity: results from two nordic lymphoma group trials with more than 10 years of follow-up. J Clin Oncol. 2018;2018:JCO1800262.
29. Moccia AA, Hayoz S, Pirosa MC, Taverna C, Novak U, Kimby E, Ghielmini M, Zucca E. Predictive value of POD24 validation in follicular lymphoma patients initially treated with chemotherapy-free regimens in a pooled analysis of three randomized trials of the Swiss Group for Clinical Cancer Research (SAKK). Hematol Oncol. 2019;37(S2):Abstract 067.
30. Friedberg JW, Byrtek M, Link BK, Flowers C, Taylor M, Hainsworth J, et al. Effectiveness of first-line management strategies for stage I follicular lymphoma: analysis of the national LymphoCare study. J Clin Oncol. 2012;30(27):3368–75.
31. Pugh TJ, Ballonoff A, Newman F, Rabinovitch R. Improved survival in patients with early stage low-grade follicular lymphoma treated with radiation: a surveillance, epidemiology, and end results database analysis. Cancer. 2010;116(16):3843–51.
32. Meignan M, Cottereau AS, Versari A, Chartier L, Dupuis J, Boussetta S, et al. Baseline metabolic tumor volume predicts outcome in high-tumor-burden follicular lymphoma: a pooled analysis of three multicenter studies. J Clin Oncol. 2016;34(30):3618–26.
33. Herfarth KB, Schnaidt S, Hohloch K, Budach V, Engelhard M, Viardot A. Engenhart-C. Rituximab with involved field irradiation for early-stage nodal follicular lymphoma. Results of the MIR study. HemaSphere. 2018;2(6):160.
34. Tsang RW, Gospodarowicz MK. Radiation therapy for localized low-grade non-Hodgkin's lymphomas. Hematol Oncol. 2005;23(1):10–7.
35. Brady JL, Binkley MS, Hajj C, Chelius M, Chau K, Balogh A, et al. Definitive radiotherapy for localized follicular lymphoma staged by (18)F-FDG PET-CT: a collaborative study by ILROG. Blood. 2019;133(3):237–45.

36. Vaughan Hudson B, Vaughan Hudson G, MacLennan KA, Anderson L, Linch DC. Clinical stage 1 non-Hodgkin's lymphoma: long-term follow-up of patients treated by the British National Lymphoma Investigation with radiotherapy alone as initial therapy. Br J Cancer. 1994;69(6):1088–93.
37. Mac Manus MP, Hoppe RT. Is radiotherapy curative for stage I and II low-grade follicular lymphoma? Results of a long-term follow-up study of patients treated at Stanford University. J Clin Oncol. 1996;14(4):1282–90.
38. Wilder RB, Jones D, Tucker SL, Fuller LM, Ha CS, McLaughlin P, et al. Long-term results with radiotherapy for stage I–II follicular lymphomas. Int J Radiat Oncol Biol Phys. 2001;51(5):1219–27.
39. Soubeyran P, Eghbali H, Bonichon F, Coindre JM, Richaud P, Hoerni B. Localized follicular lymphomas: prognosis and survival of stages I and II in a retrospective series of 103 patients. Radiother Oncol. 1988;13(2):91–8.
40. Guckenberger M, Alexandrow N, Flentje M. Radiotherapy alone for stage I–III low grade follicular lymphoma: long-term outcome and comparison of extended field and total nodal irradiation. Radiat Oncol. 2012;7:103.
41. Macmanus MPFR, Roos D, O'Brien P, Macann A, Tsang R, et al. CVP or R-CVP given after involved-field radiotherapy improves progression free survival in stage I–II follicular lymphoma: results of an international randomized trial. Hematol Oncol. 2017;35(S2):31 (Abstract 12).
42. Ruella M, Filippi AR, Bruna R, Di Russo A, Magni M, Caracciolo D, et al. Addition of rituximab to involved-field radiation therapy prolongs progression-free survival in stage I–II follicular lymphoma: results of a multicenter study. Int J Radiat Oncol Biol Phys. 2016;94(4):783–91.
43. Lowry L, Smith P, Qian W, Falk S, Benstead K, Illidge T, et al. Reduced dose radiotherapy for local control in non-Hodgkin lymphoma: a randomised phase III trial. Radiother Oncol. 2011;100(1): 86–92.
44. Luthy SK, Ng AK, Silver B, Degnan KO, Fisher DC, Freedman AS, et al. Response to low-dose involved-field radiotherapy in patients with non-Hodgkin's lymphoma. Ann Oncol. 2008;19(12):2043–7.
45. Hoskin PJ, Kirkwood AA, Popova B, Smith P, Robinson M, Gallop-Evans E, et al. 4 Gy versus 24 Gy radiotherapy for patients with indolent lymphoma (FORT): a randomised phase 3 non-inferiority trial. Lancet Oncol. 2014;15(4):457–63.
46. Zimmermann M, Oehler C, Mey U, Ghadjar P, Zwahlen DR. Radiotherapy for non-Hodgkin's lymphoma: still standard practice and not an outdated treatment option. Radiat Oncol. 2016;11(1):110.
47. Brice P, Bastion Y, Lepage E, Brousse N, Haioun C, Moreau P, et al. Comparison in low-tumor-burden follicular lymphomas between an initial no-treatment policy, prednimustine, or interferon alfa: a randomized study from the Groupe d'Etude des Lymphomes Folliculaires. Groupe d'Etude des Lymphomes de l'Adulte. J Clin Oncol. 1997;15(3):1110–7.
48. Ardeshna KM, Smith P, Norton A, Hancock BW, Hoskin PJ, MacLennan KA, et al. Long-term effect of a watch and wait policy versus immediate systemic treatment for asymptomatic advanced-stage non-Hodgkin lymphoma: a randomised controlled trial. Lancet. 2003;362(9383):516–22.
49. O'Brien ME, Easterbrook P, Powell J, Blackledge GR, Jones L, MacLennan IC, et al. The natural history of low grade non-Hodgkin's lymphoma and the impact of a no initial treatment policy on survival. Q J Med. 1991;80(292):651–60.
50. Horning SJ, Rosenberg SA. The natural history of initially untreated low-grade non-Hodgkin's lymphomas. N Engl J Med. 1984;311(23):1471–5.
51. Link BK, Maurer MJ, Nowakowski GS, Ansell SM, Macon WR, Syrbu SI, et al. Rates and outcomes of follicular lymphoma transformation in the immunochemotherapy era: a report from the University of Iowa/MayoClinic specialized program of research excellence molecular epidemiology resource. J Clin Oncol. 2013;31(26):3272–8.
52. Wagner-Johnston ND, Link BK, Byrtek M, Dawson KL, Hainsworth J, Flowers CR, et al. Outcomes of transformed follicular lymphoma in the modern era: a report from the national LymphoCare study (NLCS). Blood. 2015;126(7):851–7.
53. Young RC, Longo DL, Glatstein E, Ihde DC, Jaffe ES, DeVita VT Jr. The treatment of indolent lymphomas: watchful waiting v aggressive combined modality treatment. Semin Hematol. 1988;25(2 Suppl 2):11–6.
54. McNamara C, Davies J, Dyer M, Hoskin P, Illidge T, Lyttelton M, et al. Guidelines on the investigation and management of follicular lymphoma. Br J Haematol. 2012;156(4):446–67.
55. Bilmon IA, Ashton LJ, Le Marsney RE, Dodds AJ, O'Brien TA, Wilcox L, et al. Second cancer risk in adults receiving autologous haematopoietic SCT for cancer: a population-based cohort study. Bone Marrow Transplant. 2014;49(5):691–8.
56. van Besien K, Loberiza FR Jr, Bajorunaite R, Armitage JO, Bashey A, Burns LJ, et al. Comparison of autologous and allogeneic hematopoietic stem cell transplantation for follicular lymphoma. Blood. 2003;102(10):3521–9.
57. Robinson SP, Canals C, Luang JJ, Tilly H, Crawley C, Cahn JY, et al. The outcome of reduced intensity allogeneic stem cell transplantation and autologous stem cell transplantation when performed as a first transplant strategy in relapsed follicular lymphoma: an analysis from the lymphoma working party of the EBMT. Bone Marrow Transplant. 2013;48(11):1409–14.
58. Klyuchnikov E, Bacher U, Kroger NM, Hari PN, Ahn KW, Carreras J, et al. Reduced-intensity Allografting as first transplantation approach in relapsed/refractory grades one and two follicular lymphoma provides improved outcomes in long-

term survivors. Biol Blood Marrow Transplant. 2015;21(12):2091–9.
59. Witzig TE, Flinn IW, Gordon LI, Emmanouilides C, Czuczman MS, Saleh MN, et al. Treatment with ibritumomab tiuxetan radioimmunotherapy in patients with rituximab-refractory follicular non-Hodgkin's lymphoma. J Clin Oncol. 2002;20(15):3262–9.
60. Gordon LI, Witzig T, Molina A, Czuczman M, Emmanouilides C, Joyce R, et al. Yttrium 90-labeled ibritumomab tiuxetan radioimmunotherapy produces high response rates and durable remissions in patients with previously treated B-cell lymphoma. Clin Lymphoma. 2004;5(2):98–101.
61. Morschhauser F, Radford J, Van Hoof A, Botto B, Rohatiner AZ, Salles G, et al. 90Yttrium-ibritumomab tiuxetan consolidation of first remission in advanced-stage follicular non-Hodgkin lymphoma: updated results after a median follow-up of 7.3 years from the international, randomized, phase III first-LineIndolent trial. J Clin Oncol. 2013;31(16):1977–83.
62. Lopez-Guillermo AC, Dlouhy I, Briones J, Caballero D, Sancho JM. A randomized phase II study comparing consolidation with a single dose of 90y ibritumomab tiuxetan (Zevalin®) (Z) vs. maintenance with rituximab (R) for two years in patients with newly diagnosed follicular lymphoma (FL) responding to R-CHOP. Preliminary results at 36 months from randomization (Abstr. 369). Blood. 2013;122:389.
63. Tobinai K, Igarashi T, Itoh K, Kurosawa M, Nagai H, Hiraoka A, et al. Rituximab monotherapy with eight weekly infusions for relapsed or refractory patients with indolent B cell non-Hodgkin lymphoma mostly pretreated with rituximab: a multicenter phase II study. Cancer Sci. 2011;102(9):1698–705.
64. Rummel MJ, Al-Batran SE, Kim SZ, Welslau M, Hecker R, Kofahl-Krause D, et al. Bendamustine plus rituximab is effective and has a favorable toxicity profile in the treatment of mantle cell and low-grade non-Hodgkin's lymphoma. J Clin Oncol. 2005;23(15):3383–9.
65. Wagner LI, Zhao F, Hong F, Williams ME, Gascoyne RD, Krauss JC, et al. Anxiety and health-related quality of life among patients with low-tumor burden non-Hodgkin lymphoma randomly assigned to two different rituximab dosing regimens: results from ECOG trial E4402 (RESORT). J Clin Oncol. 2015;33(7):740–8.
66. Rummel MJ, Niederle N, Maschmeyer G, Banat GA, von Grunhagen U, Losem C, et al. Bendamustine plus rituximab versus CHOP plus rituximab as first-line treatment for patients with indolent and mantle-cell lymphomas: an open-label, multicentre, randomised, phase 3 non-inferiority trial. Lancet. 2013;381(9873):1203–10.
67. Flinn IW, van der Jagt R, Kahl B, Wood P, Hawkins T, MacDonald D, et al. First-line treatment of patients with indolent non-Hodgkin lymphoma or mantle-cell lymphoma with Bendamustine plus rituximab versus R-CHOP or R-CVP: results of the BRIGHT 5-year follow-up study. J Clin Oncol. 2019;37(12):984–91.
68. Salles G, Seymour JF, Offner F, Lopez-Guillermo A, Belada D, Xerri L, et al. Rituximab maintenance for 2 years in patients with high tumour burden follicular lymphoma responding to rituximab plus chemotherapy (PRIMA): a phase 3, randomised controlled trial. Lancet. 2011;377(9759):42–51.
69. Luminari S, Ferrari A, Manni M, Dondi A, Chiarenza A, Merli F, et al. Long-term results of the FOLL05 trial comparing R-CVP versus R-CHOP versus R-FM for the initial treatment of patients with advanced-stage symptomatic follicular lymphoma. J Clin Oncol. 2018;36(7):689–96.
70. Marcus R, Davies A, Ando K, Klapper W, Opat S, Owen C, et al. Obinutuzumab for the first-line treatment of follicular lymphoma. N Engl J Med. 2017;377(14):1331–44.
71. Morschhauser F, Fowler NH, Feugier P, Bouabdallah R, Tilly H, Palomba ML, et al. Rituximab plus lenalidomide in advanced untreated follicular lymphoma. N Engl J Med. 2018;379(10):934–47.
72. Marcus R, Imrie K, Solal-Celigny P, Catalano JV, Dmoszynska A, Raposo JC, et al. Phase III study of R-CVP compared with cyclophosphamide, vincristine, and prednisone alone in patients with previously untreated advanced follicular lymphoma. J Clin Oncol. 2008;26(28):4579–86.
73. Hiddemann W, Kneba M, Dreyling M, Schmitz N, Lengfelder E, Schmits R, et al. Frontline therapy with rituximab added to the combination of cyclophosphamide, doxorubicin, vincristine, and prednisone (CHOP) significantly improves the outcome for patients with advanced-stage follicular lymphoma compared with therapy with CHOP alone: results of a prospective randomized study of the German low-grade lymphoma study group. Blood. 2005;106(12):3725–32.
74. Herold M, Haas A, Srock S, Neser S, Al-Ali KH, Neubauer A, et al. Rituximab added to first-line mitoxantrone, chlorambucil, and prednisolone chemotherapy followed by interferon maintenance prolongs survival in patients with advanced follicular lymphoma: an east German study group hematology and oncology study. J Clin Oncol. 2007;25(15):1986–92.
75. Bachy E, Houot R, Morschhauser F, Sonet A, Brice P, Belhadj K, et al. Long-term follow up of the FL2000 study comparing CHVP-interferon to CHVP-interferon plus rituximab in follicular lymphoma. Haematologica. 2013;98(7):1107–14.
76. Federico M, Luminari S, Dondi A, Tucci A, Vitolo U, Rigacci L, et al. R-CVP versus R-CHOP versus R-FM for the initial treatment of patients with advanced-stage follicular lymphoma: results of the FOLL05 trial conducted by the Fondazione Italiana Linfomi. J Clin Oncol. 2013;31(12):1506–13.
77. Flinn IW, van der Jagt R, Kahl BS, Wood P, Hawkins TE, Macdonald D, et al. Randomized trial of bendamustine-rituximab or R-CHOP/R-CVP in

first-line treatment of indolent NHL or MCL: the BRIGHT study. Blood. 2014;123(19):2944–52.
78. Hiddemann W, Barbui AM, Canales MA, Cannell PK, Collins GP, Durig J, et al. Immunochemotherapy with Obinutuzumab or rituximab for previously untreated follicular lymphoma in the GALLIUM study: influence of chemotherapy on efficacy and safety. J Clin Oncol. 2018;36(23):2395–404.
79. Ghielmini M, Schmitz SF, Cogliatti SB, Pichert G, Hummerjohann J, Waltzer U, et al. Prolonged treatment with rituximab in patients with follicular lymphoma significantly increases event-free survival and response duration compared with the standard weekly × 4 schedule. Blood. 2004;103(12):4416–23.
80. Martinelli G, Schmitz SF, Utiger U, Cerny T, Hess U, Bassi S, et al. Long-term follow-up of patients with follicular lymphoma receiving single-agent rituximab at two different schedules in trial SAKK 35/98. J Clin Oncol. 2010;28(29):4480–4.
81. Taverna C, Martinelli G, Hitz F, Mingrone W, Pabst T, Cevreska L, et al. Rituximab maintenance for a maximum of 5 years after single-agent rituximab induction in follicular lymphoma: results of the randomized controlled phase III trial SAKK 35/03. J Clin Oncol. 2016;34(5):495–500.
82. Fowler NH, Davis RE, Rawal S, Nastoupil L, Hagemeister FB, McLaughlin P, et al. Safety and activity of lenalidomide and rituximab in untreated indolent lymphoma: an open-label, phase 2 trial. Lancet Oncol. 2014;15(12):1311–8.
83. Martin P, Jung SH, Pitcher B, Bartlett NL, Blum KA, Shea T, et al. A phase II trial of lenalidomide plus rituximab in previously untreated follicular non-Hodgkin's lymphoma (NHL): CALGB 50803 (Alliance). Ann Oncol. 2017;28(11):2806–12.
84. Zucca E, Rondeau S, Vanazzi A, Ostenstad B, Mey UJM, Rauch D, et al. Short regimen of rituximab plus lenalidomide in follicular lymphoma patients in need of first-line therapy. Blood. 2019;134(4):353–62.
85. Kahl BS, Hong F, Williams ME, Gascoyne RD, Wagner LI, Krauss JC, et al. Rituximab extended schedule or re-treatment trial for low-tumor burden follicular lymphoma: eastern cooperative oncology group protocol e4402. J Clin Oncol. 2014;32(28):3096–102.
86. Salles GA, Seymour JF, Feugier P, Offner F, Lopez-Guillermo A, Belada D, Xerri L. Long term follow-up of the PRIMA study: half of patients receiving rituximab maintenance remain progression free at 10 years. Blood. 2017;130:486.
87. Vidal L, Gafter-Gvili A, Salles G, Bousseta S, Oberman B, Rubin C, et al. Rituximab maintenance improves overall survival of patients with follicular lymphoma-individual patient data meta-analysis. Eur J Cancer. 2017;76:216–25.
88. Gyan E, Sonet A, Brice P, Anglaret B, Laribi K, Fruchart C, et al. Bendamustine and rituximab in elderly patients with low-tumour burden follicular lymphoma. Results of the LYSA phase II BRIEF study. Br J Haematol. 2018;183(1):76–86.
89. Gyan E, Foussard C, Bertrand P, Michenet P, Le Gouill S, Berthou C, et al. High-dose therapy followed by autologous purged stem cell transplantation and doxorubicin-based chemotherapy in patients with advanced follicular lymphoma: a randomized multicenter study by the GOELAMS with final results after a median follow-up of 9 years. Blood. 2009;113(5):995–1001.
90. Lenz G, Dreyling M, Schiegnitz E, Forstpointner R, Wandt H, Freund M, et al. Myeloablative radiochemotherapy followed by autologous stem cell transplantation in first remission prolongs progression-free survival in follicular lymphoma: results of a prospective, randomized trial of the German low-grade lymphoma study group. Blood. 2004;104(9):2667–74.
91. Sebban C, Mounier N, Brousse N, Belanger C, Brice P, Haioun C, et al. Standard chemotherapy with interferon compared with CHOP followed by high-dose therapy with autologous stem cell transplantation in untreated patients with advanced follicular lymphoma: the GELF-94 randomized study from the Groupe d'Etude des Lymphomes de l'Adulte (GELA). Blood. 2006;108(8):2540–4.
92. Schouten HC, Qian W, Kvaloy S, Porcellini A, Hagberg H, Johnsen HE, et al. High-dose therapy improves progression-free survival and survival in relapsed follicular non-Hodgkin's lymphoma: results from the randomized European CUP trial. J Clin Oncol. 2003;21(21):3918–27.
93. Sebban C, Brice P, Delarue R, Haioun C, Souleau B, Mounier N, et al. Impact of rituximab and/or high-dose therapy with autotransplant at time of relapse in patients with follicular lymphoma: a GELA study. J Clin Oncol. 2008;26(21):3614–20.
94. Le Gouill S, De Guibert S, Planche L, Brice P, Dupuis J, Cartron G, et al. Impact of the use of autologous stem cell transplantation at first relapse both in naive and previously rituximab exposed follicular lymphoma patients treated in the GELA/GOELAMS FL2000 study. Haematologica. 2011;96(8):1128–35.
95. Casulo C, Friedberg JW, Ahn KW, Flowers C, DiGilio A, Smith SM, et al. Autologous transplantation in follicular lymphoma with early therapy failure: a national LymphoCare study and Center for International Blood and Marrow Transplant Research Analysis. Biol Blood Marrow Transplant. 2018;24(6):1163–71.
96. Jurinovic V, Metzner B, Pfreundschuh M, Schmitz N, Wandt H, Keller U, et al. Autologous stem cell transplantation for patients with early progression of follicular lymphoma: a follow-up study of 2 randomized trials from the German low grade lymphoma study group. Biol Blood Marrow Transplant. 2018;24(6):1172–9.
97. Montoto S, Corradini P, Dreyling M, Ghielmini M, Kimby E, Lopez-Guillermo A, et al. Indications for hematopoietic stem cell transplantation in patients with follicular lymphoma: a consensus project of the

EBMT-lymphoma working party. Haematologica. 2013;98(7):1014–21.
98. Robinson KS, Williams ME, van der Jagt RH, Cohen P, Herst JA, Tulpule A, et al. Phase II multicenter study of bendamustine plus rituximab in patients with relapsed indolent B-cell and mantle cell non-Hodgkin's lymphoma. J Clin Oncol. 2008;26(27):4473–9.
99. Rummel M, Kaiser U, Balser C, Stauch M, Brugger W, Welslau M, et al. Bendamustine plus rituximab versus fludarabine plus rituximab for patients with relapsed indolent and mantle-cell lymphomas: a multicentre, randomised, open-label, non-inferiority phase 3 trial. Lancet Oncol. 2016;17(1):57–66.
100. Cheson BD, Chua N, Mayer J, Dueck G, Trneny M, Bouabdallah K, et al. Overall survival benefit in patients with rituximab-refractory indolent non-Hodgkin lymphoma who received obinutuzumab plus bendamustine induction and obinutuzumab maintenance in the GADOLIN study. J Clin Oncol. 2018;36(22):2259–66.
101. Leonard JP, Trneny M, Izutsu K, Fowler NH, Hong X, Zhu J, et al. AUGMENT: a phase III study of lenalidomide plus rituximab versus placebo plus rituximab in relapsed or refractory indolent lymphoma. J Clin Oncol. 2019;37(14):1188–99.
102. Gopal AK, Kahl BS, de Vos S, Wagner-Johnston ND, Schuster SJ, Jurczak WJ, et al. PI3Kdelta inhibition by idelalisib in patients with relapsed indolent lymphoma. N Engl J Med. 2014;370(11):1008–18.
103. Dreyling M, Santoro A, Mollica L, Leppa S, Follows GA, Lenz G, et al. Phosphatidylinositol 3-kinase inhibition by copanlisib in relapsed or refractory indolent lymphoma. J Clin Oncol. 2017;35(35):3898–905.
104. Schmidt CZ, Jurinovic V, Sökler M, Forstpointner R, Haubner S. Chemotherapy-free combination of obinutuzumab and ibrutinib in first LINE treatment of follicular lymphoma. the alternative study by the German Low Grade Lymphoma Study Group (GLSG) (Abstr. 448). Blood. 2018;132:448.
105. Ogura M, Ando K, Suzuki T, Ishizawa K, Oh SY, Itoh K, et al. A multicentre phase II study of vorinostat in patients with relapsed or refractory indolent B-cell non-Hodgkin lymphoma and mantle cell lymphoma. Br J Haematol. 2014;165(6):768–76.
106. Morschhauser F, Tilly H, Chaidos A, Phillips T, Ribrag V, Campbell P, et al. Interim update from a phase 2 multicenter study of TAZEMETOSTAT, an EZH2 inhibitor, in patients with relapsed or refractory follicular lymphoma. Hematol Oncol. 2019;37(S2):154–6.
107. Palanca-Wessels MC, Czuczman M, Salles G, Assouline S, Sehn LH, Flinn I, et al. Safety and activity of the anti-CD79B antibody-drug conjugate polatuzumab vedotin in relapsed or refractory B-cell non-Hodgkin lymphoma and chronic lymphocytic leukaemia: a phase 1 study. Lancet Oncol. 2015;16(6):704–15.
108. Davids MS, Roberts AW, Seymour JF, Pagel JM, Kahl BS, Wierda WG, et al. Phase I first-in-human study of Venetoclax in patients with relapsed or refractory non-Hodgkin lymphoma. J Clin Oncol. 2017;35(8):826–33.
109. Witzig TE, Wiernik PH, Moore T, Reeder C, Cole C, Justice G, et al. Lenalidomide oral monotherapy produces durable responses in relapsed or refractory indolent non-Hodgkin's lymphoma. J Clin Oncol. 2009;27(32):5404–9.
110. Flinn IW, Kahl BS, Leonard JP, Furman RR, Brown JR, Byrd JC, et al. Idelalisib, a selective inhibitor of phosphatidylinositol 3-kinase-delta, as therapy for previously treated indolent non-Hodgkin lymphoma. Blood. 2014;123(22):3406–13.
111. Bartlett NL, Costello BA, LaPlant BR, Ansell SM, Kuruvilla JG, Reeder CB, et al. Single-agent ibrutinib in relapsed or refractory follicular lymphoma: a phase 2 consortium trial. Blood. 2018;131(2):182–90.
112. Gopal AK, Schuster SJ, Fowler NH, Trotman J, Hess G, Hou JZ, et al. Ibrutinib as treatment for patients with relapsed/refractory follicular lymphoma: results from the open-label, multicenter, phase II DAWN study. J Clin Oncol. 2018;36(23):2405–12.
113. Kirschbaum M, Frankel P, Popplewell L, Zain J, Delioukina M, Pullarkat V, et al. Phase II study of vorinostat for treatment of relapsed or refractory indolent non-Hodgkin's lymphoma and mantle cell lymphoma. J Clin Oncol. 2011;29(9):1198–203.

7 Extranodal Marginal Zone Lymphoma of Mucosa-Associated Lymphoid Tissue (MALT Lymphoma)

Emanuele Zucca and Markus Raderer

Extranodal marginal zone lymphoma of mucosa-associated lymphoid tissue (EMZL)

Clinical outline

Mostly affects adults. Arises potentially at any extranodal site. Often multiple anatomic sites involved. The most common single location is the gastric mucosa, followed by other gastro-intestinal sites, eye adnexa, skin, lungs and salivary glands. Bone marrow and lymph nodes are infrequently involved, at least in the early phases. Patients may display the signs and symptoms of infectious or inflammatory/autoimmune conditions, which are acknowledged to underlie a substantial fraction of EMZL cases.

Cytology	Small to medium sized cells ranging in morphology from lymphocyte- and centrocyte-like to monocytoid. Features of plasmacytic differentiation may be observed.	Extranodal marginal zone lymphoma, cytology 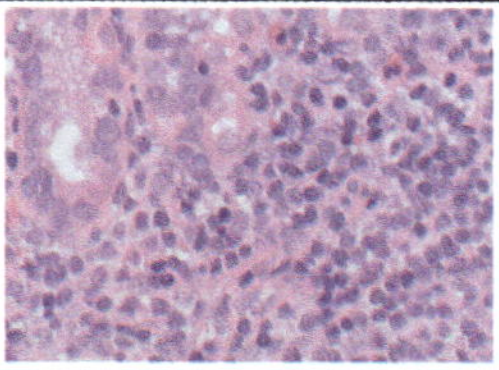
Histology	Arises in newly formed lymphoid tissue induced by chronic inflammation. Follicular structures harboring an expanded marginal zones, progressive colonization and effacement of germinal centers and diffuse infiltration with pale appearance. When present, the epithelial structures are infiltrated by lymphoma cells ("lymphoepithelial lesions"). Cutaneous forms no of little epitheliotropism. Large centroblastic/ immunoblastic cells may be numerous, but by definition should not form cohesive sheets.	Extranodal marginal zone lymphoma, hystology 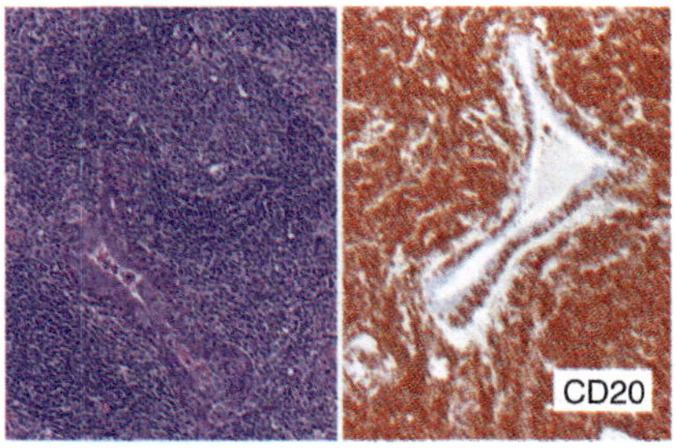

	CD20	CD5	CD23[1]	CD10	BCL6	cyclin D1	CD103	FMC7	IgM	light chains
notes	[1]partial/weak expression occacionally observed									
other marker	EMZL lacks a specific phenotype and the antibody panel primarily aims at exclusion of other lymphoma subtypes. IRTA1 and MNDA may be helpful marker but less frequently used or not widely available.									

■ = majority of cases positive ▒ = variable fraction of cases positive □ = negative

M. Dreyling, M. Ladetto (eds.), *Indolent Lymphomas*, Hematologic Malignancies,
https://doi.org/10.1007/978-3-030-55989-2_7

Main differential diagnosis	CLL (should be CD23 positive), MCL (sould be cyclin D1 positive). Subtypes of marginal zone lymphomas (extranodal, nodal, splenic, cutaneous) distinguished mainly by clinical presentation (pattern of involved organs).

Key molecular features

IGH genes are rearranged, somatic hypermutation and IGHV usage bias. NF-kB pathway often deregulated due to chromosomal translocations and mutations. Frequent translocations (frequency dependent on involved site): t(11;18)(q21;q21), t(14;18)(q32;q21), t(3;14)(p14.1;q32), t(1;14)(p22;q32) involving MALT1, BCL10 and FOXP1, respectively, Frequent copy number alterations: Trisomy 3 and 18. Del 6q23. Frequent mutations: *TNFAIP3.*

Precursor lesions

Not well defined. Chronic inflammation (autoimmune, viral by Hepatitis C, or bacterial by Helicobacter pylori) predispose to development of marginal zone lymphoma. Thus inflammation and lymphoma histologically may co-exist/overlap.

Progression

May progress/transform to diffuse large B-cell lymphoma. Definition of transformation currently purely morphologically by detection of sheets of blasts.

Key molecular features

IGH genes are rearranged, somatic hypermutation and IGHV usage bias. NF-kB pathway often deregulated due to chromosomal translocations and mutations. Frequent translocations (frequency dependent on involved site): t(11;18)(q21;q21), t(14;18)(q32;q21), t(3;14)(p14.1;q32), t(1;14)(p22;q32) involving MALT1, BCL10 and FOXP1, respectively, Frequent copy number alterations: Trisomy 3 and 18. Del 6q23. Frequent mutations: *TNFAIP3.*

Precursor lesions

Not well defined. Chronic inflammation (autoimmune, viral by Hepatitis C, or bacterial by Helicobacter pylori) predispose to development of marginal zone lymphoma. Thus inflammation and lymphoma histologically may co-exist/overlap.

Progression

May progress/transform to diffuse large B-cell lymphoma. Definition of transformation currently purely morphologically by detection of sheets of blasts.

Clinically relevant pathologic features	Relevance	Evidence
FISH for t(11;18)(q21;q21) *BIRC3/MALT1*	Predictive: in gastric MZL, identifies cases unlikely to respond to *H. pylori eradication*	**B**
Search for site specific infectious agents (histochemistry and/or PCR)	Predictive: may guide a first line eradicating approach	**B**
Increase in large cells and/or proliferative index.	Prognostic: unfavourable	**C**
Legend: A = verified in multiple studies, randomized trials and/or integrated in guidelines; B = variable between studies/ needs definitive validation; C = preliminary/discrepant results.		

E. Zucca (✉)
Division of Medical Oncology, Oncology Institute of Southern Switzerland, Bellinzona, Switzerland

Institute of Oncology Research, Bellinzona, Switzerland

Department of Medical Oncology, University Hospital, Bern, Switzerland
e-mail: Emanuele.Zucca@eoc.ch

M. Raderer
Internal Medicine I, Oncology, Medical University of Vienna, Vienna, Austria
e-mail: markus.raderer@meduniwien.ac.at

7.1 Introduction

Initially described as a special subtype of gastric lymphoma in 1983, extranodal marginal zone B-cell lymphoma of the mucosa-associated lymphoid tissue (MALT lymphoma) has been incorporated into the recent WHO classification of lymphoid malignancies [1] as a distinct subtype of marginal zone lymphoma.

MALT lymphoma is a relatively common lymphoma comprising 7–8% of newly diagnosed lymphomas making its incidence comparable to that of mantle cell lymphoma and inferior only to follicular and diffuse large B-cell lymphoma. MALT lymphoma is usually diagnosed in elderly patients (median age 65 years) and appears to be more common in women than in men, with a ratio of approximately 1.5:1 [2].

Following the initial description of gastric MALT lymphoma, it has subsequently been demonstrated that almost all organs of the human body may give rise to MALT lymphoma, including highly unusual sites such as the dura mater. In the recent WHO classification, the stomach is still defined as the most common site of origin (accounting for roughly 50% of MALT lymphomas), followed by the ocular adnexa, salivary glands and the lung. The percentage of gastric MALT lymphoma, however, seems to be declining in larger registries, with an incidence in the range of 30–40%, while most patients are being diagnosed with extragastric MALT lymphomas [3, 4].

Significant differences exist between gastric and non-gastric MALT lymphomas in terms of presentation, response to therapy and relapse rate; however, clinical and genetic data have suggested heterogeneity also within non-gastric MALT lymphomas with respect to the site of origin [5–8].

One of the most striking features of the disease is the pronounced tendency of MALT lymphoma to stay localized within mucosal environments, while showing an extremely low affinity for the bone marrow. These "homing" properties, thought to be due to the interplay between various adhesion molecules and epithelial and vascular structures were demonstrated relatively early for gastric MALT lymphoma and a tendency for multiple organ involvement has also been suggested at the molecular level. However, in terms of clinical presentation, MALT lymphomas are usually regarded as localized to a single organ [9]. Various reports using standardized staging systems have nevertheless shown gastric MALT lymphoma as a multi-organ disease in up to 25% of cases and the rate of multiorgan involvement in extragastric MALT lymphomas is even higher, occurring in up to 50% of patients [4, 10].

In view of this, it is important to recognize the individual factors and pathogenetic features giving rise to MALT lymphoma, as they are crucial to understanding and developing therapeutic strategies for this lymphoma entity, which starkly differs from nodal-based indolent B-cell lymphomas [11].

7.2 Pathology and Pathogenesis of MALT Lymphoma

7.2.1 Morphology

MALT lymphoma is diagnosed by histopathological assessment of tissue samples according to the standardized criteria outlined in the recent WHO classification, using a panel of immunohistochemical markers. As yet, molecular methods and markers do not play a role in diagnosis [1, 2].

Immunostaining is important for distinguishing MALT lymphoma from other extranodal B-cell lymphomas including follicular lymphoma, mantle cell lymphoma, extramedullary plasmocytoma or small lymphocytic lymphoma. Histopathological assessment of lymph node involvement in marginal zone lymphoma is usually unable to reliably distinguish MALT lymphoma from the much rarer nodal and splenic marginal zone lymphomas, which also require a full clinical work; this is especially necessary for defining nodal marginal zone lymphoma, which is mostly diagnosed by exclusion and its extranodal origin.

The cell of origin of MALT lymphoma is thought to be a mature B-cell related to the plasma cell. MALT lymphomas are heterogeneous in appearance; their cellular composition includes typical centrocyte-like cells, monocytoid B-cells, small lymphocytes and plasma cells, while large cells are present in varying proportions in almost all patients. In mucosal sites, the malignant clone usually infiltrates the epithelial structures to form so-called lympho-epithelial lesions, which are pathognomonic to a certain extent, but may also be absent in some locations and are thus not a prerequisite for the diagnosis of MALT lymphoma. Reactive follicles with neoplastic cells occupying the marginal-zone and the interfollicular region are also commonly seen (follicular colonization).

Lymphoma cells are positive for B-cell antigens including CD19, CD20, CD22, CD79a and CD79b, and are CD5−, CD43−/+, CD3−, CD23−, CD11c−/+ and CD10−. This immunophenotype distinguishes MALT lymphoma from other indolent B-cell lymphomas and mantle cell lymphoma, although CD5 immunoreactivity has been reported in a small proportion of cases [2], which might necessitate further tests such as testing for Cyclin D1 to distinguish MALT lymphoma from mantle cell lymphoma.

MALT lymphoma cells express surface immunoglobulins, which are more frequently IgM+ than IgG+ or IgA+, and in 30–40% of patients, monoclonal immunoglobulins can also be detected in the peripheral blood, which can sometimes be misdiagnosed as a monoclonal gammopathy of unknown significance (MGUS).

Especially in gastric MALT lymphoma, an increased number of blasts growing in sheets may be present, and in some areas, a pure diffuse large B-cell histology may be present along with the indolent MALT lymphoma component. In those cases, the diagnosis of diffuse large B-cell lymphoma (DLBCL) along with MALT lymphoma should be made. This may be present at diagnosis or may develop during the course of the disease. The risk of transformation, however, appears to be low in patients with MALT lymphoma and is thought to be in the range of 2–3% in larger series [12, 13]. While it has not been clear whether those patients are indeed transforming from MALT lymphomas or develop DLBCL at the same site due to the same underlying mechanisms such as HP-infection, recent investigations on the clonal association between MALT lymphoma and DLBCL have indeed shown a clonal relationship, i.e. transformation in the large majority of patients [13]. In agreement with these findings there are reports of successful treatment of gastric DLBCL using an antibiotic as the sole therapeutic modality [14, 15].

7.2.2 Genetics of MALT Lymphoma

While some B-cell malignancies such as follicular lymphoma and mantle cell lymphoma are characterized by a distinct genetic aberration, there is no clear-cut genetic hallmark for MALT lymphoma. Although some genetic changes result in a common activation of the NF-kB pathway, a variety of genetic features have occasionally been reported in a small percentage of patients, including t(11;18)(q21;q21), t(1;14)(p22;q32), t(14;18)(q32;q21), t(3;14)(q27;q32) and t(3;14)(p14.1;q32) translocations. Of these the t(11;18)(q21;q21) is the most commonly detected aberration occurring in up to 35% of cases. However, it is mostly found in pulmonary and gastric MALT lymphomas (24–48%). The t(11;18)(q21;q21) translocation fuses the API2 (apoptosis inhibitor-2) gene on chromosome 11 to the MALT1 (MALT lymphoma-associated translocation) gene on chromosome 18, rendering cells resistant to apoptosis. It is specific for MALT lymphoma, as it is not seen in nodal or splenic marginal zone lymphoma [8, 16].

When present, t(11;18)(q21;q21) is usually an exclusive chromosomal aberration and is associated with infection with CaGA-positive HP-strains, lymph node involvement and systemic disease, as well as unresponsiveness to HP eradication [17–19] in gastric MALT lymphoma. While t(11;18)(q21;q21) has been identified in 70% of gastric MALT lymphoma patients who did not respond to antibiotic therapy [17–19], it is rarely detected in responding patients and is not thought to predict resistance to systemic therapies including rituximab or cladribine [11]. In the current guidelines, routine assessment of t(11;18) (q21;q21) is not recommended before antibiotic therapy or for assessing the molecular persistence of the lymphoma.

Numerical aberrations including trisomy 3, 7, 12 and 18 have been reported and might be a hallmark of non-gastric gastrointestinal MALT lymphoma [20–22].

The fact that no common genetic changes have been documented throughout various localizations of MALT lymphomas further underscores the suggestion that MALT lymphoma might be composed of various clinical subtypes, an observation that is supported by the different biological behaviours and clinical course within this entity, as will be further outlined in the chapter.

7.2.3 Pathogenesis of MALT Lymphoma

The large majority of lymphoid tissue in the human body is localised in the gut, with a concentration in the so-called Peyer's patches. While the architecture of MALT lymphoma is reminiscent of those mucosal structures, MALT lymphomas almost exclusively arise in acquired mucosal lymphoid tissues developing as a result of chronic antigenic stimulation. Apart from the stomach, which has been the role model for MALT lymphoma due to the association between *Helicobacter pylori* (HP) infection and development of MALT with subsequent malignant transformation, similar processes following chronic conditions, i.e. infection and inflammation, have been reported in the lung, the skin and the ocular adnexa. Interestingly, it was reported that different types of MALT may show specialized trafficking of lymphoma cells with predominate homing to corresponding mucosal structures, which appear to vary between gastrointestinalMALT versus non-gastrointestinal mucosal lymphoid tissues [23]. These immunologic preferences to certain sites may explain the fact that different dissemination patterns exist in MALT lymphomas of various gastric and extragastric sites [4, 10, 24, 25], which may have clinical consequences for staging and treating such patients.

While MAdCAM-1 and $\alpha 4\beta 7$-integrins interacting with high endothelial venules [26–28] have been reported to be important in gastrointestinal lymphomas, more recent findings have also implicated the chemokine receptors CXCR4 and CXCR7 [29]. Receptors for CXCR4 have been found to be present not only on CLL-cells but also in 93% of patients with MALT lymphoma [30] using immunohistochemistry. Consequently, Ga68- Pentixafor-PET/MR for imaging of CXCR4 has been found to reliably visualize lymphoma involvement in a pilot series in patients with MALT lymphoma [31].

7.2.4 Infectious Agents and MALT Lymphoma

One of the most striking examples in terms of translating pathogenetic findings into therapeutic concepts was the discovery of the close link between HP-infection and gastric MALT lymphoma. Interestingly, both gastric MALT lymphoma as well as the presence of a gram-negative rod, i.e. HP able to survive in the stomach were first reported in 1983. Epidemiological reports soon disclosed a high rate of gastric lymphoma in areas with HP-infection [32], and the presence of HP in more than 90% of patients with gastric MALT lymphoma [33] raised interest in the role of the bacteria for the development of MALT and subsequent lymphoma, but also gastric cancer.

While HP-infection is commonly found, gastric MALT lymphoma is still a relatively rare condition which will occur only in a minority of HP-infected patients. Thus, MALT lymphoma development is thought to be the result of both HP-related factors, such as expression of CagA [34], but also host-related factors. In this setting, CagA not only acts as a marker for bacterial virulence, but is also able to translocate into HP-dependent MALT lymphoma cells. In an analysis of 47 samples from patients with localized gastric MALT lymphoma [35], 25 were rated as HP-dependent and studies for Cag A and other signal transduction pathways (phospho-SHP-2, phospho-ERK as well as phospho-p38 MAP-kinase, BCL2 and Bcl-x) revealed a significant association with HP-dependency and a direct role of these molecules in lymphomagenesis.

In vitro experiments have clearly demonstrated that the role of HP is specific for the particular strain of HP and the HP-specific T-cells generated within the individual patient, as removal of T-cells from cell suspensions before culturing did not result in any growth stimulus for MALT lymphoma when adding HP. Apparently, immunological specificity for HP is defined by intra-tumoural T-cells [36].

While the majority of patients with gastric MALT lymphoma are still thought to be positive for HP, the number of HP-negative gastric MALT lymphomas is apparently increasing. While up to 90% of patients with gastric MALT lymphoma were HP-positive in the 1990s [1, 33, 37, 38], recent reports have shown HP-negative patients up to 30–50% in cohorts of gastric MALT lymphoma [3, 11, 39, 40]. The reason remains unclear for the time being, but the widespread use of antibiotics in suspected HP-infection/symptoms might at least partly explain this phenomenon.

In addition to HP, also rarer infections such as *H. heilmannii* in rare cases of gastric MALT lymphoma [41] or *Campylobacter jejuni* (the latter in MALT lymphoma of the small intestine or immunoproliferative small intestinal disease IPSID occurring in the Middle East [42]) have been reported as causative agents.

Data on bacterial causes for non-gastric MALT lymphoma are relatively rare [43], and include the potential association of *Borrelia burgdorferi* with cutaneous lymphoma, *Achromobacter xylosoxidans* and *Chlamydophila psittaci* (CP) with pulmonary lymphomas and CP with ocular adnexal MALT lymphomas (OAML). In addition to indirect evidence, viable and infectious CP isolated from conjunctival swabs and peripheral blood samples of OAML patients have been successfully grown in culture [44]. However, a geographic variation was observed, as the high rate of infection reported in Italy could not be found in other countries [45]. While there is a plausible role for CP in the development of OAML in regions with high rates of infection, it is not clear whether a universal role can attributed to CP in OAML and whether the success of antibiotics in OAML is based on eradication of CP.

7.2.5 Autoimmune Disorders

An association between autoimmune diseases (ADs), especially Sjögren's syndrome (SS) and chronic autoimmune thyroiditis (CAT, Hashimoto's disease) with salivary gland and thyroid MALT lymphoma, respectively, has been shown from epidemiological series. The highly increased risk (up to 70-fold when compared to the normal population) is in line with the MALT concept of chronic antigenic stimulation within the target organ [2, 9, 46].

In addition, results from the InterLymph Non-Hodgkin Lymphoma Project [47] including 1052 cases with marginal zone lymphomas (633 MALT lymphomas, 140 splenic and 157 nodal marginal zone lymphomas), defined an increased risk for all three subtypes of marginal zone lymphoma due to underlying ADs.

In a large, single-centre retrospective analysis of 158 patients with MALT lymphoma [48], the rate of patients with AD was high at 39%. In terms of clinical impact, AD patients were significantly younger (56 versus 67 years), were predominately female (79%) and were more likely to have extragastric lymphomas. Although there was no influence on the clinical course, response to therapy and relapse rate compared to MALT lymphoma patients without AD, patients with AD were less likely to respond to HP eradication in cases of gastric MALT lymphoma, especially those with Hashimoto's thyroiditis, which affects 16% of gastric MALT lymphoma patients [49].

7.3 Clinical Presentation, Diagnosis and Staging

Due to the fact that MALT lymphoma can be diagnosed in almost every organ of the human body, presenting signs as well as diagnostic measures may broadly vary. The majority of patients are in excellent performance status and mostly asymptomatic; laboratory findings which may be abnormal in other indolent B-cell lymphomas such as beta-2-microblobulin or lactate dehydrogenase (LDH) are mostly normal [50].

While the rate of gastric lymphomas appears lower nowadays than in the last decades, the gastrointestinal tract is still the most common site, with MALT lymphomas representing 40–50% of primary gastric lymphomas.

Patients with gastric MALT lymphoma may be asymptomatic or suffer from unspecific gastritic symptoms, while bleeding, abdominal pain and weight loss, as well as B-symptoms are very uncommon [2].

Accordingly, endoscopic findings in gastric MALT lymphoma may vary from almost normal to ulcerated tumours. However, gastric MALT lymphoma is usually a multifocal disease and this needs to be taken into account when taking biopsies, which should also include mucosal regions that appear normal.

Extragastric MALT lymphoma is mostly diagnosed in the ocular adnexa followed by salivary glands and lung, thyroid gland and skin. As already stated, primary intestinal MALT lymphomas are very rare and may represent a secondary spread from undetected gastric MALT lymphomas. Symptoms vary depending on the specific site involved and in particular, diagnoses of conjunctival and pulmonary MALT lymphomas are delayed in the range of 1–135 months due to an initial suspicion of unspecific inflammatory changes [51].

For recommended staging and diagnostic procedures see Table 7.1 [11]. The special requirements for gastric MALT lymphoma are discussed below. Noteworthy is the fact that 18F-FDG-PET/CT will result in false negative findings in up to 50% of patients, and thus is not routinely recommended for work-up of patients with MALT lymphoma [11, 52].

One of the main clinical characteristics of MALT lymphoma is the propensity to remain localized for long periods, but dissemination may be present at diagnosis in 25–50% of non-gastrointestinal MALT lymphomas [53]. Bone marrow involvement, however, is very rare (i.e. <2% of cases) in recent series [3, 4, 10, 11] and does not appear to affect prognosis even in patients treated with HP eradication only. Thus, routine performance of bone marrow biopsy is not recommended in recent guidelines apart from in exceptional cases [52].

Table 7.1 Specific staging and work-up procedures for extranodal marginal zone lymphoma (EMZL) at different primary anatomic sites

Site	Exam
Stomach	• EGD: Mandatory vEndoscopic US: Optional, to evaluate the regional lymph nodes and gastric wall infiltration • IHC: Mandatory, to evaluate *Helicobacter pylori* status. Faecal antigen or breath test and serology studies are recommended when the results of histology are negative • FISH or PCR assay: Optional, to detect t(11;18) translocation
Small intestine (IPSID)	• PCR, IHC or ISH: *Campylobacter jejuni* search in the tumour biopsy
Colon	• Colonoscopy and EGD
Salivary glands	• ENT examination and echography • EGD • Anti-SSA/Ro and anti-SSB/La antibodies: To rule out association with Sjogren syndrome
Ocular adnexa	• Orbital and salivary glands imaging (MRI or CT): If clinically indicated • Head and neck imaging (MRI or CT): If clinically indicated • PCR: *Chlamydophila psittaci* search in the tumour biopsy and PBMCs (optional, according to the geographical distribution of the infection
Thyroid	• Thyroid echography • CT scan of the neck • Thyroid function tests
Lung	• Bronchoscopy and bronchoalveolar lavage • EGD
Breast	• Mammography and breast sonography • MRI (or CT scan)
Skin	• PCR: *Borrelia burgdorferi* search in the tumour biopsy

CT computed tomography, *EGD* oesophagogastroduodenoscopy, *EMZL* extranodal marginal zone lymphoma, *ENT* ear, nose and throat, *FISH* fluorescent in situ hybridisation, *IHC* immunohistochemistry, *IPSID* immunoproliferative small intestinal disease, *ISH* in situ hybridisation, *MRI* magnetic resonance imaging, *PBMC* peripheral blood mononuclear cell, *PCR* polymerase chain reaction, *US* ultrasound

7.3.1 Diagnostic Procedures for Gastric MALT Lymphoma

Diagnosis of gastric MALT lymphoma requires histopathological assessment of biopsies taken during gastric mapping, with sufficient numbers of biopsies from macroscopic lesions and normal mucosa. This is the only way to avoid a sampling bias due to insufficient material [54]. A minimum of ten biopsies are recommended from visible lesions with additional biopsies from normally appearing mucosa. In case of diagnostic doubt, insufficient or inadequate biopsy material, a repeat endoscopy is strongly recommended. HP eradication should not be started before a definite diagnosis performed by an experienced reference haemato-pathologist. Endoscopic mapping is also necessary for assessing the response to therapy in order to avoid a sampling bias.

Diagnosis of HP should be performed on biopsies taken from normal mucosa, as the rate of detection decreases with progression from HP-gastritis to MALT lymphoma, and Proton pump inhibitor (PPI) treatment should be withdrawn at least 2 weeks before endoscopy to avoid false negative results for HP diagnostic tests (with the exception of serology) [55, 56].

7.3.2 Staging Systems

Various staging systems have been developed and applied in MALT lymphoma to take into account the special clinical features of the disease such as the multifocal occurrence in paired organs including orbit [25, 52], parotid [24], lungs [57], as well as exclusive dissemination within the gastrointestinal tract.

Two distinct staging systems have been proposed for gastrointestinal MALT lymphomas, while the Ann Arbor staging based on the presence and localisation of additional non-nodal lesions and the extent of lymph node involvement is the most widely used system for extra-gastric MALT lymphomas. The modified Ann Arbor staging system by Musshoff and Radszkiewicz is one of the most commonly used for gastrointestinal lymphomas [54] and takes into account dissemination, i.e., involvement of neighbouring (II1E) and distant lymph (II2E) nodes, and the depth of infiltration into the gastric wall (involving only the mucosa and submucosa—I1E—versus also extending beyond the submucosa—I2E). The Lugano staging system for gastrointestinal lymphomas is widely used in patients with MALT lymphomas [58], and defines stage I as single or multiple lesions confined to the gastrointestinal tract, stage II1 as local and II2 as distant lymph node involvement, with stage IIE as direct extension through the serosa. There is no stage III, and disseminated extranodal involvement as well as lymph nodes in supra-diaphragmatic regions are both rated as stage IV disease. The TNM-based Paris staging system has not been validated so far and thus remains rather experimental due to various difficulties in application based on non-surgical staging [59].

7.3.3 Prognostic Factors

MALT lymphoma is an indolent lymphoma with excellent prognosis, with survival rates exceeding 10 years in almost all larger series. Both gastric as well as extragastric MALT lymphomas have a 5-year overall survival higher than 90% and a 10-year survival of 75–80% [60]. However, relapses and dissemination are common even after successful therapy and can occur decades after treatment, warranting lifelong follow-up. The median time to relapse is in the median range of 5 years in most series irrespective of therapy, and occurs in 50–60% of patients, involving the same organ in 50–60% of cases or other extranodal sites [60–62]. However, the rate of relapse appears higher in extragastric versus gastric MALT lymphomas following initial therapy [11].

Various parameters associated with a poorer prognosis have been suggested in the past, including advanced age, lower performance status, elevated lactate dehydrogenase serum levels, and/or beta-2 microglobulin levels, stage of disease and, for primary gastric MALT lymphoma, the depth of infiltration of the gastric wall as assessed by endosonography [62–64]. In addition, the presence of t(11;18)(q21;q21) has been linked to more advanced disease and a lower rate of response to HP eradication in patients with gastric MALT lymphoma.

Recently, a MALT lymphoma prognostic index (MALT-IPI) was established from the patient cohort treated within the randomized IELSG19 study [65] and subsequently validated by two large control cohorts. This index includes age >70, stage III/IV and elevated LDH-levels, and was able to stratify patients into three prognostic categories (low = 0, intermediate = one factor present, high risk = two or more factors) following systemic therapy. From the same cohort, progression of disease at 24 months (POD24) could also be defined as being prognostic for shorter survival [66]. Patients with POD24 have a higher incidence of high grade transformation [66].

7.4 Treatment of MALT Lymphoma

A large variety of therapeutic modalities have been reported in MALT lymphoma, and currently antibiotics, radiation and systemic therapy including antibodies, chemotherapy and also chemo-free combinations are the cornerstones of therapy. Surgery should only be applied in cases of localized disease in pulmonary and thyroid MALT lymphoma, while it has virtually been abandoned in gastric MALT lymphoma. In addition, the highly indolent clinical course as well as the fact that spontaneous remissions and "wax-and-wane" phenomena have been described, justify a watch-and-wait strategy in asymptomatic patients. Watch-and-wait was reported as successful in both OAML [67] and pulmonary MALT lymphomas [68]. In patients with stage I OAML time to progression, systemic dissemination, high-grade transformation, and lymphoma-related mortality, were no different from those reported with immediate radiotherapy, with a 10-year overall survival of 94% in one series [67].

In addition, also patients with gastric MALT lymphoma and microscopic residual disease after HP eradication or microscopic "relapse" (which is mostly due to sampling bias) may be safely watched, as 94% of 103 patients did not have progressive disease at a median watchful waiting period of 42 months [69].

The "choice of weapons" for patients requiring therapy is based on the primary organs involved and also on the stage of the lymphoma. Determination of the organs involved is important as infectious agents and dissemination patterns may be organ-specific. Knowledge of organ involvement is also important for gauging the potential side effects associated with irradiation of different organs. In terms of stage, limited-stage MALT lymphoma is also amenable to local therapies in addition to systemic treatment, while the latter is the standard of care for disseminated disease.

7.4.1 Anti-infective Therapy

In view of the ethiopathogenetic role of infective agents as well as the lack of relevant side effects, these therapies should be considered as frontline strategies whenever possible. In fact, recent guidelines state HP eradication as the treatment of choice in gastric MALT lymphoma irrespective of stage, and also to a certain extent, irrespective of proof of HPinfection [11, 52, 54].

In addition to HP in gastric MALT lymphoma, CP in ocular adnexal MALT lymphoma, Borrelia strains in cutaneous MALT lymphoma and in anecdotal reports *C. jejuni* in IPSID have been reported as potentially successful targets.

Following a small initial pilot study of six patients, HP eradication has been widely studied and is now the accepted standard of care for gastric MALT lymphoma [52, 54]. The choice of antibiotic therapy should be based on local guidelines and should take into account the rate of resistance to clarithromycin, which is to be best avoided when the resistance rate exceeds 15%. The duration of therapy has also been studied, and while meta-analyses data have shown improved results for treatment given for 14 days instead of 7 days, there was no significant difference between 7 and 10 days [70]. The success of HP eradication should be checked by urea breath test and be confirmed on gastric biopsies. In cases of HP persistence, further therapies should take culture results into account as well as tests for resistance to individual HP strains. Successful HP eradication usually leads to regression of the lymphoma (in more than 75% of patients, according to a meta-analysis including more than 1400 patients [71]); however, the time to best response is unpredictable and may take up to more than 2 years [72].

Assessment of response requires regular endoscopic follow-up, and definition of response should be based on the GELA-grading system [73] that defines complete remission, no change, responding residual disease (rRD) and probable minimal residual disease (pMRD). Due to the potential of histologic sampling errors during endoscopy, at least two sequential follow-up gastroscopies are necessary for definition of complete remission [54]. As already stated, the presence of t(11;18)(q21;q21) is regarded as a negative response predictor, as are involvement with lymphoma beyond the muscularis mucosae and local lymph nodes. However, neither assessment of monoclonality nor t(11;18)(q21;q21) should be done during follow-up, as they are not useful in guiding management [54] and may persist for years even in the absence of clinical lymphoma remission. This is due to data showing that more than 60% of patients have residual monoclonality or persistence of t(11;18(q21;q21) or histological residual disease but only ~6% of them will experience progressive disease [69].

A randomized trial has also shown that application of chlorambucil following HP eradication did not improve outcome in patients with gastric MALT lymphoma responsive to HP eradication [72]. In recent years, an increasing number of trials reported about lymphoma regression also in HP-negative gastric MALT lymphoma patients [11, 74]. While the mechanism as yet remains unclear, these data have led to the recommendation that antibiotic HP eradication may also be used as frontline therapy in apparently HP-negative cases of gastric MALT lymphoma.

Antibiotic therapy is also recommended in patients with OAML, and positive results have been obtained with both doxycycline and clarithromycin (for review see [75]). However, due to the sometimes prolonged mode of action, it can only be recommended for patients who are not in need of acute and fast-acting therapy [76, 77]. Interestingly, while the overall response rate to doxycycline is in the range of up to 50%, patients with both CP-positive (65%) and CP-negative (38%) lymphomas responded, resulting in a 3-year progression-free survival (PFS) of 68% in pre-treated patients. When given as first-line therapy, doxycycline has resulted in an overall response rate of 65%, and a 5-year PFS of 55% in patients with OAML in stage I [78]. The main clinical trials with antibiotic therapy in OAML are summarized in Table 7.2. Additional discussion about the use of macrolides (clarithromycin and azithromycin) will be provided later in this chapter, since their activity may be due to their intrinsic antitumour and immunomodulatory effects and not necessarily associated with the removal of an antigen drive [79].

Apart from HCV, no viral pathogens have been associated with MALT lymphoma, and results from mainly Italian studies have shown that it might constitute a therapeutic target in marginal zone lymphomas [80]. Application of pegylated IFN +/− ribavirin has resulted in a response rate of 75% in patients with marginal zone lymphoma (MZL) [81], with a 5-year PFS and OS of 78% and 92%, respectively, and anti-HCV therapy at any time was independently associated with better OS.

7.4.2 Local Therapy

Over the last decades, the use of surgery has been decreasing, and is nowadays restricted to rare emergencies such as perforation and bleeding in gastrointestinal MALT lymphomas, or to diagnostic procedures in pulmonary, thyroid and ocular adnexal MALT lymphomas. However, in those patients in whom total resection of the disease has been achieved, no additional therapies are currently recommended.

Radiotherapy is the most extensively studied treatment in localized stages of MALT lymphoma, and is considered standard therapy in

Table 7.2 Main clinical trials with antibiotic therapy in OAML

Author	Study type	*N*	Site %	Stage	Therapy	ORR, %	CR, %
Ferreri 2008 [118]	Retrospective	6	Ocular adnexa	IVE	Doxycycline po × 21 d	33	0
Han 2015 [119]	Retrospective	90	Ocular adnexa	I-IVE	Doxycycline po × 21 d	27	7
Kim 2010 [120]	Retrospective	38	Ocular adnexa	I-IVE	Doxycycline po × 21 d	47	18
Ferreri 2005 [76]	Phase II	9	Ocular adnexa	I-IVE	Doxycycline po × 21 d	44	22
Ferreri 2006 [77]	Phase II	27	Ocular adnexa	I-IVE	Doxycycline po × 21 d	48	22
Ferreri 2012 [118]	Phase II	34	Ocular adnexa	IE	Doxycycline po × 21 d	65	18
Govi 2010 [112]	Phase II	13	85 ocular adnexa, 15 other	I-IVE	Clarithromycin 1000 mg/d po for 6 mo	38	15
Ferreri 2015 [113]	Phase II	23	43 ocular adnexa, 57 other	I-IVE	High-dose clarithromycin (2000 mg po d1–14) in a 3-w cycle × 4	52	26
Ferreri 2018 [79]		55	53 ocular adenxa, 47 other	I-IVE	Clarithromycin different doses	47	23
Lagler 2019 [114]	Phase II	16	50 ocular adenxa, 50 other	I-IVE	Azithromycin 1/w	25	12

ORR overall response rate, *CR* complete response, *d* day, *po* oral administration, *mo* months, *w* week

many countries. A universally accepted radiation schedule for MALT lymphomas does not exist, but a dose of 25–30 Gy in 10–15 fractions (minimal target dose 25 Gy) has been suggested in the past [82], with consecutive dose reductions in recent years to 24 Gy, but as low as 2 × 2 Gy especially in elderly patients [83]. Response rates are high and approach 100% in most series and relapses in the radiation field are uncommon. The 5-year failure-free survival, however, ranges between 60% for ocular adnexal MALT lymphoma to 100% for thyroid MALT lymphoma [67].

In a recent series published by Teckie and coworkers, 487 patients with stage I MALT lymphomas were retrospectively analysed [84]. In line with the pattern of occurrence, the majority of patients had gastric MALT lymphoma (32%), followed by OAML and pulmonary MALT lymphoma (14% and 12%). However, a relatively high number of patients with cutaneous marginal zone lymphoma (13%) were included in the series. Overall, the median survival was excellent at 15 years, with a median follow-up time for survivors of 5 years. Five-year relapse free survival was 60% in this series, and gastric MALT lymphomas had a better outcome than non-gastric MALT lymphomas with the exception of thyroid MALT lymphomas. These findings are in line with results published by Wöhrer et al. [4], who found a 40% relapse rate at a median time of 60 months in a retrospective analysis of extragastric MALT lymphomas, which nevertheless was irrespective of therapy (i.e. local therapy vs. systemic treatment).

While local control with radiotherapy is excellent, systemic relapses are common and toxicities also have to be taken into account when analysing the (mostly retrospective) data. Especially for OAML, retrospective series from Asia have shown comparable efficacy, but lower toxicities for systemic therapies over radiation in localised OAML. However, these results were obtained with cumulative doses of 30 Gy and more, which would be considered too high according to modern standards [11]. Site-specific side effects may include cataract and local conjunctival irritation in OAML, nausea and inappetence in gastric MALT lymphoma or xerostomia for salivary gland lymphomas.

7.4.3 Systemic Therapies

When reviewing systemic therapy options for MALT lymphoma, one of the main problems is the fact that data had been restricted to advanced and disseminated disease in the last decades. In addition, the distinctive nature of MALT lymphoma as opposed to other types of indolent lymphomas or even when compared to nodal and splenic marginal zone lymphoma has not been given due consideration until recently. In view of this, patients with MALT lymphoma have been included in clinical trials for indolent lymphomas e.g. with rituximab/bendamustine or ibrutinib without the possibility of extracting information for this specific, and in most cases small cohort of patients. For the sake of this chapter, only studies on "pure" MALT lymphoma cohorts will briefly be summarized (for an overview see Table 7.3), and include mostly phase II trials or retrospective series, but also two phase III trials [72, 85–94]. One of the phase III studies, which assessed chlorambucil given after HP eradication versus no therapy has already been discussed [72], and will not be covered in this section.

The first report on systemic therapy of MALT lymphoma from 1995 included oral application of low-dose chlorambucil and cyclophosphamide [85] given for a median duration of 12 months, which resulted in CR rate of 75%.

Initial data were all obtained with classical chemotherapy, and mostly included patients with relapsing disease after local therapies or *de novo* disseminated and symptomatic disease, which might have biased results [95]. Another note of caution for older trials is the fact, that in patients with gastric MALT lymphoma, some older trials in favour of chemotherapy [96] were comparing surgery versus radiotherapy versus chemotherapy, but did not perform HP eradication, which is nowadays the standard of care. In the said study including 241 patients with stage I gastric MALT lymphoma (80 patients per arm), a significant advantage for three cycles of CHOP followed by three courses of CVP chemotherapy was found in terms of 10-year event-free survival (87% for chemotherapy versus 52% for both surgery and radiation alone, respectively); no advantage was seen for 10-year overall survival and a large majority of patients might in fact have been overtreated according to current guidelines and standards [52, 54].

In addition to alkylating agents, also bendamustine, purine analogues cladribine and fludarabine, anthracyclines and various combinations thereof have been published, which were later complemented by trials on rituximab alone or in combination, proteasome inhibitors, everolimus, ImiDs and immunomodulators such as clarithromycin. Taken together, relevant responses (sometimes up to 100%) were seen in all studies, but some therapies and combinations were associated with high toxicities that are not suitable for a sometimes asymptomatic and indolent disease, exemplified by the data obtained with R-CHOP, where a rate of neutropenia grade 3/4 in 31% of patients along with a relatively high rate of early relapses was found [11, 95].

7.4.4 Alkylating Agents and Combinations

Since the first report on its activity by Hammel and co-workers in 1995 [85] demonstrating relevant responses in a series of 24 patients (17 stage I, 7 stage IV), the oral alkylator chlorambucil has probably been the most studied agent in patients with MALT lymphoma. Characterized by a convenient oral mode of application and a mild toxicity profile, chlorambucil has widely been used especially in France and Italy, with various schedules and combinations having been studied. As monotherapy, response rates between 78% and 100% were reported, with the CR rate ranging between 55% and 100% [95]. Especially in orbital MALT lymphoma, a small series showed promising activity with 78% CR and 21% PR, with a low relapse rate [97]. Interestingly, the activity of chlorambucil was found to be independent of t(11;18)(q21;q21) status [87]. Pilot series combining chlorambucil with the anti-CD20 antibody rituximab found an increased activity of monotherapy [98, 99], with a small controlled study in gastric MALT lymphoma

Table 7.3 Chemotherapy trial for MALT lymphoma

Author	Study type	*N*	Stage	Site %	Treatment	ORR, %	CR, %
Hammel 1995 [85]	Retrospective	24	I, IVE	Gastric	Cyclophosphamide or chlorambucil continuously for 12–24 mo	100	75
Jäger 2002 [91]	Phase II	26	I, IVE	73 gastric, 27 non gastric	Cladribine (0.12 mg/kg d 1–5 every 4 w × 6)	100	84
Zinzani 2004 [93]	Phase II	31	IE	Non gastric	CVP or FM (cyclophosphamide 400 mg/m^2 d1–5, vincristine 1.4 mg/m^2 d1, and prednisone every 3 w × 6, or fludarabine 25 mg/m^2 d1–3 and mitoxantrone 10 mg/m^2 d1)	100	100
Raderer 2006 [90]	Retrospective	26	I-IVE	27 gastric, 73 non gastric	R-CNOP/R-CHOP (R 375 g/m^2 d1; cyclophosphamide 750 mg/m^2 d2, doxorubicin 50 mg/m^2 d2 or mitoxantrone 8 mg/m^2 d2, vincristine 1.4 mg/m^2, prednisone d1–5 every 3 w × 6–8)	100	77
Hancock 2009 [72]	Randomized	110	I, IIE	Gastric	Chlorambucil (6 mg/m^2 daily d1–14 in a 4-w cycle × 6) vs. observation after HP eradication	5 years relapse 21 vs. 11 ($p = 0.15$)	
Lévy 2013 [87]	Retrospective	49	I-IVE	Gastric	R monotherapy vs. R-chlorambucil (R 375 mg/m^2 d1, 8, 15, and 22, then every 4 w; chlorambucil 6 mg/m^2 d1–42 followed by d1–14 in a 4-w cycle for 4 mo)	81 vs. 93	/
Kiesewetter 2013 [89]	Retrospective	14	I-IVE	Non gastric	R-bendamustine (R 375 mg/m^2 d1; bendamustine 90 mg/m^2 d1–2 in a 3-w cycle × 6)	92	71
Troch 2013 [92]	Phase II	40	I-IVE	53 gastric, 48 non gastric	R-cladribine sc (R 375 mg/m^2 d1; cladribine 0.1 mg/kg d1–4 every 3 w × 6)	81	58
Salar 2009 [94]	Phase II	22	I-IVE	55 gastric, 46 non gastric	R-fludarabine (iv; R 375 mg/m^2 d1; fludarabine 25 mg/m^2 iv or 40 mg po d1–5 every 4 wk × 4–6)	100	90

(continued)

Table 7.3 (continued)

Author	Study type	*N*	Stage	Site %	Treatment	ORR, %	CR, %
Zucca 2017 [5]	Randomized	454	I-IVE		Chlorambucil vs. rituximab alone vs. chlorambucil (chlorambucil 6 mg/m^2 d1–42 in a 4-w cycle × 4 followed by d1–14 in a 4-w cycle × 4; R 375 mg/m^2 d1, 8, 15, and 22, then every 4 w in absence of progression)	85 vs. 78 vs. 95	63 vs. 56 vs. 79
Salar 2017 [102]	Phase II	60	I-IVE	33 gastric, 66 non gastric	R-bendamustine (R 375 mg/m^2 d1; bendamustine 90 mg/m2 d1–2 in a 3-w cycle × 4–6)	100	75
Herold 2017 [121]	Phase III	61	III-IVE	/	Rituximab-chemo vs. Obinutuzumab-chemo	78 vs. 82 (for all MZL not only MALT)	18 vs. 16 (for all MZL not only MALT)

ORR overall response rate, *CR* complete response, *MZL* marginal zone lymphoma, *MALT* mucosa-associated lymphoid tissue, *d* day, *po* oral administration, *mo* months, *w* week, *iv* intravenous, *sc* subcutaneous

showing an increase of ORR from 81% to 93% when compared to R-monotherapy [100].

In view of these promising results, chlorambucil was also the backbone for the two randomized studies performed by the International Extranodal Lymphoma Study Group on MALT Lymphoma. The first one (IELSG3/LY03), already mentioned before [72], showed that there is no benefit for the addition of single agent chlorambucil to anti-HP treatment in localized gastric MALT lymphomas. The second one (IELSG19) is the largest randomized study of front-line treatment ever conducted in MALT lymphoma [5, 86].

7.4.5 The IELSG19 Phase III Trial

This randomized multicenter trial [86] was originally designed to compare monotherapy with oral chlorambucil versus a combination of rituximab plus chlorambucil and initially included a total of 231 patients [86]. Later, it was amended with the addition of a rituximab monotherapy arm, bringing the total of patients included to 454 in order to allow further comparison of activity between rituximab and chlorambucil monotherapy.Eligible patients were initially randomly assigned (1:1 ratio) to receive either chlorambucil monotherapy (6 mg/m2/d orally on weeks 1 to 6, 9 to 10, 13 to 14, 17 to 18, and 21 to 22) or a combination of chlorambucil (same schedule as above) and rituximab (375 mg/m2 intravenously on day 1 of weeks 1, 2, 3, 4, 9, 13, 17, and 21) [86]. After the planned enrollment of 252 patients, the protocol was amended to continue with a three-arm design (1:1:6 ratio), with a new arm that included rituximab alone (same schedule as the combination arm) with a final sample size of 454 patients [5]. The main endpoint was event-free survival (EFS). At a median follow-up of 7.4 years, patients in the combination arm had significantly better EFS (hazard ratio, 0.54; 95% CI, 0.38 to 0.77). EFS at 5 years was 51% (95% CI, 42 to 60) with chlorambucil alone, 50% (95% CI, 42 to 59) with rituximab alone, and 68% (95% CI, 60 to 76) with the combination [5]. Complete response rate (CRR) and PFS were also significantly better with the combination. However, these improvements in CRR, EFS and PFS did not translate into longer overall survival (OS). In fact, 5-year OS was approximately 90% in each arm. All treatments were well tolerated, no unexpected toxicities were recorded and the rituximab chlorambucil combination is considered standard in many institutions, though there might be combinations with higher response rates seen in phase-II studies.

7.4.6 Bendamustine

While the exact nature of action of bendamustine is still unclear, it is thought to act as an aklyaltor to a certain extent. With the revival of bendamustine and proof of its efficacy in various B-cell lymphomas including follicular and mantle cell lymphoma, the combination of rituximab plus bendamustine (R-Benda) has become standard treatment particularly for elderly patients following publication of a randomized phase III trial of R-CHOP versus R-Benda [101]. In this trial, 37 patients with marginal zone lymphoma were treated in the R-Benda arm and 30 in the R-CHOP arm, with no difference for PFS for the subgroup of marginal zone lymphoma (57.2 vs. 47.2 months, $p = 0.32$). Nevertheless, extrapolation of the results to MALT lymphoma is hampered by the absence of information on specific marginal zone lymphoma subtypes.

Initial data in a small heterogeneous series have shown high activity of R-Benda (CR = 71%, PR = 21%) in pre-treated patients with MALT lymphomas of various sites of origin [89]. The most solid data so far, however, have been published by the Spanish GELTAMO group, who included 60 patients with treatment-naïve MALT lymphoma in a study of rituximab 375 mg/m^2 i.v. day 1 and bendamustine 90 mg/m^2 days 1 + 2 [82]. This trial was designed to take into account the results of interim staging; patients achieving a CR after three courses received only four cycles, while other patients had a total of six cycles. The initial response rate was high at 100% with no relapses after a median follow-up of 14 months. More recently, a publication with a median follow-up of 82 months showed no significant difference for gastric vs. extragastric MALT lymphomas, and reported an EFS of 87% after 7 years, with 5 relapses occurring in this study [102].

7.5 Nucleoside Analogues

While the nucleoside analogues fludarabine and—to a lesser extent—cladribine have been widely used in indolent lymphomas in the past, their role is currently decreasing due to potential side effects and the advent of novel agents. In MALT lymphoma, however, both agents have been tested in the past, and have shown excellent results [91–95].

An initial report of cladribine monotherapy given at a dose of 0.12 mg/kg i.v. over 2 h days 1–4 for 6 cycles has shown a high response rate, especially in the cohort of gastric MALT lymphomas [91] with a CR rate of 84%, which was significantly higher in the cohort of patients with gastric lymphoma (100%) as compared to 43% in non-gastric MALT lymphoma. A follow-up report with a median observation time of 7 years has shown no relapses in the gastric cohort, and an overall relapse rate of 27%. The combination of cladribine, albeit at a lower dose of 0.1 mg/kg given s.c. on days 1–4 combined with rituximab has resulted in ORR of 81% (CR 58%), but also gave a relatively high rate of neutropenia in 30% of patients [86]. Similarly, application of the purine analogue fludarabine either as monotherapy or in various combinations [93, 94] has shown an overall response rate approaching 100%, with a CR rate of 90%, but again haematotoxicity was substantial.

7.6 Immunotherapy and Immunomodulatory Agents

Rituximab and other anti-CD20 antibodies, as well as other small molecules and immunomodulatory agents have also been tested in MALT lymphomas, and an overview of the main studies is given in Table 7.4.

Table 7.4 Immunotherapy trial for MALT lymphoma

Author	Study type	*N*	Stage	Site, %	Treatment	ORR	CR
Conconi 2003 [103]	Phase II	35	I-IVE	43 gastric, 57 non gastric	Rituximab 375 mg/m^2 iv w × 4	73	44
Martinelli 2005 [104]	Phase II	27	I-IVE	Gastric	Rituximab 375 mg/m^2 iv w × 4	77	46
Lossos 2007 [105]	Phase II	12	I-IVE	25 gastric, 75 non gastric	Rituximab 375 mg/m^2 iv w × 4	67	17
Valencak 2009 [122]	Restros-pective	5	/	Skin	Rituximab 375 mg/m^2 iv w × 4	100	80
Troch 2009 [107]	Phase II	16	I-IVE	25 gastric, 75 non gastric	Bortezomib 1.5 mg/m^2 iv d1, 4, 8, and 11 every 3 w × 8	80	43
Troch 2009 [108]	Phase II	8	I-IIE	63 gastric, 37 non gastric	Thalidomide 100–400 mg/d po, escalated	0	
Conconi 2011 [106]	Phae II	32	I-IVE	44 gastric, 56 non gastric	Bortezomib 1.3 mg/m^2 iv d1, 4, 8, and 11 every 3 w × 6	48	31
Kiesewetter 2013 [109]	Phase II	18	I-IVE	28 gastric, 72 non gastric	Lenalidomide 25 mg po d1–21 in a 4-w cycle × 6	61	33
Kiesewetter 2015 [123]	Phase II	46	I-IVE	28 gastric, 72 non gastric	Rituximab + Lenalidomide (R 375 mg/m^2 day 1 and lenalidomide 20 mg d 1–21 in a 4-w cycle × 6–8)	80	54
Kiesewetter 2018 [124]	Phase II	16	I-IVE	31 gastric, 69 non gastric	Ofatumumab (1000 mg iv weekly × 4 followed by 4 doses at 2-mo intervals	81	50
Marangon 2019 [125]	Phase II	17	I-IVE	/	Rituximab d 1 and 8, 90Y-ibritumomab tiuxetan d 8	94	62
Thieblemont 2019 [126]	Phase III	30	I-IVE	/	Rituximab + Lenalidomide (R 375 mg/m^2 d1 and lenalidomide 20 mg d1–21 in a 4w- cycle × 12) vs. rituximab + placebo	65 vs. 44 (for all MZL not only MALT)	/
Dreyling 2017 [127]	Phase II	23	I-IVE	/	Copanlisib (60 mg iv on d 1, 8, and 15, 4 w cycle until disease progression)	70 (for all MZL not only MALT)	/
Zinzani 2019 [128]	Phase II	23	I-IVE	/	Umbralisib 800 mg po d until progression	55 (for all MZL not only MALT)	6 (for all MZL not only MALT)
Noy 2017 [129]	Phase II	32	I-IVE	/	Ibrutinib 560 mg po d until progression	50	3 (for all MZL not only MALT)

ORR overall response rate, *CR* complete response, *MZL* marginal zone lymphoma, *MALT* mucosa-associated lymphoid tissue, *d* day, *po* oral administration, *mo* months, *w* week, *iv* intravenous, *sc* subcutaneous

7.6.1 Rituximab

The anti-CD20 antibody rituximab is the prototype of immunotherapy, which has been incorporated into treatment of virtually all B-cell lymphomas, resulting in improvement of activity over chemotherapy alone. However, in MALT lymphoma, the value of rituximab has not been unequivocally proven as a mandatory addition to therapy. Initial data of single agent rituximab in several small studies have documented responses in 65–75%, but the CR rate was only between 15–45% [97–99, 103–105]. Until recently, only a retrospective SEER-medicare analysis including 347 localized gastric MALT lymphomas treated between 1997–2007 had reported a benefit for treatment with rituximab in terms of survival ($p = 0.017$), and no benefit of combined chemo-immunotherapy was found after adjusting for confounding factors [6]. The median overall survival, however, was short at only 6.7 years, and the analysis included only patients treated with either cyclophosphamide-containing regimens (CVP, CHOP) or fludarabine. Contrary to this, an improvement in terms of response rate and PFS, but not OS was seen in the randomized IELSG19 study for combining rituximab with chlorambucil when compared to either rituximab- or chlorambucil-monotherapy. For a more detailed discussion, see the previous paragraph describing the IELSG19 study. Overall, rituximab has shown good palliative effects and might be an option for relatively asymptomatic or frail patients when monotherapy is considered.

7.6.2 IMiDs

Due to the close pathogenetic relationship of MALT lymphoma to multiple myeloma, approaches used for therapy of myeloma have also been applied to patients with MALT lymphoma. One of the first agents tested was the proteasome inhibitor bortezomib which was evaluated in two relatively small studies at different doses, i.e. 1.3 mg/m^2 [106] and 1.5 mg/m^2 [107] given intravenously on days 1, 4, 8 and 11. Both schedules showed good response rates, with the higher dose giving a particularly high rate of response (81% vs. 48%), but the schedule was associated with an unacceptably high rate of neuropathy that was seen in 65% of patients, with more than 90% requiring dose reductions in this trial [107].

More recently, also IMiDs have been tested in patients with MALT lymphoma. While an initial small pilot study with thalidomide was prematurely terminated [108], the second generation lenalidomide was used either as monotherapy [109] or in combination with rituximab [110]. Not surprisingly, the response rate with the combination was higher with ORR being 80% (54% CR) than that documented in the monotherapy pilot series (ORR 61%, CR 33%). Toxicities were mild and consisted mostly of non-hematological side effects including cutaneous complaints (exanthema, itching). Evaluation of prognostic parameters, however, did not indicate the involvement of a cereblon-mediated expression of MUM-1 in responses [111].

7.6.2.1 Clarithromycin

The macrolide antibiotic has widely been used as a part of HP eradication regimens, but is being used less frequently due to high rates of resistance in certain areas. Clarithromycin, however, also displays pleiotropic immunomodulatory effects when given for a prolonged time, which are explained by inhibition of VEGF and TNF-alpha, enhancement of natural killer cells and CD8-cytotoxic T-cells, but also by interaction with cytokines such as IL-6 and inhibition of NF-kB. An ORR of 38% has been reported in a small pilot study including patients with relapsed or refractory MALT lymphoma [112]. In order to assess the direct antineoplastic activity of clarithromycin, a multi-centre trial was performed to include only patients with refractory disease and no evidence of active HP or CP infection [113]. The dose in this study was higher, with clarithromycin being given at a dose of 2 g/day in an intermittent schedule. A total of 23 patients in first or greater relapse were included, and the response rate was 52% (95% confidence interval 32–72%) with a promising 2-year PFS of 56 ± 10%. However, in an analysis of 55 consecutive patients [79], no advantage was found for the high-dose regimen (ORR 57%, 3-year PFS 42%) over a continuous intake of 2 × 500 mg over 6 months (ORR 47%, 3-year PFS 60%); the overall response rate as well as the 3-year PFS in this analysis were excellent in view of the fact that the median number of prior therapies was 2 (range; 1–7).

Interestingly, the effect of oral azithromycin, a related macrolide with favourable half-life and higher in vitro activity when compared to clarithromycin, was less pronounced, and a pilot series was terminated early due to the low efficacy of 25% ORR in 16 patients [114].

7.6.3 Radio-Immunotherapy (90-Y-Ibritumomab-Tiuxetan)

MALT lymphoma is a highly radiosensitive disease, and even low doses of radiation have been shown to result in excellent outcome (see above). Radiolabelling a CD20-ligand with 90Yttrium for radio-immunotherapy (RIT) is therefore an attractive concept in indolent B-cell malignancies including MALT lymphoma. Furthermore, MALT lymphoma is characterized by virtually absent bone marrow involvement, which is one of the contraindications against RIT. Data on the use of 90Y-ibritumomab-tiuxetan in MALT lymphoma are currently limited but results are nevertheless promising. Initial pilot series included small cohorts of mixed origin pre-treated MALT lymphomas [115], while a study of 12 patients with untreated OAML showed promising response rates (ten CR, two PR within 3 months of therapy) with low toxicities [116]. The largest series so far has included 30 heavily pre-treated patients with up to seven lines of prior therapy suffering from relapsed MALT lymphomas of various sites, who were given an activity of 0.4 mCi/kg [117]. A high ORR of 90% with a CRR of 77% after a single application of RIT was documented, and the median time to relapse was not reached at a median follow-up of 5.3 years. Toxicities were manageable and included thrombocytopenia as the major haematological toxicity, suggesting 90Y-ibritumomab tiuxetan as an active therapeutic option for patients with relapsed/refractory MALT lymphoma.

7.7 Conclusion

MALT lymphoma is a relatively common indolent B-cell lymphoma. It is a distinct clinicopathological entity, which displays unique features in terms of pathogenesis and treatment. In particular, the close association of MALT lymphoma with chronic antigenic stimulation distinguishes the disease from most other B-cell lymphomas. This has helped in understanding the underlying molecular events, and has led to a completely novel therapeutic approach, especially in gastric MALT lymphoma. The close association of gastric MALT lymphoma with HP-infection has resulted in the establishment of antibiotic therapy as first-line treatment irrespective of stage. To a lesser extent, antibiotic treatment with doxycycline or clarithromycin has also been accepted as first-line therapy for patients with ocular adnexal MALT lymphomas who are not in need of immediate response to treatment. Recently, there have been developments in the systemic treatment of MALT lymphoma with novel agents and chemo-free approaches, which have also been used in patients with localized disease. While retrospective analyses have suggested similar efficacy of systemic therapy with fewer local toxicities, particularly in OAML and in extragastric MALT lymphoma [10], no direct comparison between local and systemic therapy has yet been performed. In addition, the optimal regimen for MALT lymphoma has not been established despite many active combinations being reported in phase II studies as well as in one phase III trial. Differences in the pathogenesis, clinical presentation and genetic features of MALT lymphomas that arise in different locations further complicate data interpretation; MALT lymphomas are often included with other indolent lymphomas, or mixed together irrespective of their localisation and prior therapies. Further studies on MALT lymphomas should therefore consider their different localisations and their respectively unique features.

Acknowledgements The authors would like to thank Afua Adjeiwaa Mensah for her critical manuscript review. *Support:* Supported in part by a grant from Oncosuisse (ICP OCS-02062-03-2007).

References

1. Cook JR, Isaacson PG, Chott A, et al. Extranodal marginal zone B-cell lymphoma of mucosa-associated lymphoid tissue (MALT lymphoma). In: Swerdlow SH, Campo E, Harris NL, et al., editors. WHO classification of tumours of haematopoietic and lymphoid tissues (revised 4th edn). Lyon: IARC; 2017. p. 259–62.
2. Isaacson PG, Chott A, Nakamura S, et al. Extranodal marginal zone B-cell lymphoma of mucosa-associated lymphoid tissue (MALT lymphoma). In: Swerdlow S, Campo E, Harris NL, et al., editors. WHO classification of tumours of haematopoietic and lymphoid tissues. Lyon: IARC; 2008. p. 214–7.
3. Raderer M, Wohrer S, Kiesewetter B, et al. Antibiotic treatment as sole management of helicobacter pylori-negative gastric MALT lymphoma: a single center experience with prolonged follow-up. Ann Hematol. 2015;94:969–73.
4. Wohrer S, Kiesewetter B, Fischbach J, et al. Retrospective comparison of the effectiveness of various treatment modalities of extragastric MALT lymphoma: a single-center analysis. Ann Hematol. 2014;93:1287–95.
5. Zucca E, Conconi A, Martinelli G, et al. Final results of the IELSG-19 randomized trial of mucosa-associated lymphoid tissue lymphoma: improved event-free and progression-free survival with rituximab plus Chlorambucil versus either Chlorambucil or rituximab monotherapy. J Clin Oncol. 2017;35:1905–12.
6. Olszewski AJ, Castillo JJ. Comparative outcomes of oncologic therapy in gastric extranodal marginal zone (MALT) lymphoma: analysis of the SEER-Medicare database. Ann Oncol. 2013;24:1352–9.
7. Du MQ. MALT lymphoma: genetic abnormalities, immunological stimulation and molecular mechanism. Best Pract Res Clin Haematol. 2017;30:13–23.
8. Kwee I, Rancoita PM, Rinaldi A, et al. Genomic profiles of MALT lymphomas: variability across anatomical sites. Haematologica. 2011;96:1064–6.
9. Isaacson PG. Gastric MALT lymphoma: from concept to cure. Ann Oncol. 1999;10:637–45.
10. Raderer M, Wohrer S, Streubel B, et al. Assessment of disease dissemination in gastric compared with extragastric mucosa-associated lymphoid tissue lymphoma using extensive staging: a single-center experience. J Clin Oncol. 2006;24:3136–41.
11. Raderer M, Kiesewetter B, Ferreri AJ. Clinicopathologic characteristics and treatment of marginal zone lymphoma of mucosa-associated lymphoid tissue (MALT lymphoma). CA Cancer J Clin. 2016;66:153–71.
12. Conconi A, Franceschetti S, Aprile von Hohenstaufen K, et al. Histologic transformation in marginal zone lymphomasdagger. Ann Oncol. 2015;26:2329–35.
13. Kiesewetter B, Lamm W, Dolak W, et al. Transformed mucosa-associated lymphoid tissue lymphomas: a single institution retrospective study including polymerase chain reaction-based clonality analysis. Br J Haematol. 2019;186:448–59.
14. Ferreri AJ, Govi S, Raderer M, et al. *Helicobacter pylori* eradication as exclusive treatment for limited-stage gastric diffuse large B-cell lymphoma: results of a multicenter phase 2 trial. Blood. 2012;120:3858–60.
15. Kuo SH, Yeh KH, Wu MS, et al. *Helicobacter pylori* eradication therapy is effective in the treatment of early-stage H pylori-positive gastric diffuse large B-cell lymphomas. Blood. 2012;119:4838–44. quiz 5057
16. Rinaldi A, Mian M, Chigrinova E, et al. Genome-wide DNA profiling of marginal zone lymphomas identifies subtype-specific lesions with an impact on the clinical outcome. Blood. 2011;117:1595–604.
17. Ye H, Liu H, Attygalle A, et al. Variable frequencies of t(11;18)(q21;q21) in MALT lymphomas of different sites: significant association with CagA strains of H pylori in gastric MALT lymphoma. Blood. 2003;102:1012–8.
18. Liu H, Ye H, Dogan A, et al. T(11;18)(q21;q21) is associated with advanced mucosa-associated lymphoid tissue lymphoma that expresses nuclear BCL10. Blood. 2001;98:1182–7.
19. Liu H, Ruskon-Fourmestraux A, Lavergne-Slove A, et al. Resistance of t(11;18) positive gastric mucosa-associated lymphoid tissue lymphoma to *Helicobacter pylori* eradication therapy. Lancet. 2001;357:39–40.
20. Wotherspoon AC, Finn TM, Isaacson PG. Trisomy 3 in low-grade B-cell lymphomas of mucosa-associated lymphoid tissue. Blood. 1995;85:2000–4.
21. Dierlamm J, Pittaluga S, Wlodarska I, et al. Marginal zone B-cell lymphomas of different sites share similar cytogenetic and morphologic features. Blood. 1996;87:299–307.
22. Wotherspoon AC, Soosay GN, Diss TC, Isaacson PG. Low-grade primary B-cell lymphoma of the lung. An immunohistochemical, molecular, and cytogenetic study of a single case. Am J Clin Pathol. 1990;94:655–60.
23. Brandtzaeg P, Farstad IN, Haraldsen G. Regional specialization in the mucosal immune system: primed cells do not always home along the same track. Immunol Today. 1999;20:267–77.
24. Troch M, Formanek M, Streubel B, et al. Clinicopathological aspects of mucosa-associated lymphoid tissue (MALT) lymphoma of the parotid gland: a retrospective single-center analysis of 28 cases. Head Neck. 2011;33:763–7.
25. Kiesewetter B, Lukas J, Kuchar A, et al. Clinical features, treatment and outcome of mucosa-associated lymphoid tissue (MALT) lymphoma of the ocular

adnexa: single center experience of 60 patients. PLoS One. 2014;9:e104004.
26. Dogan A, Du M, Koulis A, et al. Expression of lymphocyte homing receptors and vascular addressins in low-grade gastric B-cell lymphomas of mucosa-associated lymphoid tissue. Am J Pathol. 1997;151:1361–9.
27. Du MQ, Xu CF, Diss TC, et al. Intestinal dissemination of gastric mucosa-associated lymphoid tissue lymphoma. Blood. 1996;88:4445–51.
28. Berlin C, Berg EL, Briskin MJ, et al. Alpha 4 beta 7 integrin mediates lymphocyte binding to the mucosal vascular addressin MAdCAM-1. Cell. 1993;74:185–95.
29. Deutsch AJ, Steinbauer E, Hofmann NA, et al. Chemokine receptors in gastric MALT lymphoma: loss of CXCR4 and upregulation of CXCR7 is associated with progression to diffuse large B-cell lymphoma. Mod Pathol. 2013;26:182–94.
30. Stollberg S, Kammerer D, Neubauer E, et al. Differential somatostatin and CXCR4 chemokine receptor expression in MALT-type lymphoma of gastric and extragastric origin. J Cancer Res Clin Oncol. 2016;142:2239–47.
31. Haug AR, Leisser A, Wadsak W, et al. Prospective non-invasive evaluation of CXCR4 expression for the diagnosis of MALT lymphoma using [(68)Ga]Ga-Pentixafor-PET/MRI. Theranostics. 2019;9:3653–8.
32. Parsonnet J, Hansen S, Rodriguez L, et al. *Helicobacter pylori* infection and gastric lymphoma. N Engl J Med. 1994;330:1267–71.
33. Wotherspoon AC, Ortiz-Hidalgo C, Falzon MR, Isaacson PG. Helicobacter pylori-associated gastritis and primary B-cell gastric lymphoma. Lancet. 1991;338:1175–6.
34. Schmausser B, Eck M, Greiner A, et al. Mucosal humoral immune response to CagA shows a high prevalence in patients with gastric MALT-type lymphoma. Virchows Arch. 2000;436:115–8.
35. Kuo SH, Yeh KH, Chen LT, et al. *Helicobacter pylori* CagA translocation is closely associated with the expression of CagA-signaling molecules in low-grade gastric mucosa-associated lymphoid tissue lymphoma. Am J Surg Pathol. 2015;39:761–6.
36. Hussell T, Isaacson PG, Crabtree JE, Spencer J. The response of cells from low-grade B-cell gastric lymphomas of mucosa-associated lymphoid tissue to helicobacter pylori. Lancet. 1993;342:571–4.
37. Choi YJ, Kim N, Paik JH, et al. Characteristics of helicobacter pylori-positive and helicobacter pylori-negative gastric mucosa-associated lymphoid tissue lymphoma and their influence on clinical outcome. Helicobacter. 2013;18:197–205.
38. Zullo A, Hassan C, Ridola L, et al. Eradication therapy in helicobacter pylori-negative, gastric low-grade mucosa-associated lymphoid tissue lymphoma patients: a systematic review. J Clin Gastroenterol. 2013;47:824–7.
39. Sena Teixeira Mendes L, Attygalle AD, Wotherspoon AC. *Helicobacter pylori* infection in gastric extranodal marginal zone lymphoma of mucosa-associated lymphoid tissue (MALT) lymphoma: a re-evaluation. Gut. 2014;63:1526–7.
40. Luminari S, Cesaretti M, Marcheselli L, et al. Decreasing incidence of gastric MALT lymphomas in the era of anti-*Helicobacter pylori* interventions: results from a population-based study on extranodal marginal zone lymphomas. Ann Oncol. 2010;21:855–9.
41. Morgner A, Lehn N, Andersen LP, et al. Helicobacter heilmannii-associated primary gastric low-grade MALT lymphoma: complete remission after curing the infection. Gastroenterology. 2000;118:821–8.
42. Mesnard B, De Vroey B, Maunoury V, Lecuit M. Immunoproliferative small intestinal disease associated with campylobacter jejuni. Dig Liver Dis. 2012;44:799–800.
43. Foster LH, Portell CA. The role of infectious agents, antibiotics, and antiviral therapy in the treatment of extranodal marginal zone lymphoma and other low-grade lymphomas. Curr Treat Options in Oncol. 2015;16:28.
44. Ferreri AJ, Dolcetti R, Dognini GP, et al. *Chlamydophila psittaci* is viable and infectious in the conjunctiva and peripheral blood of patients with ocular adnexal lymphoma: results of a single-center prospective case-control study. Int J Cancer. 2008;123:1089–93.
45. Decaudin D, Dolcetti R, de Cremoux P, et al. Variable association between *Chlamydophila psittaci* infection and ocular adnexal lymphomas: methodological biases or true geographical variations? Anti-Cancer Drugs. 2008;19:761–5.
46. Ekstrom Smedby K, Vajdic CM, Falster M, et al. Autoimmune disorders and risk of non-Hodgkin lymphoma subtypes: a pooled analysis within the InterLymph consortium. Blood. 2008;111:4029–38.
47. Bracci PM, Benavente Y, Turner JJ, et al. Medical history, lifestyle, family history, and occupational risk factors for marginal zone lymphoma: the InterLymph non-Hodgkin lymphoma subtypes project. J Natl Cancer Inst Monogr. 2014;2014:52–65.
48. Wohrer S, Troch M, Streubel B, et al. MALT lymphoma in patients with autoimmune diseases: a comparative analysis of characteristics and clinical course. Leukemia. 2007;21:1812–8.
49. Troch M, Woehrer S, Streubel B, et al. Chronic autoimmune thyroiditis (Hashimoto's thyroiditis) in patients with MALT lymphoma. Ann Oncol. 2008;19:1336–9.
50. Berger F, Felman P, Sonet A, et al. Nonfollicular small B-cell lymphomas: a heterogeneous group of patients with distinct clinical features and outcome. Blood. 1994;83:2829–35.
51. Ferreri AJ, Dolcetti R, Du MQ, et al. Ocular adnexal MALT lymphoma: an intriguing model for antigen-driven lymphomagenesis and microbial-targeted therapy. Ann Oncol. 2008;19:835–46.

52. Zucca E, Copie-Bergman C, Ricardi U, et al. Gastric marginal zone lymphoma of MALT type: ESMO clinical practice guidelines for diagnosis, treatment and follow-up. Ann Oncol. 2013;24(Suppl 6):vi144–8.
53. Zucca E, Conconi A, Pedrinis E, et al. Nongastric marginal zone B-cell lymphoma of mucosa-associated lymphoid tissue. Blood. 2003;101:2489–95.
54. Ruskone-Fourmestraux A, Fischbach W, Aleman BM, et al. EGILS consensus report. Gastric extranodal marginal zone B-cell lymphoma of MALT. Gut. 2011;60:747–58.
55. Graham DY, Opekun AR, Hammoud F, et al. Studies regarding the mechanism of false negative urea breath tests with proton pump inhibitors. Am J Gastroenterol. 2003;98:1005–9.
56. Dickey W, Kenny BD, McConnell JB. Effect of proton pump inhibitors on the detection of *Helicobacter pylori* in gastric biopsies. Aliment Pharmacol Ther. 1996;10:289–93.
57. Borie R, Wislez M, Thabut G, et al. Clinical characteristics and prognostic factors of pulmonary MALT lymphoma. Eur Respir J. 2009;34:1408–16.
58. Rohatiner A, d'Amore F, Coiffier B, et al. Report on a workshop convened to discuss the pathological and staging classifications of gastrointestinal tract lymphoma. Ann Oncol. 1994;5:397–400.
59. Ruskone-Fourmestraux A, Dragosics B, Morgner A, et al. Paris staging system for primary gastrointestinal lymphomas. Gut. 2003;52:912–3.
60. Thieblemont C, Bastion Y, Berger F, et al. Mucosa-associated lymphoid tissue gastrointestinal and non-gastrointestinal lymphoma behavior: analysis of 108 patients. J Clin Oncol. 1997;15:1624–30.
61. Bailey EM, Ferry JA, Harris NL, et al. Marginal zone lymphoma (low-grade B-cell lymphoma of mucosa-associated lymphoid tissue type) of skin and subcutaneous tissue: a study of 15 patients. Am J Surg Pathol. 1996;20:1011–23.
62. Radaszkiewicz T, Dragosics B, Bauer P. Gastrointestinal malignant lymphomas of the mucosa-associated lymphoid tissue: factors relevant to prognosis. Gastroenterology. 1992;102:1628–38.
63. Eidt S, Stolte M, Fischer R. Factors influencing lymph node infiltration in primary gastric malignant lymphoma of the mucosa-associated lymphoid tissue. Pathol Res Pract. 1994;190:1077–81.
64. Tondini C, Giardini R, Bozzetti F, et al. Combined modality treatment for primary gastrointestinal non-Hodgkin's lymphoma: the Milan Cancer institute experience. Ann Oncol. 1993;4:831–7.
65. Thieblemont C, Cascione L, Conconi A, et al. A MALT lymphoma prognostic index. Blood. 2017;130:1409–17.
66. Conconi A, Thieblemont C, Cascione L, et al. Early progression of disease (POD24) predicts shorter survival in MALT lymphoma patients receiving systemic treatment. Hematol Oncol. 2019;37:179–80.
67. Tanimoto K, Kaneko A, Suzuki S, et al. Long-term follow-up results of no initial therapy for ocular adnexal MALT lymphoma. Ann Oncol. 2006;17:135–40.
68. Troch M, Streubel B, Petkov V, et al. Does MALT lymphoma of the lung require immediate treatment? An analysis of 11 untreated cases with long-term follow-up. Anticancer Res. 2007;27:3633–7.
69. Fischbach W, Goebeler ME, Ruskone-Fourmestraux A, et al. Most patients with minimal histological residuals of gastric MALT lymphoma after successful eradication of *Helicobacter pylori* can be managed safely by a watch and wait strategy: experience from a large international series. Gut. 2007;56:1685–7.
70. Malfertheiner P, Megraud F, O'Morain C, et al. Current concepts in the management of *Helicobacter pylori* infection: the Maastricht III consensus report. Gut. 2007;56:772–81.
71. Zullo A, Hassan C, Cristofari F, et al. Effects of *Helicobacter pylori* eradication on early stage gastric mucosa-associated lymphoid tissue lymphoma. Clin Gastroenterol Hepatol. 2010;8:105–10.
72. Hancock BW, Qian W, Linch D, et al. Chlorambucil versus observation after anti-helicobacter therapy in gastric MALT lymphomas: results of the international randomised LY03 trial. Br J Haematol. 2009;144:367–75.
73. Copie-Bergman C, Wotherspoon AC, Capella C, et al. Gela histological scoring system for post-treatment biopsies of patients with gastric MALT lymphoma is feasible and reliable in routine practice. Br J Haematol. 2013;160:47–52.
74. Raderer M, Streubel B, Wohrer S, et al. Successful antibiotic treatment of *Helicobacter pylori* negative gastric mucosa associated lymphoid tissue lymphomas. Gut. 2006;55:616–8.
75. Kiesewetter B, Raderer M. Antibiotic therapy in nongastrointestinal MALT lymphoma: a review of the literature. Blood. 2013;122:1350–7.
76. Ferreri AJ, Ponzoni M, Guidoboni M, et al. Regression of ocular adnexal lymphoma after chlamydia psittaci-eradicating antibiotic therapy. J Clin Oncol. 2005;23:5067–73.
77. Ferreri AJ, Ponzoni M, Guidoboni M, et al. Bacteria-eradicating therapy with doxycycline in ocular adnexal MALT lymphoma: a multicenter prospective trial. J Natl Cancer Inst. 2006;98:1375–82.
78. Ferreri AJ, Govi S, Pasini E, et al. *Chlamydophila psittaci* eradication with doxycycline as first-line targeted therapy for ocular adnexae lymphoma: final results of an international phase II trial. J Clin Oncol. 2012;30:2988–94.
79. Ferreri AJM, Cecchetti C, Kiesewetter B, et al. Clarithromycin as a "repurposing drug" against MALT lymphoma. Br J Haematol. 2018;182:913–5.
80. Arcaini L, Vallisa D, Rattotti S, et al. Antiviral treatment in patients with indolent B-cell lymphomas associated with HCV infection: a study of the Fondazione Italiana Linfomi. Ann Oncol. 2014;25:1404–10.

81. Gisbert JP, Garcia-Buey L, Pajares JM, Moreno-Otero R. Prevalence of hepatitis C virus infection in B-cell non-Hodgkin's lymphoma: systematic review and meta-analysis. Gastroenterology. 2003;125:1723–32.
82. Ejima Y, Sasaki R, Okamoto Y, et al. Ocular adnexal mucosa-associated lymphoid tissue lymphoma treated with radiotherapy. Radiother Oncol. 2006;78:6–9.
83. Hoskin PJ, Kirkwood AA, Popova B, et al. 4 Gy versus 24 Gy radiotherapy for patients with indolent lymphoma (FORT): a randomised phase 3 non-inferiority trial. Lancet Oncol. 2014;15:457–63.
84. Teckie S, Qi S, Chelius M, et al. Long-term outcome of 487 patients with early-stage extra-nodal marginal zone lymphoma. Ann Oncol. 2017;28:1064–9.
85. Hammel P, Haioun C, Chaumette MT, et al. Efficacy of single-agent chemotherapy in low-grade B-cell mucosa-associated lymphoid tissue lymphoma with prominent gastric expression. J Clin Oncol. 1995;13:2524–9.
86. Zucca E, Conconi A, Laszlo D, et al. Addition of rituximab to chlorambucil produces superior event-free survival in the treatment of patients with extranodal marginal-zone B-cell lymphoma: 5-year analysis of the IELSG-19 randomized study. J Clin Oncol. 2013;31:565–72.
87. Levy M, Copie-Bergman C, Amiot A, et al. Rituximab and chlorambucil versus rituximab alone in gastric mucosa-associated lymphoid tissue lymphoma according to t(11;18) status: a monocentric non-randomized observational study. Leuk Lymphoma. 2013;54:940–4.
88. Salar A, Domingo-Domenech E, Panizo C, et al. First-line response-adapted treatment with the combination of bendamustine and rituximab in patients with mucosa-associated lymphoid tissue lymphoma (MALT2008-01): a multicentre, single-arm, phase 2 trial. Lancet Haematol. 2014;1:e104–11.
89. Kiesewetter B, Mayerhoefer ME, Lukas J, et al. Rituximab plus bendamustine is active in pretreated patients with extragastric marginal zone B cell lymphoma of the mucosa-associated lymphoid tissue (MALT lymphoma). Ann Hematol. 2014;93:249–53.
90. Raderer M, Wohrer S, Streubel B, et al. Activity of rituximab plus cyclophosphamide, doxorubicin/mitoxantrone, vincristine and prednisone in patients with relapsed MALT lymphoma. Oncology. 2006;70:411–7.
91. Jager G, Neumeister P, Brezinschek R, et al. Treatment of extranodal marginal zone B-cell lymphoma of mucosa-associated lymphoid tissue type with cladribine: a phase II study. J Clin Oncol. 2002;20:3872–7.
92. Troch M, Kiesewetter B, Willenbacher W, et al. Rituximab plus subcutaneous cladribine in patients with extranodal marginal zone B-cell lymphoma of mucosa-associated lymphoid tissue: a phase II study by the Arbeitsgemeinschaft Medikamentose Tumortherapie. Haematologica. 2013;98:264–8.
93. Zinzani PL, Stefoni V, Musuraca G, et al. Fludarabine-containing chemotherapy as frontline treatment of nongastrointestinal mucosa-associated lymphoid tissue lymphoma. Cancer. 2004;100:2190–4.
94. Salar A, Domingo-Domenech E, Estany C, et al. Combination therapy with rituximab and intravenous or oral fludarabine in the first-line, systemic treatment of patients with extranodal marginal zone B-cell lymphoma of the mucosa-associated lymphoid tissue type. Cancer. 2009;115:5210–7.
95. Kiesewetter B, Ferreri AJ, Raderer M. Chemoimmunotherapy for mucosa-associated lymphoid tissue-type lymphoma: a review of the literature. Oncologist. 2015;20:915–25.
96. Aviles A, Nambo MJ, Neri N, et al. Mucosa-associated lymphoid tissue (MALT) lymphoma of the stomach: results of a controlled clinical trial. Med Oncol. 2005;22:57–62.
97. Ben Simon GJ, Cheung N, McKelvie P, et al. Oral chlorambucil for extranodal, marginal zone, B-cell lymphoma of mucosa-associated lymphoid tissue of the orbit. Ophthalmology. 2006;113:1209–13.
98. Rigacci L, Nassi L, Puccioni M, et al. Rituximab and chlorambucil as first-line treatment for low-grade ocular adnexal lymphomas. Ann Hematol. 2007;86:565–8.
99. Levy M, Copie-Bergman C, Molinier-Frenkel V, et al. Treatment of t(11;18)-positive gastric mucosa-associated lymphoid tissue lymphoma with rituximab and chlorambucil: clinical, histological, and molecular follow-up. Leuk Lymphoma. 2010;51:284–90.
100. Tan D, Horning SJ, Hoppe RT, et al. Improvements in observed and relative survival in follicular grade 1–2 lymphoma during 4 decades: the Stanford University experience. Blood. 2013;122:981–7.
101. Rummel MJ, Niederle N, Maschmeyer G, et al. Bendamustine plus rituximab versus CHOP plus rituximab as first-line treatment for patients with indolent and mantle-cell lymphomas: an open-label, multicentre, randomised, phase 3 non-inferiority trial. Lancet. 2013;381:1203–10.
102. Salar A, Domingo-Domenech E, Panizo C, et al. Long-term results of a phase 2 study of rituximab and bendamustine for mucosa-associated lymphoid tissue lymphoma. Blood. 2017;130:1772–4.
103. Conconi A, Martinelli G, Thieblemont C, et al. Clinical activity of rituximab in extranodal marginal zone B-cell lymphoma of MALT type. Blood. 2003;102:2741–5.
104. Martinelli G, Laszlo D, Ferreri AJ, et al. Clinical activity of rituximab in gastric marginal zone non-Hodgkin's lymphoma resistant to or not eligible for anti-*Helicobacter pylori* therapy. J Clin Oncol. 2005;23:1979–83.
105. Lossos IS, Morgensztern D, Blaya M, et al. Rituximab for treatment of chemoimmunotherapy naive marginal zone lymphoma. Leuk Lymphoma. 2007;48:1630–2.

106. Conconi A, Martinelli G, Lopez-Guillermo A, et al. Clinical activity of bortezomib in relapsed/refractory MALT lymphomas: results of a phase II study of the International Extranodal Lymphoma Study Group (IELSG). Ann Oncol. 2011;22:689–95.
107. Troch M, Jonak C, Mullauer L, et al. A phase II study of bortezomib in patients with MALT lymphoma. Haematologica. 2009;94:738–42.
108. Troch M, Zielinski C, Raderer M. Absence of efficacy of thalidomide monotherapy in patients with extranodal marginal zone B-cell lymphoma of the mucosa-associated lymphoid tissue (MALT lymphoma). Ann Oncol. 2009;20:1446–7.
109. Kiesewetter B, Troch M, Dolak W, et al. A phase II study of lenalidomide in patients with extranodal marginal zone B-cell lymphoma of the mucosa associated lymphoid tissue (MALT lymphoma). Haematologica. 2013;98:353–6.
110. Kiesewetter B, Willenbacher E, Willenbacher W, et al. A phase 2 study of rituximab plus lenalidomide for mucosa-associated lymphoid tissue lymphoma. Blood. 2017;129:383–5.
111. Kiesewetter B, Simonitsch-Klupp I, Kornauth C, et al. Immunohistochemical expression of cereblon and MUM1 as potential predictive markers of response to lenalidomide in extranodal marginal zone B-cell lymphoma of the mucosa-associated lymphoid tissue (MALT lymphoma). Hematol Oncol. 2018;36:62–7.
112. Govi S, Dognini GP, Licata G, et al. Six-month oral clarithromycin regimen is safe and active in extranodal marginal zone B-cell lymphomas: final results of a single-centre phase II trial. Br J Haematol. 2010;150:226–9.
113. Ferreri AJ, Sassone M, Kiesewetter B, et al. High-dose clarithromycin is an active monotherapy for patients with relapsed/refractory extranodal marginal zone lymphoma of mucosa-associated lymphoid tissue (MALT): the HD-K phase II trial. Ann Oncol. 2015;26:1760–5.
114. Lagler H, Kiesewetter B, Dolak W, et al. Treatment of mucosa associated lymphoid tissue lymphoma with a long-term once-weekly regimen of oral azithromycin: results from the phase II MALT-A trial. Hematol Oncol. 2019;37:22–6.
115. Hoffmann M, Troch M, Eidherr H, et al. 90Y-ibritumomab tiuxetan (Zevalin) in heavily pretreated patients with mucosa associated lymphoid tissue lymphoma. Leuk Lymphoma. 2011;52:42–5.
116. Esmaeli B, McLaughlin P, Pro B, et al. Prospective trial of targeted radioimmunotherapy with Y-90 ibritumomab tiuxetan (Zevalin) for front-line treatment of early-stage extranodal indolent ocular adnexal lymphoma. Ann Oncol. 2009;20:709–14.
117. Vanazzi A, Grana C, Crosta C, et al. Efficacy of (9)(0)yttrium-ibritumomab tiuxetan in relapsed/refractory extranodal marginal-zone lymphoma. Hematol Oncol. 2014;32:10–5.
118. Ferreri AJ, Dognini GP, Ponzoni M, et al. Chlamydia-psittaci-eradicating antibiotic therapy in patients with advanced-stage ocular adnexal MALT lymphoma. Ann Oncol. 2008;19:194–5.
119. Han JJ, Kim TM, Jeon YK, et al. Long-term outcomes of first-line treatment with doxycycline in patients with previously untreated ocular adnexal marginal zone B cell lymphoma. Ann Hematol. 2015;94:575–81.
120. Kim TM, Kim KH, Lee MJ, et al. First-line therapy with doxycycline in ocular adnexal mucosa-associated lymphoid tissue lymphoma: a retrospective analysis of clinical predictors. Cancer Sci. 2010;101:1199–203.
121. Herold M, Hoster E, Janssens A, et al. Immunochemotherapy with obinutuzumab or rituximab in a subset of patients in the randomised GALLIUM trial with previously untreated marginal zone lymphoma (MZL). Hematol Oncol. 2017;35:146–7.
122. Valencak J, Weihsengruber F, Rappersberger K, et al. Rituximab monotherapy for primary cutaneous B-cell lymphoma: response and follow-up in 16 patients. Ann Oncol. 2009;20:326–30.
123. Kiesewetter B, Greil R, Willenbacher W, et al. AGMT MALT-2: a phase II study of rituximab plus Lenalidomide in patients with Extranodal marginal zone B-cell lymphoma of the mucosa-associated lymphoid tissue (MALT lymphoma). Blood. 2015;126:3973.
124. Kiesewetter B, Neuper O, Mayerhoefer ME, et al. A pilot phase II study of ofatumumab monotherapy for extranodal marginal zone B-cell lymphoma of the mucosa-associated lymphoid tissue (MALT) lymphoma. Hematol Oncol. 2018;36:49–55.
125. Marangon M, Morigi A, Casadei B, et al. 90Y-Ibritumomab tiuxetan in patients with extrannodal marginal zone B-cell lymphoma of mucosa associated lymphoid tissue (MALT ymphoma) – the ZENO study. Hematol Oncol. 2019;37:263–4.
126. Thieblemont C, Leonard J, Trneny M, et al. Post hoc analyses of patients with relapsed/refractory marginal zone lymphoma who received lenalidomide plus rituximab (R2) vs rituximab/placebo (AUGMENT). Hematol Oncol. 2019;37:226–7.
127. Dreyling M, Santoro A, Mollica L, et al. Long-term efficacy and safety from the Copanlisib CHRONOS-1 study in patients with relapsed or refractory indolent B-cell lymphoma. Blood. 2018;132:1595.
128. Zinzani P, Samaniego F, Jurczak W, et al. Umbralisib monotherapy demonstrates efficacy and safety in patients with relapsed/refractory marginal zone lymphoma: a multicenter, open-label, registration directed phase 2 study. Hematol Oncol. 2019;37:182–3.
129. Noy A, de Vos S, Thieblemont C, et al. Targeting Bruton tyrosine kinase with ibrutinib in relapsed/refractory marginal zone lymphoma. Blood. 2017;129:2224–32.

8 Nodal Marginal Zone Lymphoma

Luca Arcaini and Andreas Viardot

Nodal marginal zone lymphoma (NMZL)

Clinical outline
Primarily nodal disease, as localized or generalized lymphadenopathy in adults, without evidence of relevant extranodal or splenic disease.

Cytology	Small to medium sized cells ranging in morphology from lymphocyte- and centrocyte-like to monocytoid. Features of plasmacytic differentiation may be observed. Variable content of blasts.	Nodal margina zone lymphoma, cytology	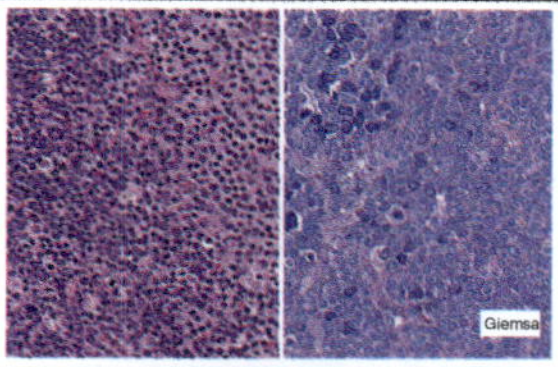
Histology	Expanded marginal zone around reactive germinal centers, which become progressively infiltrated by the neoplastic cells. Outwards growth to the paracortical zone may ultimately lead to a diffuse pattern	Nodal marginal zone lymphoma, hystology	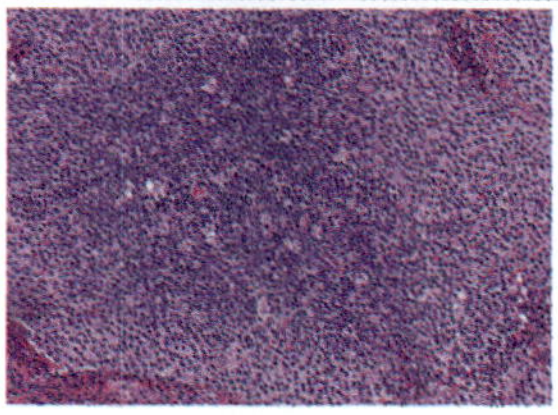

	CD20	CD5	CD23[1]	CD10	BCL6	cyclin D1	CD103	FMC7	IgM	light chains
notes	[1]partial/weak expression occacionally observed									
other marker	EMZL lacks a specific phenotype and the antibody panel primarily aims at exclusion of other lymphoma subtypes. IRTA1 and MNDA may be helpful marker but less frequently used or not widely available.									

■ = majority of cases positive ▒ = variable fraction of cases positive □ = negative

Main differential diagnosis	CLL (should be CD23 positive), MCL (sould be cyclin D1 positive). Subtypes of marginal zone lymphomas (extranodal, nodal, splenic, cutaneous) distinguished mainly by clinical presentation (pattern of involved organs). LPL (should be MYD88 mutated) needs to be excluded based on clinical findings (IgM gammopathy) and extent of bone marrow involvement (expected to be the predominant site of presentation in LPL).

M. Dreyling, M. Ladetto (eds.), *Indolent Lymphomas*, Hematologic Malignancies,
https://doi.org/10.1007/978-3-030-55989-2_8

Key molecular features		
Activation of Notch and nuclear factor kappa B pathways. IGH genes rearranged, somatic hypermutation and IGHV3 and IGHV4 usage bias. Frequent translocations: Non reported. Frequent copy number alterations: Gains of chromosome 3 and 8, loss of 6q23. Frequent mutations: *NOTCH2, MLL2/KMT2D, PTPRD, KLF2, TNFAIP3* rarer: *MYD88, CARD11*		
Precursor lesions		
Not reported. In contrast to ENMZL no association with inflammation reported.		
Progression		
May progress/transform to defuse large B-cell lymphoma. Definition of transformation currently purely morphologically by detection of sheets of blasts.		
Clinically relevant pathologic features	**Relevance**	**Evidence**
Mutations	prognostic: *KLF2* and *NOTCH2* mutations (unfavourable)	**C**
Proliferation/blasts	High proliferation and/or blast content (unfavourable)	**C**
Legend: A = verified in multiple studies, randomized trials and/or integrated in guidelines; B = variable between studies/needs definitive validation; C = preliminary/discrepant results.		

8.1 Definition

Nodal marginal zone lymphoma (NMZL) is a non-Hodgkin lymphoma of mature B-cells, with similarities to the extranodal (EMZL) or splenic marginal zone lymphoma (SMZL), but with predominant nodal involvement and without extranodal or splenic involvement [1]. Since diagnosis is made by exclusion, some inaccuracy in the distinction from other marginal zone lymphomas (MZL) or indolent lymphomas might be possible. However, there are several arguments based on immunohistological, genetic, and molecular genetic findings, suggesting that NMZL presents a distinct entity.

The NMZL was originally described as a "monocytoid" or "parafollicular" B-cell lymphoma in 1986 (historical review in [2]). Only later, the relationship to other MZL became clear. In 1994, the "nodal marginal zone lymphoma with or without monocytoid B-cells" was included as a separate entity in the REAL classification, also adopted in the WHO classification of lymphoid neoplasia of 2001 and of 2008 and in the revision of 2016.

The NMZL presents less than 2% of all lymphoid neoplasia and only a small proportion (about 10–20%) of MZL [2]. The annual incidence is 0.8 patients in 100,000 men and women

L. Arcaini (✉)
Division of Hematology, Fondazione IRCCS Policlinico San Matteo & Department of Molecular Medicine, University of Pavia, Pavia, Italy
e-mail: arcaini@unipv.it

A. Viardot
Department of Internal Medicine III, University Hospital of Ulm, Ulm, Germany
e-mail: andreas.viardot@uniklinik-ulm.de

per year. However, the incidence might be increasing in the last decade (25% from 2001 to 2009) [3]. This increase may be partly explained by a raised awareness of pathologists for this entity.

The typical age of onset is about 60 years (slightly younger than patients with SMZL), the male-to-female ratio is approximately equal. In the majority of patients, there is an advanced stage and bone marrow is involved (43%; [4]). In 10% of patients, there is a leukemic disease without marked splenic enlargement. At diagnosis, the majority of patients have a good performance status and no B symptoms [4–6].

An exception might be the pediatric NMZL, an entity included into the recent revision of the WHO classification of lymphoid neoplasia, typically in younger patients. The majority of patients are male (ratio 20–1) and have a localized stage (I or II), usually affecting cervical lymph nodes. Relapses are infrequent, even after local resection of radiotherapy [7]. There are no clear histological or molecular pathologic criteria for delineation to the adult forms. However, enlarged lymph follicle with the extension of the mantle zone and frequent CD43 expression might be characteristic but not exclusive for the pediatric NMZL [1].

8.2 Pathogenesis

Like other MZL, an association with hepatitis C virus (HCV) infection with geographical variability and chronic inflammatory disease have been reported. In a first series, 24% of patients with NMZL had a HCV infection [5, 6]. In a recent publication [8], patients with NMZL and HCV were found less frequently, in contrast to series from Asia [9]. Since the treatment of HCV infection can induce a remission of the lymphoma, screening for HCV is mandatory at diagnosis of NMZL [8].

The association with autoimmune disease is less frequently reported in comparison to EMZL; in a French series there were only four out of 47 patients (9%) with autoimmune diseases [4].

8.3 Histologic and Biologic Characteristics

The typical histopathological picture is the proliferation of small-sized lymphocytes into the marginal zone (which surrounded the reactive lymph follicle) with a secondary infiltration of the interfollicular areas of the lymph node [1]. By immunophenotyping, NMZL have typical Pan-B-cell markers like CD19 and CD20. CD23, CD5, and germinal center markers (CD10, BCL6, HGAL and LMO2) are rarely positive, Cyclin D1 is usually negative.

Like follicular lymphoma (FL), BCL2 is frequently positive; MNDA and IRTA1 are regarded as distinctive markers to differentiate FL and MZL. There is no immunological marker to differentiate to NMZL from other MZL [1, 10].

There are typical genetic markers for all MZL like gains on chromosome 3 and 18 as well as losses on chromosome arm 6q23–24. All MZL shows an activation of NFkappaB and epigenetic modifications [11]. The NMZL shares with the SMZL the lack of specific translocations like the t(11;18)(q21;q21) translocation—a hallmark of gastric EZML. Other similarities between NMZL and SMZL are the mutations of NOTCH pathway and of the transcription factor KLF2. In contrast to SMZL, deletions on chromosome arm 7q31 are unusual [11]. More specific characteristics for the NMZL may be the inactivation of PTPRD, a receptor-type protein tyrosine phosphatase (up to 20% of cases) and a high frequency of KMT2D (formerly MML-2) [12]. MYD88 L265P mutations are detected rarely in MZLs. KLF2 and NOTCH2 mutations might have a possible prognostic impact; however, larger series are necessary [12].

In a recent analysis using high-throughput sequencing, NMZL shows a higher mutational load than in EMZL. The most frequent mutated genes code for epigenetic modifiers (e.g. KMT2D 28%, CREBPA 20%, TET2 20%), followed by mutations of BRAF (17%). BRAF mutations are typically on V600E comparable to hairy cell leukemia, which might offer new therapeutic options in a subset of these patients. Moreover, this mutations seems to be restricted to MZL [13].

Similar to EMZL and SMZL, ongoing mutations and a restricted VH gene usage argue for a causal relationship to an antigenic stimulus supporting an ongoing B-cell expansion. In NMZL, the IGHV4–34 gene is used in 20–30% of cases, which is rarely reported in EMZL or SMZL with the exception of the ocular adnexal lymphoma [10].

8.4 Prognosis

Before the implementation of the CD20 antibody rituximab into the treatment, the prognosis of NMZL was considered as worse in contrast to EMZL and comparable to SMZL [14]. In recent series, this difference is not pronounced and more comparable to EZML. In the US SEER registry (Suirvellance, Epidemiology, and End Results database), the 5-year survival of patients between 1995 and 2009 was 76.5% (in contrast EZML: 79.0%) [15]. In contrast to SZML, the prognosis was improved within 15 years.

In different case series, the overall survival at 5 years was between 57% and 97% [15]. The high difference in data from epidemiological registries may be partially explained by the heterogeneity of the diagnosis due to changes in the pathological delineation and in the staging procedures, and also by changes in the treatment. Prognostic differences between EZML and NMZL can be explained by the fact that EZML is very often localized: indeed, the prognosis of EZML and NMZL in stage I is comparable [16].

For risk assessment, the international prognostic index (IPI) and the follicular lymphoma international prognostic index (FLIPI) were evaluated in a retrospective series in NMZL [17]. There are a large amount of molecular risk factors evaluated in NMZL without a clear candidate for prognostication (e.g. negative results: loss of Survivin, active Caspase 3, overexpression of Cyclin E; positive results: loss of expression of MUM1/IRF4 and Ki67 less than 5%, overview in [2]). In contrast to many hematologic neoplasia, the loss of chromosome arm 17p might be no strong prognostic factor in NMZL [11].

Recently, the progression of disease within 24 months (POD24) was established as a risk factor for relapsed marginal zone lymphoma [18]. Since NMZL represents only a small proportion of all patients of this series (10%), the impact for overall survival was not significant compared to EMZL and SMZL.

The transformation into a high-grade lymphoma is a possible event in NMZL. In a series of 340 patients with MZL, the incidence of transformation was 3% at 5 years in the group of NMZL patients [19], and possibly slightly lower than in FL or other MZL. A histological transformation is associated with a poorer prognosis: the 2-years survival after transplantation is only 57% [19].

8.5 First-Line Treatment

Due to the rarity, the heterogeneity and the diagnostic uncertainty, there are no treatment recommendations evaluated prospectively in patients with NMZL. Since NMZL and MZL were often treated in clinical trials together with other indolent lymphoma, the guidelines for treatment of FL were transferred directly to the NMZL (e.g. ESMO guidelines [20]; NCCN [21] Guidelines Non-Hodgkin's Lymphoma, Version 4.2014). Regarding to clinical trials, the NMZL were included in trials of other MZLs or indolent lymphoma.

In localized stages (stage I, II without bulky disease), involved field radiotherapy is widely accepted as a standard. However, the value of radiotherapy in contrast to "watch and wait" or systemic treatment is not well-defined. A localized NMZL in a young patient could represent a pediatric NMZL which is difficult to delineate to the adult form. In few case reports [22, 23], patients with pediatric NMZL had an excellent prognosis even after resection of the involved lymph node only. In a recent publication, there was only one patient with relapse after local resection in 20 children with pediatric NMZL [23]. Therefore, "watch and wait" might be a useful strategy as alternative to radiotherapy in (young) patients after surgical removal of the involved lymph node.

In asymptomatic patients with advanced stages, "watch and wait" is an accepted standard comparable to the strategy in FL. Symptomatic patients were treated with a combination of chemotherapy and a CD20 antibody. Like in other B-cell neoplasia, the addition of rituximab improves the outcome. Analogue to EMZL, a monotherapy with rituximab could be an alternative to the combination. However, prospective data are scarce. In the RESORT trial [24], 28 patients with NMZL and low tumor burden received a monotherapy with rituximab. The response rate in NMZL was higher than in EMZL or CLL/CL (complete response 3.8%, partial response 57.1%, others stable disease), but lower than in FL (overall response 70.8%).

There are several combination therapies, like R-CVP (rituximab, cyclophosphamide, vincristine, and prednisone), R-F (rituximab, fludarabine), R-FC (rituximab, fludarabine, cyclophosphamide), R-CHOP (rituximab, cyclophosphamide, vincristine, prednisone), or R-Benda (rituximab, bendamustine) (review in Table 8.1). In a small series, the response rates were after R-CVP, R-F, and R-FC 88%, 85, and 99%, respectively. The PFS after 3 years was 59%, 79.5%, and 90.1% [26, 27, 32]. However, treatment with fludarabine is sometimes associated with fatal complications particularly in elderly patients.

In the StIL-001 trial, 549 patients with indolent lymphomas were randomized between R-CHOP and R-Bendamustine, including 67 patients with MZL [33]. In contrast to the other subgroups, there was no difference in PFS between two arms. The toxicity was lower with R-bendamustine compared to R-CHOP, so that R-bendamustine is often used in European countries. In the GALLIUM trial, Rituximab in combination with chemotherapy (bendamustine, CVP, CHOP) was compared with the new CD20 antibody Obinutuzumab. In a subgroup analysis of 195 patients with MZL including 66 patients with NMZL, the PFS could not be improved by Obinutuzumab in contrast to the patients with FL [34]. However, there was an unexpectedly high toxicity in both arms with treatment-associated fatal events (6% in the rituximab arm, 12% in the obinutuzumab arm). The fatal events occur mostly in patients treated with the combination with bendamustine, which was observed also in the whole collective of the GALLIUM trial. The high rate of severe infections after bendamustine, and also after fludarabine, might be caused by a long-term T-cell depletion after treatment.

In an analysis of patients of the US cancer registry (SEER-Medicare; [35]), there was no significant

Table 8.1 Clinical trials of first-line treatment including patients with NMZL

Reference	Treatment	All patients/patients with MZL/with NMZL	OR/CR	Outcome
Leblond et al. [25]c	Chlorambucil	414/33/n.a.	38.6%/5.3%	mPFS 27.1 months
	Fludarabine		38.6%/2.0%	mPFS 36.1 months
Kang [26]	R-CVP	42/42/n.a.	88%/60%	3 years PFS 59%
Brown [27]	R-Fludarabine	24/24/14	85%/54%	3 years PFS 79%
Ferrario [32]	R-Fludarabine/ cyclophosphamide	46/46/6	89%/67%	3 years PFS 90.1%
Samaniego [28]	R-Pentostatin/ cyclophosphamide	83/83/n.a.	75%/70%	3 years PFS 73%
Rummel [33]	R-CHOP	463/59/n.a.	93%/42%	mPFS 31.5 months
	R-Bendamustine		93%/47%	mPFS: 69.5 months
Flinn [29]	R-CVP/R-CHOP	224/24/n.a.	91%/25%	n.a.
	R-Bendamustine		97%/31%	
Herold [34]	R-chemo	96/96/31	82%/19%	3 years PFS 78.1%
	G-chemo		83%/16%	3 years PFS 75.0%
Rummel [30]	R-Bendamustine ± R-maintenance	119/119/n.a.	91%/23%	2 years PFS 92%
Oh [31]	R-CVP + R-maintenance	45/45/15	93%/44%	3 years PFS 83%

difference between use of Rituximab-Bendamustine versus Rituximab monotherapy in 903 patients with NMZL. With all limitations and unexpected confounding factors, the authors resume to be consider the risk and benefit of the combination particularly in elderly patients.

In a subgroup analysis of the MAINTAIN-trial, including 119 patients with SMZL and NMZL, the 2-years maintenance treatment with rituximab after immunochemotherapy prolonged significantly the progression-free survival without adding any new toxicity [30].

8.6 Treatment of Relapse and New Options

In FL, the early progression within 24 months after immunochemotherapy (POD24) is regarded as a prognostic marker. POD24 was shown to be of prognostic relevance also in MZL—however the proportion of NMZL was too small (appr. 10%; [18]). However, intensive treatment options like high-dose chemotherapy with autologous stem cell support can be offered to younger patients with early progress and other high-risk factors. In later relapse, repeated immunochemotherapy is the usual standard in these patients.

In January 2017, the US Food and Drug Administration (FDA) approved the Bruton tyrosine kinase (BTK) inhibitor Ibrutinib for the treatment of patients with relapsed and refractory MZL, who had already received a CD20 antibody based pretreatment (data on novel drugs are summarized in Table 8.2). In the pivotal phase-II trial, 17 patients with NMZL were included. The overall response rate—the primary endpoint of this trial—was lower in NMZL patients than in other (41% vs. 48%), as well as the median PFS (8.3 months vs. 14.2 months [41]). Next-generation BTK inhibitors like Acalabrutinib and Zanubrutinib are under clinical investigation in MZL (NCT02180711, NCT03846427).

In the pivotal phase-II trial using the PI3Kδ inhibitors idelalisib [44], 15 patients with MZL were included, respectively. The overall response rates were approximately 50% in MZL, so that this principle may be effective. However, in contrast to FL, idelalisib is not approved for the treatment of MZL.

Copanlisib is a PI3K inhibitor which combines activity against the PI3K subunit α and δ and has a different spectrum of side effects. In a phase II trial, coplanlisib has an overall response rate of 78% in all MZLs and particularly 87% in 15 patients with NMZL. The duration of response was 17.4 months [37].

The combination of lenalidomide and rituximab (so-called R^2) may be an option in MZL with a response rate up to 89% [45]. In the AUGMENT phase III trial [40], 63 patients with MZL underwent a randomization between ritux-

Table 8.2 Novel drugs in marginal zone lymphoma

Reference	Drug	All patients/with MZL/with NMZL	OR/CR in MZL	Outcome
Wagner-Johnston [36]	Idelalisib	125/15/5	47%/6%	mPFS 6.6 months
Dreyling [37]	Copanlisib	23/23/15	83%/13%	mPFS 24.2 months
Conconi [38]	Everolimus	30/30/6	20%/3%	mPFS 14 months
Rosenthal [39]	Lenalidomide, rituximab, Cyclophosphamid, Dexamethason	33/33/5	87.9%/30.3%	mPFS: 39.7 months
Leonard [40]	R-Lenalidomide	178/31/8	65%/29%	mPFS: 20.2 months
	R-mono	180/32/10	44%/13%	mPFS: 25.2 months
Noy [41]	Ibrutinib	63/63/17	48%/3%	mPFS 14.2 months
Lossos [42]	Yttrium $^{90-}$ ibritumomab	16/16/n.a.	87.5%/56%	mPFS 47 months
Samaniego [43]	Yttrium ^{90} ibritumomab	11/11/n.a.	100%/97%	mPFS >56 months

OR overall response, *CR* complete remission, *mPFS* median progression-free survival, *R* rituximab, *CVP* cyclophophamide, vincristin, prednisone, *CHOP* cyclophosphamide, vincristine, prednisone, *n.a.* not evaluable imab monotherapy and R^2. With regard to the endpoint PFS, the whole collective, but not the subgroup of MZL shows a significant improvement. Nevertheless, the combination of lenalidomide and rituximab (R^2) was approved by FDA also for the treatment of refractory or relapsed MZL in May 2019. In contrast, the EMA approved this combination only for follicular lymphoma in January 2020.

8.7 Summary

The NMZL is a rare lymphoma entity which is partially difficult to differentiate from other indolent lymphomas. Using new techniques including high-throughput sequencing, the classification might be improved in the next years and more targeted treatment strategies might be established. Following the treatment guidelines of FL is proved of value in NMZL. However, novel drugs like BTK or PI3K inhibitor might be particularly efficient in this entity. The majority of patients with NMZL have a favorable prognosis.

References

1. Swerdlow SH, Campo E, Harris NL, et al. WHO classification of tumours of haematopoietic and lymphoid tissues. Lyon: International Agency of Cancer Research; 2016.
2. Thieblemont C, Molina T, Davi F. Optimizing therapy for nodal marginal zone lymphoma. Blood. 2016;127:2064–71. https://doi.org/10.1182/blood-2015-12-624296.
3. Khalil MO, Morton LM, Devesa SS, Check DP, Curtis RE, Weisenburger DD, Dores GM. Incidence of marginal zone lymphoma in the United States, 2001–2009 with a focus on primary anatomic site. Br J Haematol. 2014;165:67–77. https://doi.org/10.1111/bjh.12730.
4. Berger F, Felman P, Thieblemont C, Pradier T, Baseggio L, Bryon PA, Salles G, Callet-Bauchu E, Coiffier B. Non-MALT marginal zone B-cell lymphomas: a description of clinical presentation and outcome in 124 patients. Blood. 2000;95:1950–6.
5. Arcaini L, Burcheri S, Rossi A, et al. Prevalence of HCV infection in nongastric marginal zone B-cell lymphoma of MALT. Ann Oncol. 2007a;18:346–50. https://doi.org/10.1093/annonc/mdl388.
6. Arcaini L, Paulli M, Burcheri S, Rossi A, et al. Primary nodal marginal zone B-cell lymphoma: clinical features and prognostic assessment of a rare disease. Br J Haematol. 2007b;2007(136):301–4. https://doi.org/10.1111/j.1365-2141.2006.06437.x.
7. Taddesse-Heath L, Pittaluga S, Sorbara L, Bussey M, Raffeld M, Jaffe ES. Marginal zone B-cell lymphoma in children and young adults. Am J Surg Pathol. 2003;27:522–31.
8. Arcaini L, Besson C, Frigeni M, et al. Interferon-free antiviral treatment in B-cell lymphoproliferative disorders associated with hepatitis C virus infection. Blood. 2016;128:2527–32. https://doi.org/10.1182/blood-2016-05-714667.
9. Chuang SS, Liao YL, Chang ST, et al. Hepatitis C virus infection is significantly associated with malignant lymphoma in Taiwan, particularly with nodal and splenic marginal zone lymphomas. J Clin Pathol. 2010;63:595–8. https://doi.org/10.1136/jcp.2010.076810.
10. Bertoni F, Rossi D, Campo E. Recent advances in understanding the biology of marginal zone lymphoma. F1000Res. 2018;7:406. https://doi.org/10.12688/f1000research.13826.
11. Rinaldi A, Mian M, Chigrinova E, et al. Genome-wide DNA profiling of marginal zone lymphomas identifies subtype-specific lesions with an impact on the clinical outcome. Blood. 2011;117:1595–604. https://doi.org/10.1182/blood-2010-01-264275.
12. Spina V, Khiabanian H, Messina M, Monti S, Cascione L, Bruscaggin A. The genetics of nodal marginal zone lymphoma. Blood. 2016;128:1362–73. https://doi.org/10.1182/blood-2016-02-696757.
13. Pillonel V, Juskevicius D, Ng CKY, et al. High-throughput sequencing of nodal marginal zone lymphomas identifies recurrent BRAF mutations. Leukemia. 2018;32:2412. https://doi.org/10.1038/s41375-018-0082-4.
14. Thieblemont C. Improved biological insight and influence on management in indolent lymphoma. Talk 3: update on nodal and splenic marginal zone lymphoma. Hematology Am Soc Hematol Educ Program. 2017;2017:371–8.
15. Olszewski AJ, Castillo JJ. Survival of patients with marginal zone lymphoma: analysis of the surveillance, epidemiology, and end results database. Cancer. 2013;119:629–38. https://doi.org/10.1002/cncr.27773.
16. Kuper-Hommel MJ, van de Schans SA, Vreugdenhil G, van Krieken JH, Coebergh JW. Trends in incidence, therapy and outcome of localized nodal and extranodal marginal zone lymphomas: declining incidence and inferior outcome for gastrointestinal sites. Leuk Lymphoma. 2013;54:1891–7. https://doi.org/10.3109/10428194.2013.764421.
17. Heilgeist A, McClanahan F, Ho AD, Witzens-Harig M. Prognostic value of the follicular lymphoma international prognostic index score in marginal zone lymphoma: an analysis of clinical presentation and outcome in 144 patients. Cancer. 2013;119:99–106. https://doi.org/10.1002/cncr.27704.
18. Luminari S, Merli M, Rattotti S, et al. Early progression as a predictor of survival in marginal zone

lymphomas: an analysis from the FIL-NF10 study. Blood. 2019;134:798–801. https://doi.org/10.1182/blood.2019001088.
19. Conconi A, Franceschetti S, Aprile von Hohenstaufen K, Margiotta-Casaluci G, Stathis A, Moccia AA, Bertoni F, Ramponi A, Mazzucchelli L, Cavalli F, Gaidano G, Zucca E. Histologic transformation in marginal zone lymphomas†. Ann Oncol. 2015;26:2329–35. https://doi.org/10.1093/annonc/mdv368.
20. Zucca E, Arcaini L, Buske C, et al. Marginal zone lymphomas: ESMO clinical practice guidelines for diagnosis, treatment and follow-up. Ann Oncol. 2020;31:17–29. https://doi.org/10.1016/j.annonc.2019.10.010.
21. NCCN guidelines non-Hodgkin's lymphoma, version 4.2014, p 225. https://www.nccn.org/about/nhl.pdf.
22. Gitelson E, Al-Saleem T, Robu V, Millenson MM, Smith MR. Pediatric nodal marginal zone lymphoma may develop in the adult population. Leuk Lymphoma. 2010;51:89–94. https://doi.org/10.3109/10428190903349670.
23. Ronceray L, Abla O, Barzilai-Birenboim S, Bomken S, Chiang A, Jazbec J, Kabickova E, Lazic J, et al. Children and adolescents with marginal zone lymphoma have an excellent prognosis with limited chemotherapy or a watch-and-wait strategy after complete resection. Pediatr Blood Cancer. 2018;65:65. https://doi.org/10.1002/pbc.26932.
24. Williams ME, Hong F, Gascoyne RD, Wagner LI, Krauss JC, Habermann TM, Swinnen LJ, Schuster SJ, et al. Rituximab extended schedule or retreatment trial for low tumour burden non-follicular indolent B-cell non-Hodgkin lymphomas: eastern cooperative oncology group protocol E4402. Br J Haematol. 2016;173:867–75. https://doi.org/10.1111/bjh.14007.
25. Leblond V, Johnson S, Chevret S, et al. Results of a randomized trial of chlorambucil versus fludarabine for patients with untreated Waldenström macroglobulinemia, marginal zone lymphoma, or lymphoplasmacytic lymphoma. J Clin Oncol. 2013;31:301–7. https://doi.org/10.1200/JCO.2012.44.7920.
26. Kang HJ, Kim WS, Kim SJ, et al. Phase II trial of rituximab plus CVP combination chemotherapy for advanced stage marginal zone lymphoma as a first-line therapy: consortium for improving survival of lymphoma (CISL) study. Ann Hematol. 2012;91:543–51. https://doi.org/10.1007/s00277-011-1337-6.
27. Brown JR, Friedberg JW, Feng Y, et al. A phase 2 study of concurrent fludarabine and rituximab for the treatment of marginal zone lymphomas. Br J Haematol. 2009;145:741–8. https://doi.org/10.1111/j.1365-2141.2009.07677.x.
28. Samaniego F, Hagemeister F, Romaguera JE, et al. Pentostatin, cyclophosphamide and rituximab for previously untreated advanced stage, low-grade B-cell lymphomas. Br J Haematol. 2015;169(6):814–23. https://doi.org/10.1111/bjh.13367.
29. Flinn IW, van der Jagt R, Kahl BS, et al. Randomized trial of bendamustine-rituximab or R-CHOP/R-CVP in first-line treatment of indolent NHL or MCL: the BRIGHT study. Blood. 2014;123:2944–52. https://doi.org/10.1182/blood-2013-11-531327.
30. Rummel M, Koenigsmann M, Chow KU, et al. Two years rituximab maintenance vs. observation after first line treatment with bendamustine plus rituximab (B-R) in patients with marginal zone lymphoma (MZL): results of a prospective, randomized, multicenter phase 2 study (the StiL NHL7-2008 MAINTAIN trial). J Clin Oncol. 2018;36(15 Suppl):7515. https://doi.org/10.1200/JCO.2018.36.15_suppl.7515.
31. Oh SY, Kim JS, Kim WS, et al. Phase II study of R–CVP followed by rituximab maintenance therapy for patients with advanced marginal zone lymphoma: consortium for improving survival of lymphoma (CISL) study. Cancer Commun (London). 2019;39:58. https://doi.org/10.1186/s40880-019-0403-7.
32. Ferrario A, Pulsoni A, Olivero B, et al. Fludarabine, cyclophosphamide, and rituximab in patients with advanced, untreated, indolent B-cell nonfollicular lymphomas: phase 2 study of the Italian Lymphoma Foundation. Cancer. 2012;118:3954–61. https://doi.org/10.1002/cncr.26708.
33. Rummel MJ, Niederle N, Maschmeyer G, Banat GA, von Grünhagen U, Losem C, et al. Study group indolent lymphomas (StiL). Bendamustine plus rituximab versus CHOP plus rituximab as first-line treatment for patients with indolent and mantle-cell lymphomas: an open-label, multicentre, randomised, phase 3 non-inferiority trial. Lancet. 2013;381:1203–10. https://doi.org/10.1016/S0140-6736(12)61763-2.
34. Herold M, Hoster E, Janssens A, et al. Immunochemotherapy with obinutuzumab or rituximab in patients with previously untreated marginal zone lymphoma (MZL) in the randomised GALLIUM trial. IMCL (abstract). J Clin Oncol. 2017;36(23):239.
35. Olszewski AJ, Ollila TA, Reagan JL. Bendamustine-rituximab does not improve survival over rituximab monotherapy for older patients with nodal or splenic marginal zone lymphoma. Blood. 2019;134(Suppl_1):2824.
36. Wagner-Johnston N, Schuster S, de Vos S, et al. Long-term follow-up of Idelalisib monotherapy in patients with double-refractory marginal zone lymphoma or lymphoplasmacytic lymphoma/Waldenstrom's macroglobulinemia. Blood. 2019;134(Suppl_1):4006. https://doi.org/10.1182/blood-2019-121936.
37. Dreyling M, Panayiotidis P, Follows GA, et al. Long-term efficacy and safety of Copanlisib in multiply relapsed or refractory patients with marginal zone lymphoma. Blood. 2019;134(Suppl 1):1531.
38. Conconi A, Raderer M, Franceschetti S, et al. Clinical activity of everolimus in relapsed/refractory marginal zone B-cell lymphomas: results of a phase II study of the international Extranodal Lymphoma Study Group. Br J Haematol. 2014;166:69–76. https://doi.org/10.1111/bjh.12845.
39. Rosenthal A, Dueck AC, Ansell S, et al. A phase 2 study of lenalidomide, rituximab, cyclophosphamide, and dexamethasone (LR-CD) for untreated low-grade

non-Hodgkin lymphoma requiring therapy. Am J Hematol. 2017;92:467–72. https://doi.org/10.1002/ajh.24693.

40. Leonard JP, Trneny M, Izutzu K, et al. AUGMENT: a phase III study of Lenalidomide plus rituximab versus placebo plus rituximab in relapsed or refractory indolent lymphoma. J Clin Oncol. 2019;37:1188–99. https://doi.org/10.1200/JCO.19.00010.
41. Noy A, de Vos S, Thieblemont C, Martin P, Flowers CR, Morschhauser F, et al. Targeting Bruton tyrosine kinase with ibrutinib in relapsed/refractory marginal zone lymphoma. Blood. 2017;129:2224–32. https://doi.org/10.1182/blood-2016-10-747345.
42. Lossos IS, Fabregas JC, Koru-Sengul T, Miao F, Goodman D, Serafini AN, Hosein PJ, Stefanovic A, Rosenblatt JD, Hoffman JE. Phase II study of (90) Y Ibritumomab tiuxetan (Zevalin) in patients with previously untreated marginal zone lymphoma. Leuk Lymphoma. 2015;56:1750–5. https://doi.org/10.3109/10428194.2014.975801.
43. Samaniego F, Berkova Z, Romaguera JE, Fowler N, Fanale MA, Pro B, Shah JJ, McLaughlin P, Sehgal L, Selvaraj V, Braun FK, Mathur R, Feng L, Neelapu SS, Kwak LW. 90Y-ibritumomab tiuxetan radiotherapy as first-line therapy for early stage low-grade B-cell lymphomas, including bulky disease. Br J Haematol. 2014;167:207–13. https://doi.org/10.1111/bjh.13021.
44. Gopal AK, Kahl BS, de Vos S, Wagner-Johnston ND, Schuster SJ, Jurczak WJ, et al. PI3Kδ inhibition by idelalisib in patients with relapsed indolent non-Hodgkin lymphoma refractory to both rituximab and an alkylating agent. N Engl J Med. 2014;370:1008–18. https://doi.org/10.1056/NEJMoa1314583.
45. Fowler NH, Davis RE, Rawal S, Nastoupil L, Hagemeister FB, McLaughlin P, et al. Safety and activity of lenalidomide and rituximab in untreated indolent lymphoma: an open-label, phase 2 trial. Lancet Oncol. 2014;15:1311–8. https://doi.org/10.1016/S1470-2045(14)70455-3.

9 Splenic Marginal Zone Lymphoma

Emilio Iannitto and Catherine Thieblemont

Splenic marginal zone lymphoma (SMZL)

Clinical outline
Primarily the spleen, peripheral blood and bone marrow. Lymph nodes and extranodal sites usually spared. Cytopenia and autoimmune manifestations frequent. Association with HCV infection observed in Southern Europe.

Cytology	In peripheral blood "villous" lymphocytes (small cell with short, polar cytoplasmic projections). In the tissues, range in morphology from centrocyte-like to monocytoid, with variable degree of lymphoplasmacytic differentiation. Few or no blasts.	Splenic marginal zone lymphoma, cytology	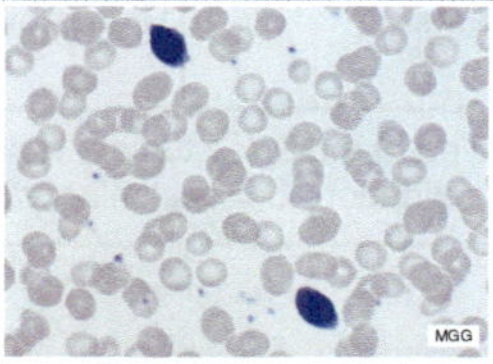
Histology	In bone marrow biopsies, characteristic sinusoidal pattern of infiltration. Splenic histology, effaced white pulp with a biphasic picture (pale ring around residual follicles) and extension into to the red pulp. Frequent infiltration large vessel walls. In lymph nodes, SMZL resembles nodal MZL.	Splenic marginal zone lymphoma, hystology	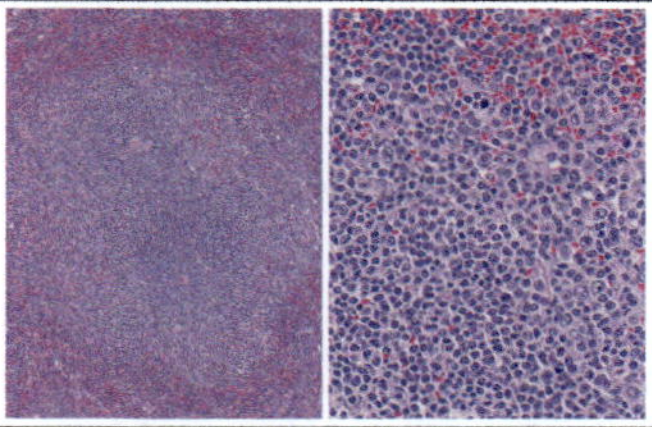

	CD20	CD5[1]	CD23[1]	CD10	BCL6	cyclin D1	CD103	FMC7	IgM	light chains
notes	[1]usually partially and/or weak.									
other marker	SMZL lacks a specific phenotype and the antibody panel should be primarily aimed at the exclusion of other lymphoma subtypes.									

■ = majority of cases positive   ▒ = variable fraction of cases positive   □ = negative

Main differential diagnosis	HCL (should be CD103 and BRAF V600E positive), CLL (should be CD23 and CD5 positive), MCL (should be cyclin D1 positive). Subtypes of marginal zone lymphomas (extranodal, nodal, splenic, cutaneous) distinguished mainly by clinical presentation (pattern of involved organs).

M. Dreyling, M. Ladetto (eds.), *Indolent Lymphomas*, Hematologic Malignancies,
https://doi.org/10.1007/978-3-030-55989-2_9

Key molecular features		
Activation of NOTCH and nuclear factor kappa B pathways IGH genes rearranged, somatic hypermutation and IGHV3 and IGHV4 usage bias. Frequent translocations: Non reported. Frequent copy number alterations: Loss of 7q. Frequent mutations: *NOTCH2, KLF2, TNFAIP3, MLL2/KMT2D, MYD88, CARD11*		
Precursor lesions		
Some cases appear be preceded by monoclonal B-cell lymphocytosisof the non-CLL type (CD5-negative).		
Progression		
10-15% progress to high grade lymphoma, typically of the diffuse large B-cell subtype.		
Clinically relevant pathologic features	**Relevance**	**Evidence**
IGHV mutation status	Prognostic: unmutated (unfavorable)	C
Mutations	Prognostic: *NOTCH2, TP53* (unfavorable)	C
Hepatitis C	predictive: may respont to anti-viral therapy	
Proliferation/blasts	High proliferation and/or blast content (unfavourable)	B
Legend: A = verified in multiple studies, randomized trials and/or integrated in guidelines; B = variable between studies/ needs definitive validation; C = preliminary/discrepant results.		

9.1 Epidemiology

SMZL is a rare B-cell neoplasm, accounting for less than 2% of all lymphomas and about 20% of the marginal zone lymphoma (MZL) subset [1, 2], yet it embodies the most common primary malignancy of the spleen [3]. Gender prevalence varies in different series [4–6], but these differences are lost in large retrospective registries [7]. The median age at diagnosis is 68 years, and nearly all patients are aged greater than 50 years [7, 8]. The overall age-adjusted incidence is 0.13 per 100,000 persons per year, with increasing trends among patients who are white, male, or age ≥70 years. However, the incidence is likely to be underestimated because splenectomy is not routinely performed in all cases of splenic lymphoma, and establishing a precise diagnosis without the examination of splenic tissue may be challenging [9]. Epidemiological data have postulated a possible association between hepatitis C virus (HCV) infection and lymphoproliferative disorders, particularly MZL [10, 11]. Subsequently, the presence of a higher risk of developing lymphoma, particularly MZL or DLBCL, has been confirmed both in areas of high (Overall Relative Risk:2.4; 95% CI: 2.0–3.0) and low HCV infection prevalence (OR:1.6; 95% CI: 1.3–1.9) [12–14]. Also, several groups reported regression or even remission of the lymphoma after successful treatment of HCV chronic infection [15–17]. These findings

E. Iannitto
Haematology and BMT Unit, Department of Oncology, Casa di Cura La Maddalena, Palermo, Italy

C. Thieblemont (✉)
APHP, Saint-Louis Hospital, Hemato-Oncology – Paris Diderot University, Paris, France
e-mail: catherine.thieblemont@aphp.fr

strengthen the hypothesis that HCV might play a role in the lymphomagenesis by driving a chronic antigen stimulation triggered by the virus glycoprotein E2, which in turn stimulates CD81 in B-cells [13]. Other factors reported linked to an increased risk are autoimmune diseases, asthma and permanent use of hair dyes [18].

9.2 Clinical Manifestation

Clinical presentation often consists of isolated splenomegaly with or without cytopenia(s) and or mild lymphocytosis [5, 6, 8, 19, 20]. About one-third of patients are genuinely asymptomatic, and the diagnosis is made by chance after the incidental detection of splenomegaly amidst clinical assessment for unrelated causes [9]. Splenomegaly is usually massive (median longitudinal diameter 20 cm), but in a subset of patients the spleen is relatively small [21]. A small subset of patients presents with an isolated, slight to moderate, lymphocytosis showing the morphology and immunophenotype consistent with the diagnosis of SMZL [22]. This clinical picture overlaps with that of monoclonal B-cell lymphocytosis with marginal zone phenotype (MBL-MZ) [23]. Whether this presentation embodies an indolent SMZL variant or a pre-lymphomatous condition is still an open issue [22–24]. Symptoms, if present, are mostly related to massive splenomegaly, such as abdominal discomfort, early satiety or left flank pain. Slight to moderate anaemia and thrombocytopenia are detected in 50%, 20% and 24% of cases, respectively, mostly due to hypersplenism or autoimmunity, rarely to bone marrow infiltration [25, 26]. Exceptionally, the degree of thrombocytopenia is severe enough to account for haemorrhagic symptoms; neutropenia is definitively rare, usually mild and clinically inconsequential. A leukemic component (defined as the presence of absolute lymphocytosis or >5% neoplastic lymphocytes in peripheral blood) is present in 52–75% of cases [6, 20, 26]. A moderate increase of LDH and beta2 microglobulin concentrations are found in about 30% and 60% of patients, respectively. A small (less than 2 g/dL) monoclonal component (MC), mainly μ (IgM) isotype, is detected in approximately one-third of patients. These patients also frequently display haemolytic anaemia, immune thrombocytopenia or coagulation disorders [4]. In the Mediterranean basin, up to 19% of SMZL patients are carriers of a chronic HCV infection and may show a distinctive presentation trait comprising higher incidence of CM mainly μ (IgM), type II cryoglobulinemia and nodal disease [26]. Saadun reported the association of HCV infection, cryoglobulinemia along with the presence of villous lymphocytes in peripheral blood and proposed it could represent a distinct entity [27]. About 20% of patients show autoimmune manifestations [4, 28]. Autoimmune haemolytic anaemia (AHA), autoimmune thrombocytopenia (AITP) and cold agglutinin disease are the most frequently reported autoimmune disorders and are generally present on diagnosis [6, 20]. Moreover, some patients may show a positive direct antiglobulin test (DAT) without signs of overt AHA. Among other autoimmune manifestations associated with SMZL, the most clinically relevant are acquired C1q deficiency and angioedema [29], acquired coagulation disorders [4], and acquired antiphospholipid antibodies and thrombophilic syndrome [30]. By clinical examination, little can be inferred other than signs related to splenomegaly, because clinically significant peripheral lymphadenopathies are exceptionally detected, and moderate hepatomegaly is reported in only one-third of patients [4, 6, 22].

9.3 Peripheral Blood Cytology

A leukemic component, in the form of slight to moderate lymphocytosis, is quite common. At variance with other lymphoid tumours, leukemic neoplastic cells display a marked morphological heterogeneity shown by the simultaneous presence of small lymphocytes without specific features, lymphoplasmacytic cells, lymphocytes with nuclear clefts, medium-sized lymphomonocytic cells with relative abundant pale cytoplasm and villous lymphocytes [22, 31–33]. In some cases, the prevalent morphology is that of villous lymphocytes, small lymphocytes with round nucleus with thickened chromatin and basophilic cytoplasm characterised by the presence of short villi unevenly distributed or concentrated at one of the two poles of the cell [33]. Villi are lost after a few hours of storage of blood; then they can hardly be seen if a peripheral blood smear is not set up timely.

9.4 Bone Marrow

Bone marrow (BM) infiltration is a constant finding in SMZL [2]. Particularly in the early phases of the disease, BM infiltration may be very subtle and difficult to recognise on routine morphologic sections. The BM infiltration pattern may be almost exclusively intrasinusoidal [34], but concurrently with the progression of the disease or after splenectomy a nodular and or interstitial involvement of the intertrabecular space become apparent [35]. Rare and scattered reactive germinal centres surrounded by a rim tumour cells can be found. Neoplastic cells comprise rather monomorphic small- to medium-sized lymphocytes showing round to oval nucleus with regular contour and a small rim of cytoplasm. However, plasmacytoid features with a morphological differentiation gradient from lymphocyte to a plasmacytic cell can be observed in about 20% of cases [2]. While none of the infiltration patterns and morphological aspects described are specific to SMZL, their combination is rather characteristic [36].

9.5 Spleen

The cut surface of the spleen displays a micronodular white miliary-like pattern as a result of the neoplastic infiltration centred on pre-existing follicles. Microscopic examination shows pre-existing lymphoid follicles infiltrated or substituted by small B-lymphocytes with round or slightly irregular nuclei effacing the follicle mantle zone. In the outer peripheral part of the follicle, the marginal zone, neoplastic cells are of medium size and have a clear pale cytoplasm giving rise to a distinctive biphasic picture [2, 37]. Scattered transformed blasts outline the follicle marginal zone and can infiltrate the red pulp intermingled with small B-lymphocytes and marginal zone-like cells [38]. A variable degree of lymphoplasmacytic differentiation can be found with micronodular or patchy infiltration pattern in the marginal zone, characteristically in germinal centres, and the red pulp [39].

9.6 Immunophenotype

SMZL clonal B-cells do not express a specific immunophenotype. All neoplastic cells consistently express CD20, CD79a, BCL2 and variably DBA44 and are negative for CD10, BCL6, cyclin D1/BCL1, CD43 and annexin A1. SMZL cells carry surface immunoglobulin IgM and IgD with moderate to strong intensity [2, 40]. About 15% of cases are CD5 positive, and 20% of cases may express CD23. CD5 expression correlates with higher lymphocytosis and diffuse infiltration pattern of the bone marrow [41]. The Matutes flow cytometry score [42] is low in SMZL, ranging from 0 to 2.

9.7 Genetic and Biomolecular Landscape

SMZL displays a high genomic complexity [43]; genetic aberrations are documented in over 70% of patients and are complex in 53% of cases (defined as ≥3 aberrations or ≥2 clones). Although no specific genetic alteration has been described so far, deletions of chromosome 7q are quite characteristic [44, 45], occurring with significantly higher frequency (30–40%) in SMZL than in other lymphoid neoplasms. Also, there are a plethora of recurring abnormalities shared with other MZL subtypes. These include gains of 3q, 9q, 12q and 18q, and losses of 6q, 8p, 14q and 17p- [43, 46]. At variance with most other B-cell lymphomas, in SMZL, specific recurrent chromosomal translocations are not described. The immunoglobulin heavy chain variable region (IGVH) genes mutational analysis show that only 15% of cases carry truly unmutated IGVH. In mutated cases, the load of somatic hypermutation ranges from minimal (97–99.9% germline identity) to pronounced [47–50]. Furthermore, the analysis of immunoglobulin genes shows a highly restricted gene repertoire and biased use of the IGVH allele IGHV1–2*04 in 25–40% of cases [47, 51]. Most of these rearrangements (95%) have a low mutational load (97–99.9% germline identity) of conservative nature and restricted distribution. A parallel picture has emerged from the investigation of the clonotypic immunoglobulin light chains revealing restrictions in both kappa (IGKV) and lambda (IGLV) variable gene repertoires [52]. Most of these rearrangements display a minimal mutational load (97–99.9% germline identity) and a long CDR3 sequence with common motifs. Moreover, a stereotyped configuration of the B-cell receptor (BCR) has been detected in 10% of cases [53]. Overall, these findings strongly point to a possible selection of T-cell-independent MZ B-cells by superantigens and suggest that an antigenic drive might play a role in SMZL development [54, 55]. Whole-exome sequencing in SMZL reveals an expression signature consistently characterised by upregulation of genes involved in MZ cell differentiation and circulation between the functional compartments of the lymphoid tissues [56–60]. Recurring mutations in SMZL can be classified into three main groups: NOTCH signalling, nuclear factor kB (NF-kB) pathway, chromatin remodelling and the cytoskeleton [54, 61]. Inactivating mutations of the Krüppel-like factor 2 (KLF2) zinc finger gene occur in 20–40% of SMZL cases [56, 57], resulting in the most frequent somatic change detected in SMZL. Mutated KLF2 delocalises from the nucleus into the cytoplasm and is not able to inhibit the NF-κB activation by upstream signalling, including the BCR and TLR pathways. Interestingly, KLF2 lesions frequently co-occur with IGHV1–2*04 usage, NOTCH2 mutations, and 7q deletions. NOTCH2 and NOTCH1 genes are mutated in 10–25% and 5% of SMZLs, respectively; mutations and truncations cluster in the C-terminal PEST domain thus leading to enhanced stability of the active NOTCH intracellular domains [58, 59]. Overall, considering mutations in negative regulators of NOTCH signalling (such as SPEN, DTX1, and MAML2), upregulation of the NOTCH pathway by genetic events occurs in up to 40% of SMZLs. Since NOTCH2 mutations appear to be very rare in other B-cell lymphomas except for DLBCL (5%), in an appropriate clinical contest they turn out to be specific for SMZL. Mutations activating NF-κB signalling are reported in 34% of cases and are mutually exclusive with that of NOTCH pathway. Mutations occur both in genes of canonical and non-canonical NF-kB pathways (TRAF3, MAP3K14, TNFAIP3, IKBKB, BIRC3) and of coding members of upstream pathways of the BCR (CARD11), and TLR (MYD88) [62]. Mutations were also found in chromatin remodeler genes such as MLL2 (6/40 cases), ARID1A (2/40), and SIN3A (3/40), and more frequently in CREBBP and TP53 (15% of cases) [59]. Methylation changes described in SMZL are associated with silencing of diverse tumour suppressor genes and over-expression of genes involved in BCR/PI3K/AKT/ NF-κB signalling [61, 63]. Finally, an SMZL miRNA signature has been described, targeting some of the key genes and pathways involved in NF-kB activation and B-cell survival. The pattern of miRNA expression is different in HCV positive cases, also showing downregulation of miR-26b, a miRNA with tumour suppressor activity [64].

9.8 Diagnosis

A vast and heterogeneous array of lymphoid neoplasms may show limited or prevalent homing and growth in the spleen. The definition of splenic lymphomas encompasses cases with splenic involvement and in which the disease may also extend to the BM, peripheral blood and the liver, in the absence of prominent lymph node involvement [65]. Some lymphoid neoplasms typically occur confined to the spleen, whereas for others, this presentation is a possible and rare clinical variant (Table 9.1). While presenting clinical, laboratory, pathologic and immunophenotypic features of such lymphomas display significant overlaps, clinical course, biological characteristics and outcomes differ significantly ranging from indolent to very aggressive [9]. Thus, to establish an accurate diagnosis of SMZL is of

Table 9.1 Primary splenic lymphomas (PSL)

(a) Lymphomas commonly presenting as PSL
• Splenic marginal zone lymphoma
• lymphoma/leukemia unclassifiableSplenic diffuse red pulp B-cell lymphomaHairy-cell leukemia variant
• Hairy cell leukemia
• Lymphoplasmacytic lymphoma
• B-cell prolymphocytic leukemia
• T-cell large granular lymphocytic leukemia
• Hepatosplenic T-cell lymphoma
(b) Primary nodal lymphomas occasionally presenting as PSL
• Mantle cell lymphoma
• Follicular lymphoma
• Diffuse large B-cell lymphoma not otherwise specified
• Micronodular T-cell/histiocyte rich large B-cell lymphoma

Splenic lymphomas encompass cases with splenic involvement and in which the disease may also extend to the bone marrow, peripheral blood, and the liver, in the absence of prominent lymph node involvement

Table 9.2 Criteria for coding clinical response in SMZL

Response to splenectomy	
	All the following: • At least 50% improvement on the blood counts • Non-progressive lymphocytosis • No change or improvement in the degree of BM infiltration
Response to systemic treatment	
PR	*50% or greater improvement in the disease manifestations*: • Resolution or decrease in spleen size • Improvement on cytopenias • Resolution or decrease in lymphadenopathy if present • BM should show a decrease in the level of lymphoid infiltration and improvement of the hemopoietic reserve
CR	*All the following*: • Resolution of organomegaly • Normalization of the blood counts § • No evidence of circulating clonal B cells • No evidence or minor BM infiltration detected by immunohistochemistry
NR	Less than 10% improvement on the disease manifestations or deterioration of the above, respectively.

PR partial remission, *CR* complete remission, *NR* no response

[a]Haemoglobin >120 g/L; platelets > 100×10^9 L^{-1}; neutrophils >1.5×10^9 L and no evidence of circulating clonal B cells)

paramount importance for the different appropriate treatment strategies, prognosis and outcomes of these other lymphomas. Spleen histology still is the reference for the diagnosis of SMZL. However, splenectomy is a major surgical procedure with morbidity mostly due to perioperative complications, late infections and even mortality [66, 67]. On the clinical ground, in a substantial proportion of splenic lymphomas, splenectomy could be not advised and or not have a therapeutic role [68]. The SMZL study group (SMZLSG) provided an expert guideline aimed to establish the diagnosis of SMZL when information on the spleen histology is not available [22]. Indeed, consistent integration of BM histological and immunohistochemical findings with the results of the various clinical, laboratory investigations, including peripheral blood morphology, immunophenotype, genetics and molecular biology, usually allows for diagnosis with a reasonably high level of confidence. The differential diagnosis in some instances is particularly challenging, such as that between SMZL and lymphoplasmacytic lymphoma in patients that have a serum IgM monoclonal paraprotein and or show lymphoplasmacytic differentiation. Yet after such a thorough and integrated examination, in some cases only a generic diagnosis of B-cell chronic lymphoproliferative disorder can be reached [9, 36, 69]. In such instances, if the differential diagnostic problem should affect treatment choices and outcome expectations, it is required to resort to splenectomy to reach a definite diagnosis.

9.9 Staging and Prognostic Scores

SMZL has a peculiar way of presentation, diffusion and evolution. The criteria for staging and evaluation of the response to therapy proposed by the SMZLSG still constitute a reference (Table 9.2). SMZL is not conceived as a fluorodeoxyglucose avid disease [70] and should routinely be staged through computed tomography. The use of fdg-PET scans could be clinically useful whenever an evolution towards aggressive histology is suspected. Nevertheless, the role of fdg-PET [71] and new imaging techniques, such as whole-body MRI [72] in staging and response assessment, has not been specifically investigated yet. SMZL is a neoplasm with a rather favourable prognosis given that about two-thirds of patients are alive five years after the diagnosis [26, 73] and about 20% do not need any therapy for several years. However, around 20% of patients experience a more aggressive course and shorter survival. Understandably, the different and particular features of presentation and diffusion make the prognostic scores built for the other lymphoproliferative neoplasms unsuited for SMZL. The first specifically conceived clinical scoring system was developed by the Intergruppo Italiano linfomi (IIL, now Federazione Italiana Linfomi: FIL) on 309 SMZL patients with a 5-year cause-specific survival (CSS) rate of 76%. The prognostic score was built by selecting the three variables with the highest hazard ratios for a shorter CSS, (haemoglobin <12 g/dL, elevated LDH and albumin <35 g/dL). By using these variables, three prognostic groups were identified: low-risk (no adverse factor), intermediate-risk (one adverse factor) and high-risk (two or more adverse factors) with statistically different 5-year CSS ($P = 0.001$) of 88%, 73% and 50%, respectively [26]. Interestingly, the high-risk group intercepted 54% of all lymphoma deaths. Subsequently, the SMZLSG proposed a risk stratification system based on the assessment of four variables developed on a large series of 593 patients [25]. The score was named HPLL, after the determinant factors H (haemoglobin), P (platelet count), L (LDH) and L (extra-hilar lymphadenopathy) found in correlation with a shorter lymphoma specific survival (LSS). According to the number of variables, three groups were identified: A (no adverse factor), B (1 or 2 adverse factors) and C (3 or 4 adverse factors) with survival at five years of 95%, 87% and 68%, respectively. In the HPLL score both haemoglobin and platelets are accounted as a continuous variable to obtain the best fit, and the application of the score requires a calculation by a formula; thus a simplified version of the prognostic score was developed to make more comfortable its use in daily clinical practice [74]. To this end, the same four risk factors were used, and clinically acceptable cut-off points of 9.5 g/dL for haemoglobin level and 80×10^9 L^{-1} for platelet count were established. Patients with 0, 1, 2, 3 or 4 factors were separated in a final set of three groups: A: 198 patients (0); B: 311 patients (1 or 2); C: 41 patients (3 or 4) with 5-year LSS significantly different among the three risk groups. Recently, Kalpadakis et al. have validated this simplified HPLL score in an independent series of SMZL patients, confirming its ability in identifying subgroups of SMZL patients with a significantly different outcome [75]. However, clinical scores are surrogate markers which imperfectly intercept disease outcome differences. Thus, a great effort has been focused on studies aimed to explore the prognostic value of biomolecular markers. Parameters that have been associated with adverse outcomes are p53 mutation, 7q deletion, NOTCH2 mutation and the absence of somatic mutation in IgVH genes and aberrant promoter methylation [43, 47, 58, 76–78]. However, other studies have reported conflicting results [59, 79].

9.10 Therapy

Diverse therapeutic options, including splenectomy, chemotherapy, rituximab monotherapy and chemoimmunotherapy, produce clinical responses and effective control of SMZL-related symptoms. However, no prospective randomised study specifically designed for SMZL has been conducted so far, and there is no clue that any of the proposed therapies can appreciably modify the natural history of the disease [73, 74, 80]. Furthermore, the comparison of retrospective studies is made particularly difficult by the lack of prospectively validated prognostic scores and uniform criteria for initiation of therapy. According to the recently updated ESMO guidelines [81], and expert statements [9, 22, 54], only symptomatic patients should receive treatment. Currently, effective palliation should be pursued by rituximab monotherapy or with splenectomy if it is deemed necessary also for diagnostic purposes [81].

9.11 Watchful Waiting

About 20–30% of newly diagnosed SMZL patients are asymptomatic [4–6], can remain stable for several years and there is no evidence that they would benefit from early therapeutic intervention. In the large retrospective series of SMZLSG [25], 161 patients (27%) had not received any treatment and only three of them (1.8%) ultimately died of lymphoma. These data support the reliability and safety of adopting a watchful and waiting strategy in asymptomatic patients and suggest avoiding splenectomy for mere diagnostic purposes. Patients in vigilant waiting policy may be followed every 3–6 months with a physical examination, blood counts and biochemistry [9, 22]. SMZL patients showing an active HCV infection constitute the exception to the "no move" strategy described for asymptomatic patients, and antiviral treatment should be considered as a first-line treatment [81, 82].

9.12 HCV Antiviral Treatment

In a seminal observation, Hermine et al. showed that interferon-based antiviral treatment (AVT) can induce haematological response along with virological clearance in patients with HCV-associated splenic lymphoma with villous lymphocytes [15]. Subsequently, the association of interferon with ribavirine has been confirmed effective in several series of HCV-associated lymphomas, and particularly MZL [83]. Further, a recent a meta-analysis on 20 studies of IFN-based antiviral therapy (AVT) in patients with HCV-associated B-NHL showed that the response rate was 73% in all patients and up to 83% in those who attained a sustained virological response (SVR) [84]. A better lymphoma response was shown in MZL compared to no-MZL (81% vs.71%). A direct anti-lymphoma activity of interferon cannot be ruled out, particularly in MZL. Nevertheless, recent data on the efficacy of new IFN-free regimens with direct-acting antivirals (DAA) in a retrospective series of 46 HCV-associated lymphoproliferative disorders suggest their anti-lymphoma activity [85]. The median duration of DAA therapy was 12 weeks (range, 6–24 weeks). An SVR after finishing DAAs was obtained in 45 patients (98%): the overall lymphoproliferative disease response rate (LDR) was 67%, including 12 patients (26%) who achieved a complete response. The LDR rate was 73% among patients with MZL, whereas no response was observed in CLL/SLL patients. Seven patients cleared cryoglobulins out of 15 who were initially positive. After a median follow-up of 8 months, 1-year progression-free and overall survival rates were 75% (95% confidence interval [CI], 51–88) and 98% [95% CI, 86–100], respectively. DAA therapy induces a high LDR rate in HCV-associated indolent lymphomas. These data strongly support a causative role of HCV in lymphomagenesis and prospective trials with DAAs in this setting are underway.

9.13 Who Needs Anti-neoplastic Treatment?

Treatment should be initiated in patients with symptomatic splenomegaly, cytopenia(s), systemic symptoms or progressive nodal disease [22, 81]. These criteria are clinically sound but have not been prospectively validated yet. Noteworthy, three of these criteria (lymphatic adenopathy, anaemia and thrombocytopenia) are independently associated with LSS and were incorporated in the HPLL risk stratification for SMZL. Consensus guidelines suggest that autoimmune cytopenias should be specifically treated and antiviral treatment should be considered in patients with concurrent active HCV chronic infection with HCV-related hepatitis who do not need immediate conventional treatment against the lymphoma [81, 85].

9.14 Splenectomy

Splenectomy provides the tissue for diagnosis and has been considered the first-choice treatment for SMZL in the pre-rituximab era [32, 80] Indeed, after surgery, a quick relief from pressure-and volume-related symptoms (abdominal discom-

Table 9.3 Series of SMZL reporting splenectomy as first-line therapy

Year-author	# of pts	ORR	PFS % (at *n* years)	OS % (at *n* years)	Surgery related deaths
1991-Mulligan et al.	20	96	Median 4 years	NR	1
1996-Troussard et al.	28	75	NR	71 (5)	1
2002-Chacon et al.	60	93	Median 40 months	65 (5)	NR
2002-Thieblemont et al.	48	100	Median 4 years	NR	NR
2003-Parry-Jones et al.	33	NR	NR	95 (10)	NR
2004-Iannitto et al.	21	91	Median 4 years	NR	NR
2006-Tsimberidou et al.	10	60	Median 4 years	83 (3)	0
2012-Olszewski et al.	652	NR	80 (3)	67.8 (5)	NR
2013-Kalpadakis et al.	27	86	58 (5)	77 (5)	1
2014-Lenglet et al.	100	97	61 (5)	84 (5)	0
2015-Xing et al.	52	NR	39 (10)	61 (10)	0
2015-Pata et al.	41	90	35 (5)	75 (5)	0

ORR overall response rate, *PFS* progression-free survival, *OS* overall survival

fort, early satiety) and complete or partial recovery of cytopenia(s) are expected in all and up to 90% of patients, respectively [4, 6, 86, 87]. Though clinical responses to splenectomy are not complete since extra-splenic disease persists, they are durable; published series report a 5-year PFS of approximately 35–61% and OS ranging from 61% to 75% (Table 9.3). However, these data should be taken cautiously because in many series of splenectomised patients post-splenectomy chemotherapy has been delivered in a significant proportion of cases. Furthermore, splenectomy does not modify the natural history of the disease, and particularly the risk of histologic transformation into DLBCL, which ranges between 11% and 14% in the largest series [43, 86]. Finally, splenectomy is a major surgical procedure and is associated with morbidity and even a low-risk of mortality. Perioperative complications in surgical series on SMZL occur in 25–35% of patients and are mostly due to pulmonary dysfunction and major bleeding [88, 89]. Although perioperative mortality is <1%, significant long-term mortality of about 5% due to infectious complications is reported [86, 87]. Therefore, a possible indication for the therapeutic splenectomy should be limited to patients complaining of symptoms related to the presence of splenomegaly (abdominal discomfort and or hypersplenism), minimal bone marrow disease, absent nodal involvement and without lung comorbidities. Immunisation against encapsulated bacteria is mandatory in all patients at least 2 weeks before elective surgery and sepsis prevention measures must be maintained throughout life [90].

9.15 Chemotherapy

Single-agent chemotherapy has been used in the past mainly in patients relapsed to splenectomy and or with advanced disease, often extended to lymph nodes and analysed in small retrospective series; a detailed and comprehensive analysis on this topic is reported elsewhere [31]. Alkylating agents proved to be not effective, while purine analogues produced a significant number of complete clinical responses though at the expense of haematological and infectious toxicity. These data are now outdated by rituximab therapy, and chemotherapy alone is no longer recommended as first-line treatment.

9.16 Rituximab Monotherapy

Bennet's 2005 report on the efficacy of the anti CD20 monoclonal antibody rituximab in a series of 11 SMZL patients has paved a new way in the treatment of SMZL [91]. Several other retrospective series have subsequently shown that rituximab monotherapy yields up to 90% of clinical responses, half these responses being complete even at molecular level, with minimal toxicity (Table 9.4). Furthermore, in many cases after relapse, rituximab re-treatment is still effective. On these premises, according to the ESMO guidelines, rituximab monotherapy is a reasonable first-line treatment as effective and less traumatic than splenectomy [81]. The Italian Society of Hematology guidelines specifies that rituximab monotherapy is the therapy of choice for patients without disseminated disease who need treatment and unfit for splenectomy [85]. In a large series of consecutively treated patients, Kalpadakis et al. [92] first reported that the 5-year overall and progression-free survival (PFS) rates for rituximab-treated and splenectomised patients were comparable: 92% and77% ($p = 0.09$) and 73% and 58% ($p = 0.06$), respectively, and that 2-year maintenance therapy with rituximab resulted in a longer duration of response (at 5 years, PFS was 84% for patients receiving maintenance and 36% for patients without maintenance, $p =$ 0001). This study has been recently updated and extended to 108 patients [93]. The overall response rate after the end of induction treatment was 92% (CR 44%; Cru 21%; PR 27%). Rituximab maintenance therapy, one shot every two months for two years, improved the quality of response in 16/77 patients: 14/22 (64%) patients in PR achieved either CR (n5) or Cru (n11). The outcomes were remarkable: the 5- and 10-year FFP rates were 71% and 64%; the 5- and 10-year OS rates were 93% and 85%, and the 5- and 10-year LSS rates were 99% and 90%, respectively. PFS was significantly better in patients who received maintenance (7-year PFS 75% for patients who received maintenance vs. 39% for those who did not, $p < 0.0004$) but no difference in OS was noticed between patients who received maintenance and those who did not.

9.17 Chemoimmunotherapy

Rituximab in combination with chemotherapy (R-chemo) is the standard of care for the treatment of indolent lymphomas, but due to toxicity concerns, the indication for SMZL is currently limited to fit patients with suspected histological transformation and or with constitutional symptoms [81, 85] or disseminated disease. Seven clinical studies, five retrospective [94–98] and two prospective [99, 100], dedicated to investigating the role of R-chemo in SMZL have been published so far (Table 9.5). Overall, the accumulated experience on a total of 302 patients suggests that the R-chemo yields higher CR rates and comparable duration of response and PFS [96, 97, 99, 100] rates than rituximab monotherapy [93, 94]. In 2015, the FIL group published the first multicentre prospective study dedicated to SMZL. Fifty-one patients with SMZL were treated with a modified R-CHOP: rituximab, cyclophosphamide, vincristine, non-pegylated liposomal doxorubicin and prednisone (R-COMP). The ORR and

Table 9.4 Rituximab monotherapy

Year-author	# pts	Patients Status	ORR	CRR	PFS % (at *n* years)	OS % (at *n* years)
2005-Bennet et al.	11	RR	91	NR	60 (5)	60 (5)
2006-Tsimberidou et al.	25	First-line	88	31	86 (3)	86 (3)
2007-Kalpadakis et al.	16	First-line	100	69	92 (2.4)	92 (2.4)
2012-Else et al	10	RR and First-line	100	90	89 (3)	89 (3)
2013-Kalpadakis et al.	58	First-line	95	45	73 (5)	73 (59)
2018-Kalpadakis et al	104	First-line	92	47	64 (10)	88 (10)

RR relapsed or resistant, *ORR* overall response rate, *CRR* complete response rate, *PFS* progression-free survival, *OS* overall survival

Table 9.5 Rituximab plus chemotherapy

Year-author	Patients status	Schema	# pts	Response		Survival	
				ORR, %	CRR, %	FFS/PFS/DOR (at *n* years)	OS (at *n* years)
2006-Tsimberidou	First-line	R-chemo	6	83	34	FFS 100% at 3 years	100% at 5 years
2010-Cervetti	RR and First-line	R-2CdA	47	87	62	PFS 80% at 5 years	83% at 3 years
2012-Else	RR and First-line	R-chemo	33	100	70	DSF 71% at 3 years	NR
2015-Iannitto[a]	First-line	R-COMP	51	84	65	PFS 54% at 6 years	72% at 6 years
2017-Cervetti	First-line	R-CTX	30	87	70	20 months (median)	(10)
2017-Castelli	First-line	R-Benda	70	86	70	DOR 18 months (median)	NR
2018-Iannitto[a]	First-line	R-Benda	65	91	73	PFS 90 at 3 years	96% at 3 years

[a]Prospective study; *ORR* overall response rate, *CRR* complete remission rate, *OS* overall survival, *FFS* failure-free survival, *mth* months, *PFS* progression-free survival, *DOR* duration of response, *R* rituximab, *benda* bendamustine, *Chemo* chemotherapy, *CTX* cytoxan, *COMP* cytoxan, oncovin, myocet, prednisone, *2CdA* 2-chlodesoxyadenosine

CR rates were 84% and 65%, respectively; 6-year PFS was 54% and OS was 72%. Overall, toxicity was R-CHOP alike, moderate and manageable but two toxic deaths were recorded (grade >3 neutropenia, 26%; grade >3 infections, 8%; two deaths as a result of infection). A large amount of data indicates the association bendamustine-rituximab (BR) as an effective regimen with an acceptable toxicity profile on almost the entire spectrum of indolent lymphomas [101]. Recently, two studies have explored the role of this association in SMZL [97, 101]. In a retrospective analysis of 70 consecutive SMZL patients treated with BR, 60 patients (86%) achieved a complete response (CR), and seven (10%) a partial response (PR). Three patients (4.3%) experienced disease progression (PD). The median duration of remission was 18 months. Side effects were generally mild [97]. These promising results were prospectively confirmed by the IELSG36/BRISMA study [101]. Sixty-five patients received BR at standard doses q28 and were restaged after three cycles: those patients in CR received a further BR cycle as consolidation while those in PR completed the entire six-course cycles. The OR and CR rates were 91% and 73%, respectively. DOR, PFS and OS at 3 years were 93% (95CI 81–98), 90% (95CI 77–96) and 96% (95CI 84–98), respectively. Toxicity was mostly haematological. Neutropenia G ≥ 3 was recorded in 43% of patients, infections and febrile neutropenia in 5.4% and 3.6%. Most of the non-haematological toxicities were G ≤ 2. Furthermore, more than half of the patients examined achieved molecular remission. A molecular marker was found in 43/54 (80%) cases and MRD negativisation rates were 47% at interim restaging (BM: 13/32; PB: 21/36), 54% at completion of treatment (BM: 10/23; PB: 18/22) and 61% after 1 year (BM:14/22; PB: 19/29) [102].

References

1. Khalil MO, Morton LM, Devesa SS, Check DP, Curtis RE, Weisenburger DD, et al. Incidence of marginal zone lymphoma in the United States, 2001–2009 with a focus on primary anatomic site. Br J Haematol. 2014;165(1):67–77.
2. Piris MA, Isaacson PG, Swerdlow SH, Thieblemont C, Pittaluga S, Rossi D, et al. Splenic marginal zone lymphoma. In: Swerdlow SH, Campo E, Harris NL, Jaffe ES, Pileri SA, Stein H, et al., editors. WHO classification of tumours of haematopoietic and lymphoid tissues. 2nd ed. Lyon: IARC Press; 2017. p. 223–5.
3. Sohani AR, Zukerberg LR. Small B-cell lymphomas of the spleen: how to tell them apart. J Hematop. 2014;7(3):109–21.

4. Thieblemont C, Felman P, Berger FF, Dumontet C, Arnaud P, Hequet O, et al. Treatment of splenic marginal zone b-cell lymphoma: an analysis of 81 patients. Clin Lymphoma. 2002;3(1):41–7. http://www.ncbi.nlm.nih.gov/pubmed/12141954.
5. Iannitto E, Ambrosetti A, Ammatuna E, Colosio M, Florena AMAM, Tripodo C, et al. Splenic marginal zone lymphoma with or without villous lymphocytes: hematologic findings and outcomes in a series of 57 patients. Cancer. 2004;101(9):2050–7.
6. Parry-Jones N, Matutes E, Gruszka-Westwood AM, Swansbury GJ, Wotherspoon AC, Catovsky D. Prognostic features of splenic lymphoma with villous lymphocytes: a report on 129 patients. Br J Haematol. 2003;120(5):759–64. http://www.ncbi.nlm.nih.gov/pubmed/12614206.
7. Liu L, Wang H, Chen Y, Rustveld L, Liu G, Du XL. Splenic marginal zone lymphoma: a population-based study on the 2001–2008 incidence and survival in the United States. Leuk Lymphoma. 2013;54(7):1380–6.
8. Oscier D, R.Owen SJ. Splenic marginal zone lymphoma. Blood Rev. 2005;19:39–51.
9. Iannitto E, Tripodo C. How I diagnose and treat splenic lymphomas. Blood. 2011;117(9):2585–95. http://www.ncbi.nlm.nih.gov/pubmed/21119113.
10. Sriskandarajah P, Dearden CE. Epidemiology and environmental aspects of marginal zone lymphomas. Best Pract Res Clin Haematol. 2017;30(1–2):84–91. https://doi.org/10.1016/j.beha.2016.07.002.
11. Arcaini L, Burcheri S, Rossi A, Paulli M, Bruno R, Passamonti F, et al. Prevalence of HCV infection in nongastric marginal zone B-cell lymphoma of MALT. Ann Oncol. October 2006;2007:346–50.
12. Iqbal T, Mahale P, Turturro F, Kyvernitakis ATH. Prevalence and association of hepatitis C virus infection with different types of lymphoma. Int J Cancer. 2016;138(4):1035–7.
13. Couronné L, Bachy E, Roulland S, Nadel B, Davi F, Armand M, Canioni DMJ, Visco C, Arcaini L, Besson CHO. From hepatitis C virus infection to B-cell lymphoma. Ann Oncol. 2018;28(1):92–100.
14. Pozzato G, Mazzaro C, Maso LD, Mauro E, Zorat F, Moratelli G, et al. Hepatitis C virus and non-Hodgkin's lymphomas: meta-analysis of epidemiology data and therapy options. World J Hepatol. 2016;8(2):107–16.
15. Hermine O, Lefrère F, Bronowicki JP, Mariette X, Jondeau K, Eclache-Saudreau V, et al. Regression of splenic lymphoma with villous lymphocytes after treatment of hepatitis C virus infection. N Engl J Med. 2002;347(2):89–94.
16. Arcaini L, Besson C, Frigeni M, Fontaine H, Goldaniga M, Casato M, et al. Interferon-free antiviral treatment in B-cell lymphoproliferative disorders associated with hepatitis C virus infection. Blood. 2016;128(21):2527–32. https://ashpublications.org/blood/article/128/21/2527/35718/Interferonfree-antiviral-treatment-in-Bcell.
17. Vallisa D, Bernuzzi P, Arcaini L, Sacchi S, Callea V, LA Marasca R, Trabacchi E, Anselmi E, Arcari AL, Moroni C, Bertè R, Lazzarino MCL. Role of anti-hepatitis C virus (HCV) treatment in HCV-related, low-grade, B-cell, non-Hodgkin's lymphoma: a multicenter Italian experience. J Clin Oncol. 2005;23(3):468–73.
18. Bracci PM, Benavente Y, Turner JJ, Paltiel O, Slager SL, Vajdic CM, et al. Medical history, lifestyle, family history, and occupational risk factors for marginal zone lymphoma: the interLymph non-Hodgkin lymphoma subtypes project. J Natl Cancer Inst Monogr. 2014;48:52–65.
19. Franco V, Florena AM, Iannitto E. Splenic marginal zone lymphoma. Blood. 2003;101(7):2464–72. http://www.ncbi.nlm.nih.gov/pubmed/12446449.
20. Berger F, Felman P, Thieblemont C, Pradier T, Baseggio L, Bryon PA, et al. Non-MALT marginal zone B-cell lymphomas: a description of clinical presentation and outcome in 124 patients. Blood. 2000;95(6):1950–6.
21. Perrone S, D'Elia GM, Annechini G, Ferretti A, Tosti ME, Foà R, et al. Splenic marginal zone lymphoma: prognostic factors, role of watch and wait policy, and other therapeutic approaches in the rituximab era. Leuk Res. 2016;44:53–60. https://doi.org/10.1016/j.leukres.2016.03.005.
22. Matutes E, Oscier D, Montalban C, Berger F, Callet-Bauchu E, Dogan A, et al. Splenic marginal zone lymphoma proposals for a revision of diagnostic, staging and therapeutic criteria. Leukemia. 2008;22(3):487–95. http://www.nature.com/doifinder/10.1038/sj.leu.2405068.
23. Xochelli A, Kalpadakis C, Gardiner A, Baliakas P, Vassilakopoulos TP, Mould S, et al. Clonal B-cell lymphocytosis exhibiting immunophenotypic features consistent with a marginal-zone origin: is this a distinct entity? Blood. 2014;123(8):1199–206. https://ashpublications.org/blood/article/123/8/1199/32835/Clonal-Bcell-lymphocytosis-exhibiting.
24. Parker H, McIver-Brown NR, Davis ZA, Parry M, Rose-Zerilli MJJ, Xochelli A, et al. CBL-MZ is not a single biological entity: evidence from genomic analysis and prolonged clinical follow-up. Blood Adv. 2018;2(10):1116–9.
25. Montalbán C, Abraira V, Arcaini L, Domingo-Domenech E, Guisado-Vasco P, Iannitto E, et al. Risk stratification for splenic marginal zone lymphoma based on haemoglobin concentration, platelet count, high lactate dehydrogenase level and extrahilar lymphadenopathy: development and validation on 593 cases. Br J Haematol. 2012;159(2):164–71. http://www.ncbi.nlm.nih.gov/pubmed/22924582.
26. Arcaini L, Lazzarino M, Colombo N, Burcheri S, Boveri E, Paulli M, et al. Splenic marginal zone lymphoma: a prognostic model for clinical use. Blood. 2006;107(12):4643–9.
27. Saadoun D, Suarez F, Lefrere F, Valensi F, Mariette X, Aouba A, et al. Splenic lymphoma with villous

lymphocytes, associated with type II cryoglobulinemia and HCV infection: a new entity? Blood. 2005;105(1):74–6.
28. Teixeira Mendes LS, Wotherspoon A. Marginal zone lymphoma: associated autoimmunity and autoimmune disorders. Best Pract Res Clin Haematol. 2017;30(1–2):65–76. https://doi.org/10.1016/j.beha.2016.07.006.
29. Sbattella M, Zanichelli A, Ghia P, Gattei V, Suffritti C, Teatini T, et al. Splenic marginal zone lymphomas in acquired C1-inhibitor deficiency: clinical and molecular characterization. Med Oncol. 2018;35(9):118. https://doi.org/10.1007/s12032-018-1183-7.
30. Gebhart J, Lechner K, Skrabs C, Sliwa T, Müldür E, Ludwig H, et al. Lupus anticoagulant and thrombosis in splenic marginal zone lymphoma. Thromb Res. 2014;134(5):980–4. https://linkinghub.elsevier.com/retrieve/pii/S0049384814004575.
31. Matutes E. Splenic marginal zone lymphoma: disease features and management. Expert Rev Hematol. 2013;6(6):735–45. http://www.tandfonline.com/doi/full/10.1586/17474086.2013.845522.
32. Mulligan SP, Matutes E, Dearden C, Catovsky D. Splenic lymphoma with villous lymphocytes: natural history and response to therapy in 50 cases. Br J Haematol. 1991;78(2):206–9. https://doi.org/10.1111/j.1365-2141.1991.tb04417.x.
33. Troussard X, Valensi F, Duchayne E, Garand R, Felman P, Tulliez M, et al. Splenic lymphoma with villous lymphocytes: clinical presentation, biology and prognostic factors in a series of 100 patients. Groupe Francais d'Hématologie Cellulaire (GFHC). Br J Haematol. 1996;93(3):731–6. http://www.ncbi.nlm.nih.gov/pubmed/8652403.
34. Franco V, Florena AM, Campesi G. Intrasinusoidal bone marrow infiltration: a possible hallmark of splenic lymphoma. Histopathology. 1996;29(6):571–5. https://onlinelibrary.wiley.com/doi/abs/10.1046/j.1365-2559.1996.d01-536.x.
35. Franco V, Florena AM, Stella M, Rizzo A, Iannitto E, Quintini G, et al. Splenectomy influences bone marrow infiltration in patients with splenic marginal zone cell lymphoma with or without villous lymphocytes. Cancer. 2001;91(2):294–301. http://www.ncbi.nlm.nih.gov/pubmed/11180074.
36. Ponzoni M, Kanellis G, Pouliou E, Baliakas P, Scarfò L, Ferreri AJM, et al. Bone marrow histopathology in the diagnostic evaluation of splenic marginal-zone and splenic diffuse red pulp small B-cell lymphoma. Am J Surg Pathol. 2012;36(11):1609–18. https://insights.ovid.com/crossref?an=00000478-201211000-00003.
37. Schmid C, Kirkham N, Diss T, Isaacson PG. Splenic marginal zone cell lymphoma. Am J Surg Pathol. 1992;16(5):455–66. https://insights.ovid.com/crossref?an=00000478-199205000-00004.
38. Lloret E, Mollejo M, Mateo MS, Villuendas R, Algara P, Martínez P, et al. Splenic marginal zone lymphoma with increased number of blasts: an aggressive variant? Hum Pathol. 1999;30(10):1153–60. https://linkinghub.elsevier.com/retrieve/pii/S004681779990031X.
39. Van Huyen J-PD, Molina T, Delmer A, Audouin J, Le Tourneau A, Zittoun R, et al. Splenic marginal zone lymphoma with or without plasmacytic differentiation. Am J Surg Pathol. 2000;24(12):1581–92. https://insights.ovid.com/crossref?an=00000478-200012000-00001.
40. Rancoita MV, Campos CP, De Forconi F, Ponzoni M, Govi S, Andrés JM, et al. High-grade transformation in splenic marginal zone lymphoma with circulating villous lymphocytes: the site of transformation influences response to therapy and prognosis. Br J Haematol. 2008;143(1):71–4. https://doi.org/10.1016/j.humpath.2009.09.007.
41. Baseggio L, Traverse-Glehen A, Petinataud F, Callet-Bauchu E, Berger F, Ffrench M, et al. CD5 expression identifies a subset of splenic marginal zone lymphomas with higher lymphocytosis: a clinico-pathological, cytogenetic and molecular study of 24 cases. Haematologica. 2010;95(4):604–12. http://www.haematologica.org/cgi/doi/10.3324/haematol.2009.011049.
42. Matutes E, Owusu-Ankomah K, Morilla R, Garcia Marco J, Houlihan A, Que TH, et al. The immunological profile of B-cell disorders and proposal of a scoring system for the diagnosis of CLL. Leukemia. 1994;8(10):1640–5. http://www.ncbi.nlm.nih.gov/pubmed/7523797.
43. Salido M, Baró C, Oscier D, Stamatopoulos K, Dierlamm J, Matutes E, et al. Cytogenetic aberrations and their prognostic value in a series of 330 splenic marginal zone B-cell lymphomas: a multicenter study of the Splenic B-Cell Lymphoma Group. Blood. 2010;116(9):1479–88.
44. Mateo M, Mollejo M, Villuendas R, Algara P, Sanchez-Beato M, Martínez P, et al. 7q31-32 allelic loss is a frequent finding in splenic marginal zone lymphoma. Am J Pathol. 1999;154(5):1583–9. https://linkinghub.elsevier.com/retrieve/pii/S0002944010654119.
45. Watkins AJ, Huang Y, Ye H, Chanudet E, Johnson N, Hamoudi R, et al. Splenic marginal zone lymphoma: characterization of 7q deletion and its value in diagnosis. J Pathol. 2010;220(4):461–74. https://doi.org/10.1002/path.2665.
46. Troussard M, Radford-Weiss R, Valensi G, et al. Genetic analysis of splenic lymphoma with villous lymphocytes: a Groupe Français d'Hématologie Cellulaire (GFHC) study. Br J Haematol. 1998;101(4):712–21. https://doi.org/10.1046/j.1365-2141.1998.00764.x.
47. Algara P, Mateo MS, Sanchez-Beato M, Mollejo M, Navas IC, Romero L, et al. Analysis of the IgVH somatic mutations in splenic marginal zone lymphoma defines a group of unmutated cases with frequent 7q deletion and adverse clinical course. Blood. 2002;99(4):1299–304.
48. Stamatopoulos K, Belessi C, Papadaki T, Kalagiakou E, Stavroyianni N, Douka V, et al. Immunoglobulin

heavy- and light-chain repertoire in splenic marginal zone lymphoma. Mol Med. 2004;10(7–12):89–95. https://molmed.biomedcentral.com/articles/10.2119/2005-00001.Stamatopoulos.
49. Kalpadakis C, Pangalis GA, Dimitriadou E, Angelopoulou MK, Siakantaris MP, Kyrtsonis M-C, et al. Mutation analysis of IgVH genes in splenic marginal zone lymphomas : correlation with clinical characteristics and outcome. Blood. 2009;42(5):1811–6. http://www.ncbi.nlm.nih.gov/pubmed/19443409.
50. Zhu D, Orchard J, Oscier DG, Wright DH, Stevenson FK. V H gene analysis of splenic marginal zone lymphomas reveals diversity in mutational status and initiation of somatic mutation in vivo. Blood. 2002;100(7):2659–61. https://ashpublications.org/blood/article/100/7/2659/106207/VH-gene-analysis-of-splenic-marginal-zone.
51. Traverse-Glehen A, Davi F, Ben Simon E, Callet-Bauchu E, Felman P, Baseggio L, et al. Analysis of VH genes in marginal zone lymphoma reveals marked heterogeneity between splenic and nodal tumors and suggests the existence of clonal selection. Haematologica. 2005;90(4):470–8. http://www.ncbi.nlm.nih.gov/pubmed/15820942.
52. Bikos V, Darzentas N, Hadzidimitriou A, Davis Z, Hockley S, Traverse-Glehen A, et al. Over 30% of patients with splenic marginal zone lymphoma express the same immunoglobulin heavy variable gene: ontogenetic implications. Leukemia. 2012;26(7):1638–46.
53. Zibellini S, Capello D, Forconi F, Marcatili P, Rossi D, Rattotti S, et al. Stereotyped patterns of B-cell receptor in splenic marginal zone lymphoma. Haematologica. 2010;95(10):1792–6.
54. Arcaini L, Rossi D, Paulli M. Splenic marginal zone lymphoma: from genetics to management. Blood. 2016;127(17):2072–81.
55. Xochelli A, Bikos V, Polychronidou E, Galigalidou C, Agathangelidis A, Charlotte F, et al. Disease-biased and shared characteristics of the immunoglobulin gene repertoires in marginal zone B cell lymphoproliferations. J Pathol. 2019;247(4):416–21.
56. Piva R, Deaglio S, Famà R, Buonincontri R, Scarfò I, Bruscaggin A, et al. The Krüppel-like factor 2 transcription factor gene is recurrently mutated in splenic marginal zone lymphoma. Leukemia. 2015;29(2):503–7.
57. Clipson A, Wang M, De Leval L, Ashton-Key M, Wotherspoon A, Vassiliou G, et al. KLF2 mutation is the most frequent somatic change in splenic marginal zone lymphoma and identifies a subset with distinct genotype. Leukemia. 2015;29(5):1177–85.
58. Kiel MJ, Velusamy T, Betz BL, Zhao L, Weigelin HG, Chiang MY, et al. Whole-genome sequencing identifies recurrent somatic NOTCH2 mutations in splenic marginal zone lymphoma. J Exp Med. 2012;209(9):1553–65. https://rupress.org/jem/article/209/9/1553/41267/Wholegenome-sequencing-identifies-recurrent.
59. Rossi D, Trifonov V, Fangazio M, Bruscaggin A, Rasi S, Spina V, et al. The coding genome of splenic marginal zone lymphoma: activation of NOTCH2 and other pathways regulating marginal zone development. J Exp Med. 2012;209(9):1537–51. https://rupress.org/jem/article/209/9/1537/41269/The-coding-genome-of-splenic-marginal-zone.
60. Martínez N, Almaraz C, Vaqué JP, Varela I, Derdak S, Beltran S, et al. Whole-exome sequencing in splenic marginal zone lymphoma reveals mutations in genes involved in marginal zone differentiation. Leukemia. 2014;28(6):1334–40. http://www.nature.com/articles/leu2013365.
61. Bertoni F, Rossi D, Zucca E, Bertoni F, Rossi D. Recent advances in understanding the biology of marginal zone lymphoma. F1000Res. 2018;7:1–10.
62. Rossi D, Deaglio S, Dominguez-Sola D, Rasi S, Vaisitti T, Agostinelli C, et al. Alteration of BIRC3 and multiple other NF-κB pathway genes in splenic marginal zone lymphoma. Blood. 2011;118(18):4930–4.
63. Arribas AJ, Gómez-Abad C, Sánchez-Beato M, Martinez N, Dilisio L, Casado F, et al. Splenic marginal zone lymphoma: comprehensive analysis of gene expression and miRNA profiling. Mod Pathol. 2013;26(7):889–901.
64. Peveling-Oberhag J, Crisman G, Schmidt A, Döring C, Lucioni M, Arcaini L, et al. Dysregulation of global microRNA expression in splenic marginal zone lymphoma and influence of chronic hepatitis C virus infection. Leukemia. 2012;26(7):1654–62.
65. Gobbi PG, Grignani GE, Pozzetti U, Bertoloni D, Pieresca C, Montagna G, et al. Primary splenic lymphoma: does it exist? Haematologica. 1994;79(3):286–93. http://www.ncbi.nlm.nih.gov/pubmed/7926983.
66. Baccarani U, Terrosu G, Donini A, Zaja F, Bresadola F, Baccarani M. Splenectomy in hematology. Current practice and new perspectives. Haematologica. 1999;84(5):431–6.
67. Rodeghiero F, Ruggeri M. Short- and long-term risks of splenectomy for benign haematological disorders: should we revisit the indications? Br J Haematol. 2012;158(1):16–29.
68. Fallah J, Olszewski AJ. Diagnostic and therapeutic splenectomy for splenic lymphomas: analysis of the National Cancer Data Base. Hematology (UK). 2019;24(1):378–86.
69. Piris MA, Onaindía A, Mollejo M. Best practice & research clinical haematology splenic marginal zone lymphoma. Best Pract Res Clin Haematol. 2017;30(1–2):56–64. https://doi.org/10.1016/j.beha.2016.09.005.
70. Cheson BD, Fisher RI, Barrington SF, Cavalli F, Schwartz LH, Zucca E, et al. Recommendations for initial evaluation, staging, and response assessment of Hodgkin and non-Hodgkin lymphoma: the Lugano classification. J Clin Oncol. 2014;32(27):3059–68. http://ascopubs.org/doi/10.1200/JCO.2013.54.8800.
71. Carrillo-Cruz E, Marín-Oyaga VA, de la Cruz VF, Borrego-Dorado I, Ruiz Mercado M, Acevedo Báñez

I, et al. Role of 18F-FDG-PET/CT in the management of marginal zone B cell lymphoma. Hematol Oncol. 2015;33(4):151–8.
72. Petralia G, Padhani AR. Whole-body magnetic resonance imaging in oncology: uses and indications. Magn Reson Imaging Clin N Am. 2018;26(4):495–507. http://www.ncbi.nlm.nih.gov/pubmed/30316463.
73. Olszewski AJ, Castillo JJ. Survival of patients with marginal zone lymphoma: analysis of the surveillance, epidemiology, and end results database. Cancer. 2013;119(3):629–38. https://doi.org/10.1002/cncr.27773.
74. Montalban C, Abraira V, Arcaini L, Domingo-Domenech E, Guisado-Vasco P, Iannitto E, et al. Simplification of risk stratification for splenic marginal zone lymphoma: a point-based score for practical use. Leuk Lymphoma. 2014;55(4):929–31. http://www.ncbi.nlm.nih.gov/pubmed/23799931.
75. Kalpadakis C, Pangalis GA, Angelopoulou MK, Sachanas S, Kontopidou F, Moschogiannis M, et al. Validation of the simplified prognostic score for splenic marginal zone lymphoma of the Splenic Marginal Zone Lymphoma Working Group. Leuk Lymphoma. 2014;55(11):2640–2.
76. Parry M, Rose-Zerilli MJJ, Ljungström V, Gibson J, Wang J, Walewska R, et al. Genetics and prognostication in splenic marginal zone lymphoma: revelations from deep sequencing. Clin Cancer Res. 2015;21(18):4174–83.
77. Arribas AJ, Rinaldi A, Mensah AA, Kwee I, Cascione L, Robles EF, et al. DNA methylation profiling identifies two splenic marginal zone lymphoma subgroups with different clinical and genetic features. Blood. 2015;125(12):1922–31.
78. Gruszka-Westwood AM, Hamoudi RA, Matutes E, Tuset E, Catovsky D. p53 abnormalities in splenic lymphoma with villous lymphocytes. Blood. 2001;97(11):3552–8. http://www.ncbi.nlm.nih.gov/pubmed/11369650.
79. Hockley SL, Else M, Morilla A, Wotherspoon A, Dearden C, Catovsky D, et al. The prognostic impact of clinical and molecular features in hairy cell leukaemia variant and splenic marginal zone lymphoma. Br J Haematol. 2012;158(3):347–54. http://www.ncbi.nlm.nih.gov/pubmed/22594855.
80. Olszewski AJ, Ali S. Comparative outcomes of rituximab-based systemic therapy and splenectomy in splenic marginal zone lymphoma. Ann Hematol. 2014;93(3):449–58. http://link.springer.com/10.1007/s00277-013-1900-4.
81. Zucca E, Arcaini L, Buske C, Johnson PW, Ponzoni M, Raderer M, et al. Marginal zone lymphomas: ESMO clinical practice guidelines for diagnosis. Ann Oncol. 2020;31(1):17–29. https://doi.org/10.1016/j.annonc.2019.10.010.
82. Zignego AL, Ramos-Casals M, Ferri C, Saadoun D, Arcaini L, Roccatello D, et al. International therapeutic guidelines for patients with HCV-related extrahepatic disorders. A multidisciplinary expert statement. Autoimmun Rev. 2017;16(5):523–41. https://doi.org/10.1016/j.autrev.2017.03.004.
83. Merli M, Carli G, Arcaini L, Visco C. Antiviral therapy of hepatitis C as curative treatment of indolent B-cell lymphoma. World J Gastroenterol. 2016;22(38):8447. http://www.wjgnet.com/1007-9327/full/v22/i38/8447.htm.
84. Peveling-Oberhag J, Arcaini L, Bankov K, Zeuzem S, Herrmann E. The anti-lymphoma activity of antiviral therapy in HCV-associated B-cell non-Hodgkin lymphomas: a meta-analysis. J Viral Hepatol. 2016;23(7):536–44. https://doi.org/10.1111/jvh.12518.
85. Tarella C, Arcaini L, Baldini L, Barosi G, Billio A, Marchetti M, et al. Italian Society of Hematology, Italian Society of Experimental Hematology, and Italian Group for Bone Marrow Transplantation guidelines for the management of indolent, nonfollicular B-cell lymphoma (marginal zone, lymphoplasmacytic, and small lymphocytic). Clin Lymphoma Myeloma Leuk. 2015;15(2):75–85. https://linkinghub.elsevier.com/retrieve/pii/S2152265014002626.
86. Lenglet J, Traullé C, Mounier N, Benet C, Munoz-Bongrand N, Amorin S, et al. Long-term follow-up analysis of 100 patients with splenic marginal zone lymphoma treated with splenectomy as first-line treatment. Leuk Lymphoma. 2014;55(8):1854–60. http://www.tandfonline.com/doi/full/10.3109/10428194.2013.861067.
87. Xing KH, Kahlon A, Skinnider BF, Connors JM, Gascoyne RD, Sehn LH, et al. Outcomes in splenic marginal zone lymphoma: analysis of 107 patients treated in British Columbia. Br J Haematol. 2015;169(4):520–7. https://doi.org/10.1111/bjh.13320.
88. Pata G, Bartoli M, Damiani E, Solari S, Anastasia A, Pagani C, et al. Still a role for surgery as first-line therapy of splenic marginal zone lymphoma? Results of a prospective observational study. Int J Surg. 2017;41:143–9. https://doi.org/10.1016/j.ijsu.2017.03.077.
89. Wu Z, Zhou J, Wang X, Li Y, Bin, Niu T, Peng B. Laparoscopic splenectomy for treatment of splenic marginal zone lymphoma. World J Gastroenterol. 2013;19(24):3854–60.
90. Davies JM, Lewis MPN, Wimperis J, Rafi I, Ladhani S, Bolton-Maggs PHB. Review of guidelines for the prevention and treatment of infection in patients with an absent or dysfunctional spleen: prepared on behalf of the British Committee for Standards in Haematology by a Working Party of the Haemato-Oncology Task Force. Br J Haematol. 2011;155(3):308–17.
91. Bennett M, Sharma K, Yegena S, Gavish I, Dave HP, Schechter GP. Rituximab monotherapy for splenic marginal zone lymphoma. Haematologica. 2005;90(6):856–8. http://www.ncbi.nlm.nih.gov/pubmed/15951303.
92. Kalpadakis C, Pangalis GA, Angelopoulou MK, Sachanas S, Kontopidou FN, Yiakoumis X, et al.

Treatment of splenic marginal zone lymphoma with rituximab monotherapy: progress report and comparison with splenectomy. Oncologist. 2013;18(2):190–7. http://www.ncbi.nlm.nih.gov/pubmed/23345547.
93. Kalpadakis C, Pangalis GA, Sachanas S, Tsirkinidis P, Kontopidou FN, Moschogiannis M, et al. Rituximab monotherapy in splenic marginal zone lymphoma: prolonged responses and potential benefit from maintenance. Blood. 2018;132(6):666–70. https://ashpublications.org/blood/article/132/6/666/39401/Rituximab-monotherapy-in-splenic-marginal-zone.
94. Tsimberidou AM, Catovsky D, Schlette E, O'Brien S, Wierda WG, Kantarjian H, et al. Outcomes in patients with splenic marginal zone lymphoma and marginal zone lymphoma treated with rituximab with or without chemotherapy or chemotherapy alone. Cancer. 2006;107(1):125–35. http://www.ncbi.nlm.nih.gov/pubmed/16700034.
95. Else M, Marín-Niebla A, de la Cruz F, Batty P, Ríos E, Dearden CE, et al. Rituximab, used alone or in combination, is superior to other treatment modalities in splenic marginal zone lymphoma. Br J Haematol. 2012;159(3):322–8. http://www.ncbi.nlm.nih.gov/pubmed/23016878.
96. Castelli R, Bergamaschini L, Deliliers GL. First-line treatment with bendamustine and rituximab, in patients with intermediate-/high-risk splenic marginal zone lymphomas. Med Oncol. 2018;35(2):15. https://doi.org/10.1007/s12032-017-1076-1.
97. Cervetti G, Galimberti S, Pelosini M, Ghio F, Cecconi N, Petrini M. Significant efficacy of 2-chlorodeoxyadenosine± rituximab in the treatment of splenic marginal zone lymphoma (SMZL): extended follow-up. Ann Oncol. 2013;24(9):2434–8.
98. Cervetti G, Galimberti S, Sordi E, Buda G, Orciuolo E, Cecconi N, et al. Significant efficacy of 2-CdA with or without rituximab in the treatment of splenic marginal zone lymphoma (SMZL). Ann Oncol. 2010;21(4):851–4. http://www.ncbi.nlm.nih.gov/pubmed/19825880.
99. Iannitto E, Luminari S, Tripodo C, Mancuso S, Cesaretti M, Marcheselli L, et al. Rituximab with cyclophosphamide, vincristine, non-pegylated liposomal doxorubicin and prednisone as first-line treatment for splenic marginal zone lymphoma: a Fondazione Italiana Linfomi phase II study. Leuk Lymphoma. 2015;56(12):3281–7. http://www.ncbi.nlm.nih.gov/pubmed/25791121.
100. Iannitto E, Bellei M, Amorim S, Ferreri AJM, Marcheselli L, Cesaretti M, et al. Efficacy of bendamustine and rituximab in splenic marginal zone lymphoma: results from the phase II BRISMA/IELSG36 study. Br J Haematol. 2018;183(5):755–65.
101. Cheson BD, Brugger W, Damaj G, Dreyling M, Kahl B, Kimby E, et al. Optimal use of bendamustine in hematologic disorders: Treatment recommendations from an international consensus panel – an update. Leuk Lymphoma. 2016;57(4):766–82. http://www.tandfonline.com/doi/full/10.3109/10428194.2015.1099647.
102. Ferrero S, Ladetto M, Beldjord K, Drandi D, Stelitano C, Bernard S, et al. First application of minimal residual disease analysis in splenic marginal zone lymphoma trials: preliminary results from BRISMA/IELSG36 phase II study. Hematol Oncol. 2019;37:224–5. https://doi.org/10.1002/hon.39_2630.

10 Waldenstrom's Macroglobulinemia

Christian Buske and Véronique Leblond

Lymphoplasmacytic lymphoma (LPL)/Waldenstrom macroglobulinaemia (WM)

Clinical outline
Primary bone marrow disease of adults. Partly involvement of spleen, rarely lymph nodes, extranodal sites or leukemic spread. WM is a clinical condition of the adults, characterized by the coexistence of monoclonal gammopathy of the IgM type in a patient with LPL.

Cytology	Small lymphocytes admixed with lymphoid cells with plasmacytoid features and mature plasma cells, associated with a variable amount of well differentiated mast cells.	Lymphoplasmacytic lymphoma, cytology	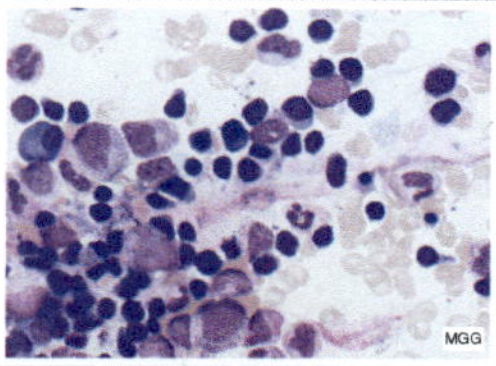
Histology	Infiltration by small to medium sized lymphoid cells with plasmacytoid differentiation growing with an interstitial, perivascular, nodular or diffuse pattern. Variable extent of plasma cells, occasionally with immunoglobulin inclusions (Dutcher and Russell bodies). Prominent mast cells. Infiltration of other tissues from LPL may mimic marginal zone lymphoma.	Lymphoplasmacytic lymphoma, histology	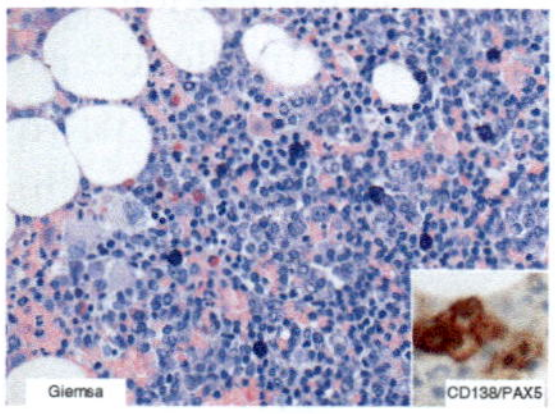

	CD20[1]	CD5	CD23	CD10[2]	BCL6	cyclin D1	CD103	FMC7	IgM	light chains
notes	[1] plasma cell component may be negative, [2] few positive cases reported									
other marker	CD25 may be +; plasma cells component may be CD38+, CD138+ and retain PAX5 expression. Overall, LPL lacks a specific phenotype and the antibody panel should be primarily aimed at the exclusion of other lymphoma subtypes.									

■ = majority of cases positive ▒ = variable fraction of cases positive □ = negative

Main differential diagnosis	Marginal zone lymphomas with plasmacytic differentiation (should be less frequently *MYD88* mutated. Clinical disease distribution: LPL is primarily bone marrow). Infiltration pattern in bone marrow (sinusoidal argues for splenic marginal zone lymphoma) IgM myeloma (should be negative for *MYD88* mutation)

M. Dreyling, M. Ladetto (eds.), *Indolent Lymphomas*, Hematologic Malignancies,
https://doi.org/10.1007/978-3-030-55989-2_10

Key molecular features		
IGH genes are rearranged, somatic hypermutation not ongoing. The most recurrent chromosomal anomaly is isolated del(6q). Recurrent mutations target *MYD88* (L265P mutation, present in >90% patients) and *CXCR4* (~30–40% cases). Frequent translocations: none reported.		
Precursor lesions		
IgM type monoclonal gammopathy of uncertain significance, with *MYD88* with/without additional *CXCR4* mutation.		
Progression		
Uncommon, but patterns of transformation include DLBCL.		
Clinically relevant pathologic features	**Relevance**	**Evidence**
Mutations	Prognostic: lack of *MYD88* mutation predicts lower survival	B
	Predictive: *MYD88* mutated cases show better response to ibrutinib single agent; CXCR4 mut predicts shorter progression free survival upon treatment with ibrutinib single agent.	B
Legend: A = verified in multiple studies, randomized trials and/or integrated in guidelines; B = variable between studies/ needs definitive validation; C = preliminary/discrepant results.		

10.1 Epidemiology

WM is an uncommon disease, accounting for 1–2% of hematological neoplasm, with a reported age-adjusted incidence rate of 3.4 per million among males and 1.7 per million among females in the USA [1]. The median age of diagnosis is around 70 years with a male predominance [2]. The incidence increases sharply with advancing age until the age 60–69 years, after which, there is a slower increase in incidence [3]. The incidence rate for WM is higher among Caucasians, with African descendants representing only 5% of all patients. Genetic factors appear to be important for the pathogenesis of WM, with numerous reports of familiar clustering of individuals with WM alone, and with other B-cell lymphoproliferative diseases [2, 4].

Familial predisposition is common in WM as up to 20% of WM patients have a first-degree relative with either a WM or closely related B-cell disorders [4]. Family studies have provided evidence for not only genetic but also environmental factors contributing to WM predisposition [5, 6].

Clinical-based studies are, however, likely to be subjected to selection bias and could overestimate the familial component in WM. In a large population-based case-control study on 2144 LPL/WM patients (1539 WM [72%] and 605 LPL patients) there was a 20-fold increased risk of developing LPL/WM and furthermore, an increased risk of developing non-Hodgkin lymphoma, chronic lymphocytic leukemia, and MGUS (monoclonal gammopathy of undetermined significance). There was, however, no excess risk of multiple myeloma or Hodgkin lymphoma. There was a similar excess risk among parents, siblings, and offspring, which favors the operation of dominant or codominant gene effects, rather than recessive genes [2, 7].

C. Buske (✉)
University Hospital Ulm, CCC Ulm – Institute of Experimental Cancer Research, Ulm, Germany
e-mail: christian.buske@uni-ulm.de

V. Leblond
Haematology, Sorbonne University-Pitié Salpêtrière Hospital, Paris, France
e-mail: veronique.leblond@aphp.fr

A large international study of 374 WM/LPL cases and 23,096 controls found a 64% increased risk for developing WM/LPL in individuals with a first-degree relative diagnosed with a hematologic malignancy [7].

Recently, a two-stage genome-wide association study of WM/LPL in 530 unrelated cases and 4362 controls of European ancestry identified two high-risk loci associated with WM/LPL at 6p25.3 and 14q32.13. Both risk alleles are observed at a low frequency among controls (~2–3%) and occur in excess in affected cases within families. Although further studies are needed to fully elucidate underlying biological mechanisms, together these loci explain 4% of the familial risk and provide insights into genetic susceptibility to this malignancy [5, 6].

Frequent familiar association with other immunological disorders in healthy relatives, including hypogammaglobulinemia and hypergammaglobulinemia (particularly polyclonal IgM), autoantibody (particularly to thyroid) production, and manifestation of hyperresponsive B cells have also been reported [8].

An increased risk of solid tumors has been reported in WM patients analogous to observations in forms of indolent lymphoproliferative disorders. The Italian group reported an increased incidence of second cancers in a retrospective study of WM patients either untreated or treated with alkylating agents with a cumulative incidence of solid cancers of 12% at 10 years and 17% at 15 years [9]. The Surveillance, Epidemiology and End Results program (SEER multiple primary data base) yielded 1618 WM patients for analysis with population and age-matched controls. The results were consistent with the Italian results regarding the increased risk of acute leukemia and non-Hodgkin lymphoma but did not support an increased risk of brain cancer. However, the larger SEER sample yielded evidence that there was an increased risk of myeloma, melanoma, and cancers of colon, uterus, lung, and kidney [10]. A more recent study based on the SEER data found that WM patients had a 49% higher risk of secondary malignancy than the general population and the median time from diagnosis to a second malignancy was 3.7 years. The risk was significant for lungs, urinary tract, thyroid, melanoma, aggressive, lymphoma, and acute leukemia [11].

The greatest risk factor for the development of WM is that having an MGUS. These patients have a 46 times greater risk of developing WM than the general population [12]. Approximately 10–20% of individuals with MGUS have the IgM subtype, associated with an increased risk of developing Waldenström's macroglobulinemia or other lymphoid malignancies [13]. An independent study from Sweden reported similar outcomes for patients with IgM MGUS. Amongst 728 individuals with MGUS, 116 (16%) had IgM MGUS. With up to 30 years of follow-up, these patients had approximately 15-fold higher risk of progression to lymphoid malignancies, particularly Waldenstrom's macroglobulinemia [14].

The role of environmental factors in WM remains to be clarified, an etiological role for hepatitis C virus (HCV) infection has been suggested, though in one study no association could be established using both serological and molecular diagnostic studies for HCV infection in 100 consecutive WM patients [15].

10.2 Clinical Features

It should be noted that most patients with WM will have limited and nonspecific symptoms at diagnosis, such as fatigue. In a large retrospective study in 454 patients, the most frequent reasons for starting front-line treatment were anemia (in 328 [72%] patients) and constitutional symptoms (in 264 [58%] patients) [16]. The morbidity associated with WM is caused by the concurrence of two main components: tissue infiltration by neoplastic cells and, more importantly, the physicochemical and immunological properties of the monoclonal IgM.

As shown in Table 10.1, the monoclonal IgM can produce clinical manifestations through several different mechanisms related to its physicochemical properties, non-specific interactions with other proteins, antibody activity, and tendency to deposit in tissues [17–19].

Table 10.1 Physicochemical and immunological properties of the monoclonal IgM protein in Waldenstrom's macroglobulinemia

Properties of IgM monoclonal protein	Diagnostic condition	Clinical manifestations
Pentameric structure	Hyperviscosity	Headaches, blurred vision, epistaxis, retinal hemorrhages, leg cramps, impaired mentation, intracranial hemorrhage
Precipitation on cooling	Cryoglobulinemia (type I)	Raynaud's phenomenon, acrocyanosis, ulcers, purpura, cold urticaria
Autoantibody activity to myelin-associated glycoprotein (MAG), ganglioside M1 (GM1), sulfatide moieties on peripheral nerve sheaths	Peripheral neuropathies	Sensorimotor neuropathies, painful neuropathies, ataxic gait, bilateral foot drop
Autoantibody activity to IgG	Cryoglobulinemia (type II)	Purpura, arthralgias, renal failure, sensorimotor neuropathies
Autoantibody activity to red blood cell antigens	Cold agglutinins	Hemolytic anemia, Raynaud's phenomenon, acrocyanosis, livedo reticularis
Tissue deposition as amorphous aggregates	Organ dysfunction	Skin: Bullous skin disease, papules, Schnitzler's syndrome GI: Diarrhea, malabsorption, bleeding Kidney: Proteinuria, renal failure (light chain component)
Tissue deposition as amyloid fibrils (light chain component most commonly)	Organ dysfunction	Fatigue, weight loss, edema, hepatomegaly, macroglossia, organ dysfunction of involved organs: Heart, kidney, liver, peripheral sensory and autonomic nerves

10.3 Morbidity Mediated by the Physicochemical Properties of IgM

10.3.1 Hyperviscosity Syndrome

Observed in 15% of patients at diagnosis, blood hyperviscosity is caused by increased red cell aggregation and decreased red cell deformability, induced by the monoclonal IgM. The possible presence of cryoglobulins can contribute to increasing blood viscosity as well as to the tendency to induce erythrocyte aggregation. Usually, these symptoms are observed when the serum IgM level is >30 g/L, but there is an individual variability. Clinical manifestations are related to circulatory disturbances that can be best appreciated by ophthalmoscopy, which shows distended and tortuous retinal veins, exudates such as cotton-wool spots, hemorrhages, and papilledema. The most common symptoms are oronasal bleeding, visual disturbances due to retinal bleeding, and dizziness that may rarely lead to coma. Heart failure can be aggravated, particularly in the elderly, owing to increased blood viscosity, expanded plasma volume, and anemia. Inappropriate transfusion can exacerbate hyperviscosity and may precipitate cardiac failure [20]. Gustine et al. conclude that serum IgM level >60 g/L is a criterion for plasmapheresis initiation in an asymptomatic WM patient. Indeed, this level leads to a 370-fold higher risk of developing symptomatic hyperviscosity, and showed an association with CXCR4 mutation status [21]. Furthermore, plasma exchange can be discussed in asymptomatic patients with multiple vascular comorbidities, when transfusion of red cells is necessary or in preoperative situations.

10.3.2 Type I Cryoglobulinemia

Monoclonal IgM can have the property to precipitate upon cooling and then induces type I cryoglobulinemia (10–20%). This is symptomatic in less than 5% of the cases, and it is dependent on the monoclonal IgM concentration. Symptoms result from impaired blood flow in small vessels and include Raynaud's phenomenon, acrocyanosis, and necrosis of the regions most exposed to cold such as the tip of the nose, ears, fingers, and toes, malleolar ulcers, purpura, cold urticaria, and neuropathy. Renal manifestations may occur but are infrequent [22].

10.3.3 Tissue Deposition

The monoclonal protein can deposit in several tissues as amorphous aggregates. Linear deposition of monoclonal IgM along the skin basement membrane is associated with bullous skin disease. Amorphous IgM deposits in the dermis determine the so-called IgM storage papules on the extensor surface of the extremities—macroglobulinemia cutis [23]. The deposition of monoclonal light chain as fibrillar amyloid deposits (AL amyloidosis) is uncommon in patients with WM. Amyloidosis develops in 2% of patients with monoclonal IgM and is caused by the deposition of monoclonal light chain (mostly kappa) as fibrillar amyloid deposits (AL amyloidosis). In a French series of 72 patients, a peculiar pattern of relatively frequent lymph node (31%) and lung (10%) involvement was noted in patients with systemic AL amyloidosis. A prognostic factor predicting worse outcome remains cardiac involvement [24]. In a large series of 997 WM patients from the Mayo Clinic, 75 (7.5%) had coexisting AL amyloidosis. In 40 (53%) patients, AL amyloidosis was diagnosed concurrently with WM (AL amyloidosis established within 2 months of the diagnosis of WM), whereas 35 (47%) patients developed it subsequently after a median of 2.7 years (95% CI: 1.3–4.5 years) from the diagnosis of WM. Clinical expression and prognosis are similar to those of other AL patients with involvement of heart (61%), kidneys (45%), liver (18%), lungs (10%), peripheral/autonomic nerves (38%), and soft tissues (18%) [25].

10.3.4 Interaction with Circulating Proteins

The monoclonal IgM protein can interact with circulating proteins, including several coagulation factors, mainly factor VIII von Willebrand and fibrinogen, and may cause prolonged clotting times. The macroglobulin can coat platelets, may impair their adhesion and aggregation, and may result in prolonged bleeding time. Acquired von Willebrand syndrome is described in patients with WM. Assessment of ristocetin cofactor activity (VWF: RCo) and von Willebrand factor (VWF) antigen (VWF: Ag) in patients with 72 WM showed a negative relation between VWF levels <130 U/dL and both monoclonal immunoglobulin M concentration (mIgMC) and viscosity. Ten patients with VWF: RCo <50 U/dL (<40 for patients with blood group O) fulfilled the acquired von Willebrand syndrome criteria. They had higher mIgMC and viscosity. Reduction in mIgMC was associated with increase in VWF levels. The low VWF: RCo/VWF:Ag ratio suggested that high viscosity might be associated with increased shear force and cleavage of multimers [26].

10.4 Morbidity Mediated by the Immunological Effects of IgM

10.4.1 Autoantibody Activity

Monoclonal IgM may exert its pathogenic effects through specific recognition of autologous antigens, the most notable being nerve constituents, immunoglobulin determinants, and red blood cell antigens [20, 21].

10.4.2 Type II Cryoglobulinemia

In Type II or mixed cryoglobulins, monoclonal IgM is an autoantibody to the Fc portion of polyclonal IgG. They are rheumatoid factor-positive and often present at a high titer. The cryoprecipitating phenomenon is caused by the immune complex, as separation of the reactants yields clear solution. The manifestations are the same as previously described in type I. Renal manifestation particularly membranoproliferative glomerulonephritis can be observed. Hepatitis C infection must be researched.

10.4.3 IgM-Related Neuropathy

The presence of peripheral neuropathy has been estimated to range from 5% to 38% in WM patients [27–29]. The first step in evaluation is to determine if the monoclonal gammopathy is the likely cause of peripheral neuropathy or if it is a coincidental finding related to other causes of peripheral neuropathy such as diabetes mellitus, alcoholism, and drugs. In WM patients, the nerve damage is mediated by diverse pathogenetic mechanisms: the electrophysiological features that suggest demyelination and include slowed motor conduction velocities are observed with IgM antibody activity; rare cases show characteristics of classic chronic inflammatory demyelinating polyradiculoneuropathy (CIDP) with conduction block, whereas axonal findings are associated with endoneurial granulofibrillar deposits of IgM, amyloidosis, IgM cryoglobulin, and neoplastic infiltration.

Half of the patients with IgM neuropathy have a distinctive clinical syndrome that is associated with antibodies against a minor 100-kDa glycoprotein component of nerve, myelin-associated glycoprotein (MAG). Anti-MAG antibodies are generally monoclonal IgMκ, and usually also exhibit reactivity with other glycoproteins or glycolipids that share antigenic determinants with MAG [30]. The anti-MAG-related neuropathy is typically distal and symmetrical, affecting both motor and sensory functions; it is slowly progressive with a long period of stability. Most patients present with sensory complaints (paresthesias, aching discomfort, dysesthesias, or lancinating pains), imbalance and gait ataxia, owing to lacking proprioception, and leg muscles atrophy in advanced stage [31]. Patients with predominantly demyelinating sensory neuropathy in association with monoclonal IgM to gangliosides with disialosyl moieties, such as GD1b, GD3, GD2, GT1b, and GQ1b, have also been reported. Anti- GD1b and anti-GQ1b antibodies were significantly associated with predominantly sensory ataxic neuropathy. These antiganglioside monoclonal IgMs present core clinical features of chronic ataxic neuropathy with variably present ophthalmoplegia and/or red blood cell cold agglutinating activity (CANOMAD) [32]. The disialosyl epitope is also present on red blood cell glycophorins, thereby accounting for the red cell cold agglutinin activity of anti-Pr2 specificity Monoclonal IgM proteins that bind to gangliosides with a terminal trisaccharide moiety, including GM2 and GalNac-GD1A, are associated with chronic demyelinating neuropathy and severe sensory ataxia, unresponsive to corticosteroids. Motor neuron disease has been reported in patients with WM, and monoclonal IgM with anti-GM1 and sulfoglucuronyl paragloboside activity [33]. Clinically, multifocal motor neuropathy affects predominantly distal muscles and the upper limbs and definite motor conduction blocks are observed in the majority of patients [34].

Monoclonal IgMs behaving as cryoglobulins cause severe painful neuropathy that may present with multifocal distribution also involving cranial nerves. Moreover, cryoglobulinemia may be associated with arthralgia, glomerulonephritis, and dermatological findings such as skin ulceration or purpura. IgM amyloid light-chain (AL) amyloidosis is a rare axonal neuropathy that may complicate WM, often associated with pain, autonomic dysfunction (orthostatic hypotension, gastrointestinal dysmotility, pupils abnormalities, genitourinary, and sexual dysfunction), and systemic involvement with organ failure (heart, kidneys, and liver) and weight loss [35].

Neuropathy associated with tumoral infiltration, though rare, has also been described. Histology of nerve biopsy (with immunolabeling with anti CD20 and polymerase chain reaction-based gene rearrangement analysis of either the IGHV) is the gold standard for the diagnosis, but the neuroimaging has greatly contributed to the diagnostic workup. Magnetic resonance neurography can reveal enlarged nerves or masses that are usually isointense on T1 and hyperintense on T2, often present disruption of the normal fascicular morphology on T1 images and enhance with gadolinium [36].

For the neurologist and hematologist, diagnosing WM neuropathies is challenging because of their heterogeneous presentation. Yet it is crucially important to identify the mechanism involved in order to adapt the therapeutic strategy [35, 37].

10.4.4 Cold Agglutinin Hemolytic Anemia

Primary chronic cold agglutinin disease (CAD) is a well-defined clinicopathologic entity in which a specific, clonal lymphoproliferative B-cell bone marrow disorder results in autoimmune hemolytic anemia [38]. The monoclonal component is usually an IgMκ and reacts most commonly with I/i antigens, with complement fixation and activation. The agglutination of RBCs in the cooler peripheral circulation also causes Raynaud's syndrome, acrocyanosis, and livedo reticularis [38].

The immune hemolysis is entirely complement-dependent, predominantly mediated by activation of the classical pathway and phagocytosis of erythrocytes opsonized with complement protein C3b. The VH4–21 gene segment is necessary to encode anti- I specificity. The *MYD88 L265P* somatic mutation could not be detected by polymerase chain reaction in any of the 17 samples from patients with CAD tested for this mutation in a Norwegian study, as compared to 96% of control samples from patients with typical LPL/WM CAD is now regarded as a well-defined clinicopathologic entity and should be called a disease not syndrome and is a distinct entity from WM [39].

10.5 Manifestations Related to Tissue Infiltration by Neoplastic Cells

Tissue infiltration by neoplastic cells is rare and can involve various organs and tissues, from the bone marrow to the liver, spleen, lymph nodes, and possibly the lungs, gastrointestinal tract, kidneys, skin, eyes, and central nervous system. Pulmonary involvement in the form of masses, nodules, diffuse infiltrate, or pleural effusions is relatively rare, since the overall incidence of pulmonary and pleural findings reported for WM is only 3–5%. Malabsorption, diarrhea, bleeding, or obstruction may indicate involvement of the gastrointestinal tract at the level of the stomach, duodenum, or small intestine. The skin can be the site of dense lymphoplasmacytic infiltrates, similar to that seen in the liver, spleen, and lymph nodes, forming cutaneous plaques and, rarely, nodules [40]. Chronic urticaria and IgM gammopathy are the two cardinal features of the Schnitzler syndrome, which is not usually associated initially with clinical features of WM, although evolution to WM is not uncommon. Skin IgM deposits are observed in 25% of the patients. The efficacy of Il-1beta inhibitors identifies Il-1beta as a pivotal mediator [41].

Invasion articular and periarticular structures by WM malignant cells is rarely reported. The neoplastic cells can infiltrate the periorbital structures, lacrimal gland, and retro-orbital lymphoid tissues, resulting in ocular nerve palsies [42]. Direct infiltration of the central nervous system by monoclonal lymphoplasmacytic cells as infiltrates or as tumors constitutes the rarely observed Bing–Neel syndrome, characterized clinically by confusion, memory loss, disorientation, and motor dysfunction [43–45].

10.6 Laboratory Investigations and Findings

10.6.1 Laboratory Assessment

Essential laboratory parameters for the evaluation of patients with WM has been defined at the eighth international workshop on WM [46]. Complete blood count is mandatory: anemia is the most common finding in patients with symptomatic WM and is caused by a combination of factors: mild decrease in red cell survival, impaired erythropoiesis, hemolysis, moderate plasma volume expansion, and blood loss from the gastrointestinal tract. Blood smears are usually normocytic and normochromic, and rouleaux formation is often pronounced. Leukocyte and platelet counts are usually within the reference range at presentation, although patients may occasionally present with severe thrombocytopenia. Monoclonal B-lymphocytes expressing surface IgM and late-differentiation B-cell markers are detected in blood by flow cytometry. A raised erythrocyte sedimentation rate is almost constantly observed in WM and may be the first clue to the presence of the macroglobulin. The clotting abnormality detected most frequently is prolongation of thrombin time.

High-resolution electrophoresis combined with immuno-fixation of serum and urine are recommended for identification and characterization of the IgM monoclonal protein. The light chain of the monoclonal IgM is κ in 75–80% of patients. A few WM patients have more than one M-component. The concentration of the serum monoclonal protein is very variable but in most cases lies within the range of 15–45 g/L. Densitometry should be adopted to determine IgM levels for serial evaluations because nephelometry is unreliable and shows large intralaboratory as well as interlaboratory variation. The presence of cold agglutinins or cryoglobulins may affect determination of IgM levels and, therefore, testing for cold agglutinins and cryoglobulins should be performed at diagnosis. If present, subsequent serum samples should be analyzed under warm conditions for determination of serum monoclonal IgM level. Although Bence-Jones proteinuria is frequently present, it exceeds 1 g/24 h in only 3% of cases. While IgM levels are elevated in WM patients, IgA and IgG levels are most often depressed and do not demonstrate recovery even after successful treatment suggesting that patients with WM harbor a defect which prevents normal plasma cell development and/or Ig heavy chain rearrangements [47]. In patients with symptomatic neuropathy anti-MAG, antiganglioside and anti-sulfatide antibodies are sought.

10.6.2 Genomic Features

The common cytogenetic abnormality associated with WM is the 6q deletion, observed in 50% of patients. Other less frequent abnormalities have been described in WM patients: del13q, Trisomy 4, del17p. The 17p deletion was associated with a shorter time to first treatment and a poor outcome [48, 49].

The *L265P* mutation of the "myeloid primary differentiation 88" gene (MYD88) has been first reported in more than 90% of MW by Treon using whole-genome sequencing and was rapidly confirmed by others [50, 51]. The *MYD88* activating mutation is responsible of enhancement of cell survival through increase in NF-KB activity, JAK-STAT3 signaling and consequently cytokine production.

The identification of this mutation has been a major development in WM because it can have diagnostic, therapeutic, and prognostic implications [50, 52]. Mutations in the CXCR4 gene have been detected in 40% of patients with WM. More than 30 CXCR4 mutations have been identified and can be frameshift or nonsense. These mutations have not been associated with worse survival outcome but can affect the response to ibrutinib [53]. Other less common mutations have been described as ARID1A, CD79A/B, TP53, and SPi1. Their clinical value is under investigation [54, 55].

10.6.3 Serum Viscosity

Because of its large size (almost 1,000,000 Da), most IgM molecules are retained within the intravascular compartment and can exert an undue effect on serum viscosity. Therefore, serum viscosity should be measured if the patient has signs or symptoms of hyperviscosity syndrome [20].

10.6.4 Prognosis

WM typically presents as an indolent disease though considerable variability in prognosis can be seen. WM is preceded by asymptomatic WM (AWM), for which the risk of progression to overt disease is not well defined. Bustoros et al. studied 439 patients with AWM, who were diagnosed and observed at Dana-Farber Cancer Institute between 1992 and 2014. During the 23-year study period, with a median follow-up of 7.8 years, 317 patients progressed to symptomatic WM (72%). IgM 4500 mg/dL or greater, bone marrow lymphoplasmacytic infiltration 70% or greater, β2-microglobulin 4.0 mg/dL or greater, and albumin 3.5 g/dL or less were all identified as independent predictors of disease progression. A proportional hazards model using bone marrow infiltration, immunoglobulin M, albumin, and beta-2 microglobulin values as continuous measures divided the cohort into three distinct risk groups: a high-risk group with a median time to progression (TTP) of 1.8 years, an intermediate-risk group with a median TTP of 4.8 years, and a low-risk group with a median TTP of 9.3 years [56].

The median survival reported in several large series has ranged from 8 to 10 years [57–59]. Most studies have focused on overall survival from diagnosis to last follow-up, but others have analyzed survival after initiation of treatment in patients with symptomatic WM [60, 61]. Indeed, a high proportion of patients died from unrelated causes, because of their advanced age at diagnosis. The rate of death unrelated to WM was estimated at 20% [62].

Many prognostic factors influencing overall survival have been described: age, constitutional signs, hemoglobin, platelet, serum albumin, beta 2 microglobulin, 6q deletion, 17p deletion, MyD88 status, etc.

Table 10.2 summarizes the prognostic scoring systems in Waldenstrom's macroglobulinemia. The International Prognostic Scoring System for WM (IPSSWM), was developed a decade ago for patients with Waldenström's macroglobulinemia (WM) in order to improve prognostication of symptomatic WM patients. It stratified patients into three risk groups with 5-year survival rates of 87%, 68%, and 36% in the low, intermediate- and high-risk group, respectively [58]. However, IPSSWM formulation was based on the data of 587 patients of which very few (4%) had received primary therapy with rituximab, while survival data did not differentiate deaths due to WM or other non-WM related causes, which is not uncommon among elderly WM patients. Furthermore, LDH, which is a well-identified prognostic factor in lymphomas, was not included in this model although several publications had suggested a significant prognostic role in WM [63]. Furthermore, there have been significant changes in the treatment of WM with the intro-

Table 10.2 Prognostic scoring systems in Waldenstrom's macroglobulinemia

Study	Adverse prognostic factors	Number of groups	Survival
Gobbi et al. [61]	Hb <9 g/dL Age >70 years Weight loss Cryoglobulinemia	0–1 Prognostic factors	Median: 48 months
		2–4 prognostic factors	Median: 80 months
Dhodapkar et al. [60]	B2-microglobulin (β_2M) ≥3 g/dL Hb <12 g/dL IgM <4 g/dL	$\beta_2M < 3$ mg/dL + Hb ≥ 12 g/dL	5 year: 87%
		$\beta_2M < 3$ mg/dL + Hb < 12 g/dL	5 year: 63%
		$\beta_2M \geq 3$ mg/dL + IgM ≥ 4 g/dL	5 year: 53%
		$\beta_2M \geq 3$ mg/dL + IgM < 4 g/dL	5 year: 21%
International prognostic scoring system for WM Morel et al. [58]	Age >65 year Hb <11.5 g/dL Platelets <100 × 10^9/L $\beta_2M > 3$ mg/L IgM > 7 g/dL	0–1 Prognostic factors[a]	5 year: 87%
		2 prognostic factors[b]	5 year: 68%
		3–5 prognostic factors	5 year: 36%
Revised IPSSWM Kastritis et al. [59]	Age (≤65 vs. 66–75 vs. ≥76 years), B2-microglobulin ≥4 mg/L, serum albumin <3.5 g/dL LDH ≥ 250 IU/L (ULN < 225)	0 Prognostic factor	5 year: 95%; 10 year: 84%
		1 Prognostic factor	5 year: 86%; 10 year 59%
		2 Prognostic factors	5 year: 78%; 10 year 37%
		3 Prognostic factors	5 year: 47%; 10 year: 19%
		4–5 Prognostic factors	5 year: 36%; 10 year: 9%

[a]Excluding age
[b]Age >65 years

duction of rituximab-based therapies, proteasome inhibitors and targeted therapies. Kastritis et al. reported a revised system based on data from 492 symptomatic patients with at least 3 years and a median of 7 years of follow-up, while an independent validation cohort included 229 symptomatic patients. Age (≤65 vs. 66–75 vs. ≥76 years), b_2-microglobulin ≥4 mg/L, serum albumin <3.5 g/dL and LDH ≥250 IU/L (ULN < 225) stratified patients in five different prognostic groups with a 3-year WM-related death rate of 0%, 10%, 14%, 38%, and 48% ($p < 0.001$) and 10-year survival rate of 84%, 59%, 37%, 19%, and 9% ($p < 0.001$). This revised IPSSWM could improve WM patient risk stratification, is easily available, and may be used in the everyday practice to provide prognostic information [59].

10.7 Treatment of Waldenström's Macroglobulinemia

10.7.1 Asymptomatic Patients

WM is an indolent B-cell lymphoma which is not curable by treatment approaches available today. In addition, there are no prospective data documenting survival benefit for patients treated immediately versus treated after a watch and wait period until emergence of lymphoma related symptoms. Based on this, there is consensus that only patients suffering from lymphoma-related symptoms should start treatment [64, 65]. In the case of WM this includes symptoms caused by circulating IgM paraprotein such as hyperviscosity, amyloidosis, symptomatic cryoglobulinemia, cold agglutinin disease, neuropathy, or disease-related hemoglobin level less than 10 g/dL or platelet count less than $100 \times 10^9\ L^{-1}$. On the other hand, monoclonal IgM per se is not a reason to initiate treatment [65]. Close observation is appropriate for these patients.

10.7.2 Treatment Options

In the last years the introduction of the BTK inhibitor ibrutinib has led to major changes in the clinical management of WM, combining oral application with avoidance of chemotherapy for these mostly elderly patients [66]. Nevertheless, rituximab-chemotherapy is still a backbone of treatment in WM in many clinical situations, also reflected by the most recent ESMO treatment guidelines for WM [67]. Alkylating agents still play a major role and there are two regimens widely used in WM, which is rituximab in combination with Bendamustine (B-R) and the combination dexamethasone, rituximab, and cyclophosphamide (DRC). Fludarabine is not recommended anymore in WM because of partly severe toxicity. R-CHOP (rituximab, cyclophosphamide, vincristine, prednisone) can cause neurotoxicity and is therefore also considered not to be first choice in WM. The proteasome inhibitor bortezomib is an important option, but also carries the risk to cause neurotoxicity. In the following section, treatment options are described in more detail.

10.7.3 Immunochemotherapy

10.7.3.1 DRC

A very interesting regimen was introduced by Dimopoulos et al. consisting of dexamethasone 20 mg followed by rituximab 375 mg/m^2 IV on day 1 and cyclophosphamide 100 mg/m^2 orally bid on days 1 to 5 (DRC). This regimen was highly effective in a phase II trial in 72 previously untreated patients with symptomatic WM. An objective response was documented in 83% of patients, including 7% with CR, 67% with PR. Furthermore, the median time to response was 4.1 months. The 2-year progression-free survival rate for the total patient group was 67%, for responding patients 80% (Fig. 10.2). This remarking activity was paralleled by only moderate myelotoxicity with only 9% of patients experiencing grade 3 or 4 hematologic neutropenia and none experiencing grade 3 or 4 thrombocytopenia [68]. The final analysis of this trial confirmed the high activity of this immunochemotherapy paralleled by a favorable toxicity profile [69].

10.7.3.2 Rituximab-Bendamustine (B-R)

Bendamustine is a chemotherapeutic drug which chemically displays characteristics both of a purine nucleoside analog as well as an alkylating agent. Developed in the 60s of the last century in the postwar communist Eastern part of Germany as a competitor to established alkylating drugs such as cylophosphamide, it has experienced a rebirth based on its high efficacy in follicular lymphoma and its favorable toxicity profile. This rediscovery was largely based on a multicenter, randomized, open-label, noninferiority German trial, which randomized patients with newly diagnosed stage III or IV indolent or mantle-cell lymphoma between R-CHOP and B-R (Bendamustine 90 mg/m^2 on days 1 and 2 of a 4-week cycle) for a maximum of six cycles. The primary endpoint was progression-free survival, with a noninferiority margin of 10%. Two-hundred and seventy-four patients were assigned to bendamustine plus rituximab (261 assessed) and 275 to R-CHOP (253 assessed). At a median follow-up of 45 months, median PFS was significantly longer in the B-R arm compared to the R-CHOP group with 69.5 vs. 31.2 months (hazard ratio 0.58; $p < 0.0001$). B-R had a different toxicity profile than R-CHOP with lower rates of alopecia, less myelotoxicity, infections, and peripheral neuropathy. A subgroup analysis comprising 41 evaluable patients with WM documented high response rates in both arms with 96% for B-R and 94% for R-CHOP. Both treatments were not able to induce complete remissions. However, the median PFS was longer for B-R with a median of 69.5 versus 28.1 months for R-CHOP after a median follow-up of 46 months for the total patient population [70]. Although this was a subgroup analysis with a limited number of patients, these early results pointed to a remarkable activity of B-R in WM and indicated that B-R is another highly attractive treatment option in this often elderly group of patients. In a phase II study outcome of 30 relapsed/refractory WM patients after bendamustine-containing therapy was reported. Patients received B-R (24 pts) or ofatumumab with bendamustine in the case of rituximab intolerance. The median number of treatment cycles was 5. Overall response rate was 83.3%, with 5 VGPR and 20 PR. The median estimated PFS for all patients was 13 months. There were cases of prolonged myelosuppression in patients who received prior nucleoside analogs [71].

10.7.3.3 Bortezomib

Among the proteasome inhibitors bortezomib has been tested most in WM. Several phase II trials have confirmed the efficacy of bortezomib used as a single agent in WM [72, 73]. The combination of bortezomib with rituximab was analysed in a phase II trial: 37 patients with relapsed or refractory WM were treated with Bortezomib 1.6 mg/m^2 day 1, 8, 15 in a 28 day cycle for six cycles combined with rituximab 375 mg/m^2 day 1,8, 15, 22 cycles 1 and 4. The median number of treatment was three and 78% of the patients completed the treatment. This combination induced an OR of 81% with 5% CR and 46% PR. Grade 3 or 4 toxicity was acceptable with 16% leucocytopenia, 11% anemia and 5% neuropathy. One patient died by pneumonia, emphasizing that severe infectious complications might occur in this patient population [74]. The same regimen was tested in 26 untreated WM patients with 88% minor responses, 58% partial response and 8% complete response or near-complete response. The 1-year event -free survival was 79% and importantly no grade 3/4 neuropathy was documented [74]. A lower incidence of peripheral neuropathy was observed using once a week bortezomib as compared to the incidence of grade 3 neuropathy (30%) in a study which utilized a twice a week schedule for bortezomib administration at 1.3 mg/m^2 [75]. The impact of once versus twice weekly bortezomib administration on PFS remains to be clarified. It is still an open question, however, whether adding Bortezomib to Rituximab/chemotherapy increases efficacy without enhancing toxicity. This important question has to be addressed in future clinical trials. Another open question is, whether Bortezomib acts independent of the MYD88 and CXCR4 mutational status. There are no prospective data yet, but in a retrospective analysis comprising 63 patients with WM treated with bortezomib/rituximab in the upfront or relapsed/refractory setting as part of a phase 2 clinical trial PFS and OS was independent of the CXCR4 mutational status in MYD88 mutated patients. In this retrospective analysis 43 patients were evaluable for CXCR mutations with 17 patients being CXCR4 mutated. All CXCR4 mutated patients carried also the MYD88 L265P mutation. Thus, this study did not allow to test the efficacy in MYD88 nonmutated WM [76].

10.7.4 Chemotherapy-Free Approaches

10.7.4.1 Rituximab

Rituximab single agent was the first widely used chemotherapy-free approach, in particular in the US before the introduction of ibrutinib. Rituximab single-agent therapy is less effective in WM than in follicular lymphoma and four weekly infusions of Rituximab achieve overall response rates of about 20–30%. However, extended rituximab applications enhance response rates up to 50% [77]. Response is often slow after rituximab single-agent therapy and in particular in patients with signs of hyperviscosity or patients with high IgM values there is the danger of the so-called IgM flare, a transient increase of serum IgM immediately following initiation of rituximab treatment [78]. Patients with baseline serum IgM levels of >50 g/dL or serum viscosity of >3.5 cp may be particularly at risk for a hyperviscosity related event, and in such patients plasmapheresis should be considered or rituximab should be omitted for the first few cycles of therapy until IgM levels decline to safer levels. Importantly, the IgM flare in response to rituximab does not predict treatment failure with most patients returning to baseline serum IgM level by 12 weeks.

10.7.4.2 BTK Inhibitors

Targeting the BTK in WM cells has emerged as a key therapeutic concept in this disease. In the pivotal phase II study 63 symptomatic patients with Waldenström's macroglobulinemia who had received at least one previous treatment, were treated with Ibrutinib at a daily oral dose of 420 mg until disease progression or the development of unacceptable toxicity. Efficacy data characterized ibrutinib as the most effective single agent in the treatment of WM with an overall response rate of 90.5% and a major response rate of 73%. However, responses were dependent on the mutational status of MYD88 and CXCR4 with highest responses in the $MYD88^{Mut}/CXCR4^{WT}$, intermediate responses in the $MYD88^{Mut}/CXCR4^{Mut}$ and lowest responses in the $MYD88^{WT}/CXCR4^{WT}$ cases. The estimated 2-year progression-free and overall survival rates among all patients were 69.1% and 95.2%, respectively. Treatment-related toxic effects of grade 2 or higher included neutropenia (in 22% of the patients) and thrombocytopenia (in 14%), which were more common in heavily pretreated patients; there was postprocedural bleeding in 3% and atrial fibrillation associated with a history of arrhythmia in 5% of cases [50, 52, 66]. These data were confirmed for patients with untreated WM in a prospective study comprising 30 patients. All patients were MYD88 mutated and 47% had additional CXCR4 mutations. Overall and major responses for all patients were 100% and 83%, respectively, but again depending on the mutational status with a drop in major (94% vs. 71%) and very good partial (31 vs. 7%) responses for patients with mutated CXCR4 and delayed time to major responses in this patient group (1.8 vs. 7.3 months; $p = 0.01$) [79]. Based on the observation that ibrutinib single agent has less activities in CXCR4 mutated patients and in patients with nonmutated MYD88 and CXCR4, a large international prospective study was initiated randomizing 150 patients with treatment naive or pretreated WM between ibrutinib plus rituximab or placebo plus rituximab. Primary endpoint was PFS, which was significantly superior in the ibrutinib arm at 30 months (82% with ibrutinib–rituximab versus 28% with placebo–rituximab; hazard ratio for progression or death, 0.20; $p < 0.001$) (Fig. 10.1). Of note, the combination showed efficacy largely independent of the mutational status of MYD88 and CXCR4, demonstrating that addition of rituximab to ibrutinib can increase response, time to response and PFS in WM with double-mutated MYD88 and CXCR4 as well as in WM with both genes non-mutated (Fig. 10.2). Atrial fibrillation and hypertension of grade 3 or higher occurred more frequently with ibrutinib–rituximab than with placebo–rituximab (12% vs. 1% and 13% vs. 4%, respectively); in contrast, infusion reactions and any grade of IgM flare occurred less frequently in the ibrutinib arm (1% vs. 16% and 8% vs. 47%, respectively). Based on these data ibrutinib in combination with rituximab was approved for treatment naive and relapsed patients with WM by the FDA and the EMA [80]. As rituximab is still widely used as part of the initial treatment of WM first line, the question whether ibrutinib acts in rituximab-refractory patients is clinically relevant. In a small prospective observational study comprising 31 rituximab refractory WM patients,

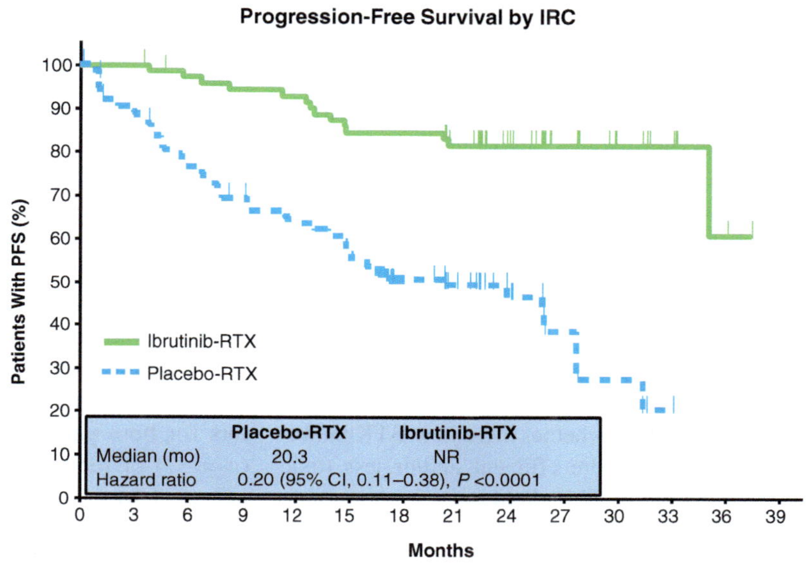

Fig. 10.1 Progression-free survival among all patients receiving either ibrutinib/rituximab or placebo/rituximab (Reprinted from Dimopoulos et al. with permission from the New England Journal of Medicine [80])

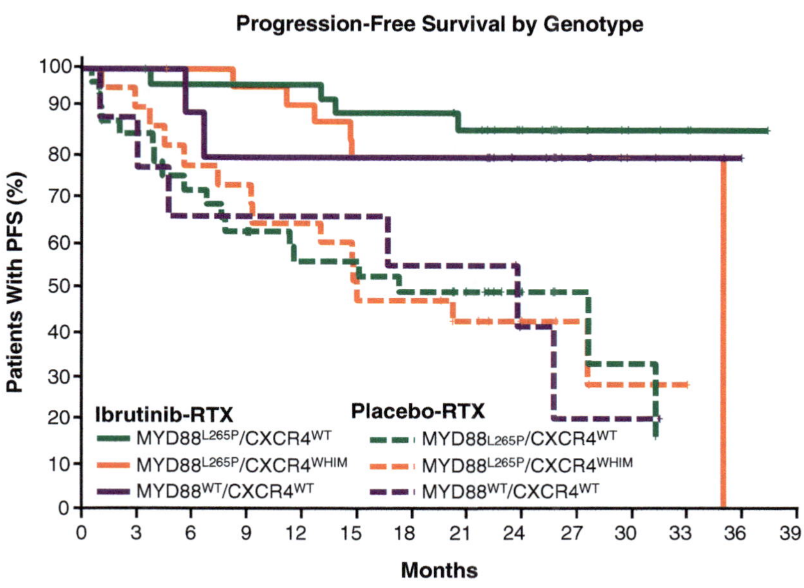

Fig. 10.2 Progression-free survival according to genotypes among all patients receiving either ibrutinib/rituximab or placebo/rituximab (Reprinted from Dimopoulos et al. with permission from the New England Journal of Medicine [80])

ibrutinib single agent demonstrated comparable activity as shown in the pivotal trial for relapsed patients, underlining that in this patient population ibrutinib is a valid treatment option [81].

Second-generation BTK inhibitors are characterized by less off-target effects and aim at increasing efficacy and reducing side effects seen with ibrutinib. More recently, a randomized Phase II trial reported excellent results in 102 patients with treatment naive or relapsed WM with single-agent acalabrutinib, given 100 mg twice a day until progression or nontolerated toxicity. After a median follow-up of 27 4 months response rate was 93% for treatment naive patients and 93% for relapsed/refractory patients. There seemed to be less atrial fibrillation compared historically to ibrutinib [82]. Zanubrutinib, another second-generation BTK inhibitor has shown encouraging data in CLL and in a limited number of WM patients and is currently tested in a randomized phase III trial in MYD88 mutated patients in a head-to-head comparison with single-agent ibrutinib (ClinicalTrials.gov: NCT03053440) [83]. Longer follow-up of the aforementioned study is needed to confirm whether these new BTK inhibitors are indeed more efficient and/or less toxic compared to ibrutinib in WM.

10.7.5 Maintenance Therapy

A role for maintenance rituximab in WM patients following response to a rituximab containing regimen was raised in a study examining the outcome of 248 WM rituximab naïve patients who were either observed or received maintenance rituximab.[157] In this retrospective study, categorical responses improved in 16/162 (10%) of observed patients, and in 36/86 (41.8%) of patients who received maintenance rituximab following induction therapy. Both progression-free (56.3 vs. 28.6 months) and overall survival (>120 vs. 116 months) were longer in patients who received maintenance rituximab [71]. In a recently reported randomized phase III study, treatment naive WM patients were randomized between rituximab maintenance every 8 weeks for 2 years versus observation after initial rituximab-bendamustine induction therapy. There was no significant difference in PFS, the primary endpoint of the study, between the two groups, so that rituximab maintenance is not generally recommended outside of clinical trials in this disease [84].

10.8 High-Dose Therapy and Stem Cell Transplantation

Autologous stem cell transplantation and allogenic stem cell transplantation (SCT) is a valid treatment option in clinically aggressive WM: the European Bone Marrow Transplant (EBMT) registry reported on 158 patients who underwent autologous SCT with a 5-year PFS and OS of 39.7% and 68.5%, respectively. Non-relapse mortality at 1 year was 3.8%. Chemorefractory disease and the number of prior lines of therapy at time of the autologous SCT were the most important prognostic factors for both parameters. Either myeloablative (n = 37) or reduced-intensity (n = 49) allogeneic SCT was associated in a total of 86 patients with a relapse rate at 3 years of 11% for myeloablative, and 25% for reduced-intensity conditioning regimens. Five year PFS and OS was 56% and 62% for myeloablative, and 49% and 64%, for received reduced intensity conditioning, respectively. The occurrence of chronic graft-versus-host disease was associated with improved progression-free survival, indicating a clinically relevant graft-versus-WM effect. A consensus document on the role of transplantation in WM was reported recently, stating that autologous SCT is not appropriate as part of first-line therapy in patient responding to induction therapy, but is a treatment option following second or subsequent relapses in high-risk patients with chemosensitive disease and that allogeneic SCT should not be considered in patients, not treated with BTK inhibitors so far [85, 86].

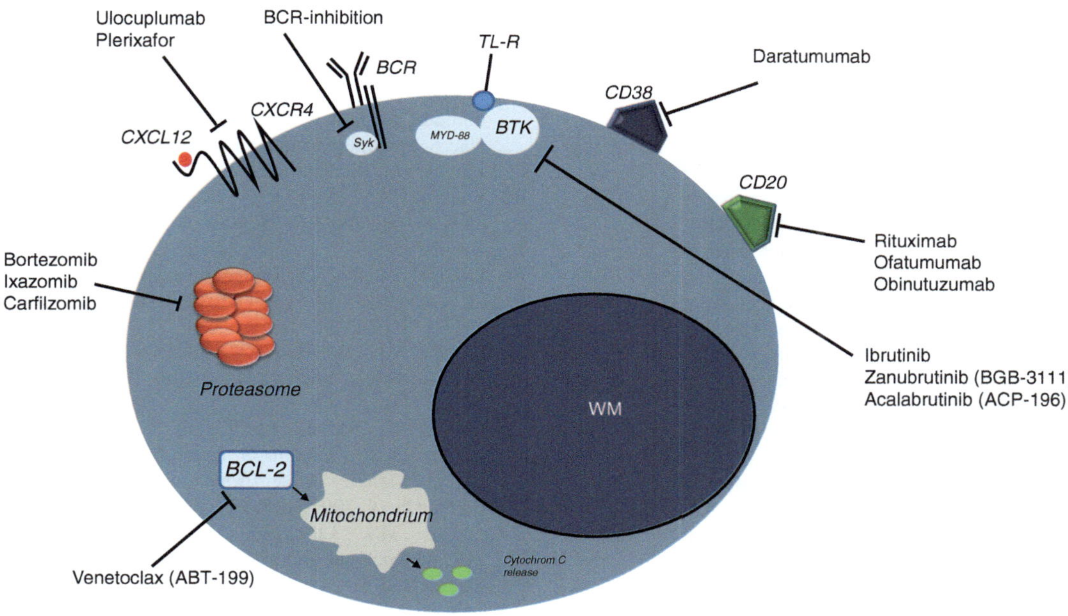

Fig. 10.3 Schematic representation of a WM cell with established and experimental drug targets. *CXCL12* C-X-C motif chemokine ligand 12, *CXCR4* C-X-C motif chemokine receptor 4, *Bcl-2* B-cell lymphoma 2, *BCR* B-cell receptor, *SYK* spleen tyrosine kinase, *BTK* Bruton tyrosine kinase, *MYD88* myeloid differentiation factor 88, *TL-R* toll-like receptor, *CD* cluster of differentiation, *WM* Waldenström's macroglobulinemia

10.9 Future Developments

WM is an example, which demonstrates that insights into the biology has been successfully translated into clinical concepts as shown for the class of BTK inhibitors. Following this line and in the light of activating CXCR4 mutations in up to 40% of patients, clinical trials have been initiated with CXCR4 antagonists with the idea to optimize treatment outcome particularly in patients with the MYD88^{mut} /CXCR4^{mut} genotype. WM comprises a cellular compartment with plasmacytic differentiation, being responsible for the IgM production of the malignant clone. These cells are positive for CD38, and trials are ongoing testing daratumumab in patients with WM. BCL-2 is highly expressed in WM cells largely independent of the genotype, and first data have shown promising activity of the BCL-2 inhibitor venetoclax in relapsed/refractory MYD88^{mut} WM. In addition, proteasome inhibitors, which are orally available and have less neurotoxicity, are tested in this disease (Fig. 10.3). All these examples demonstrate that in WM new treatment approaches are rapidly emerging, promising establishment of therapies which are highly efficient and avoid chemotherapy—associated side effects.

References

1. Groves FD, Travis LB, Devesa SS, Ries LA, Fraumeni JF. Waldenström's macroglobulinemia: incidence patterns in the United States, 1988–1994. Cancer. 1998;82(6):1078–81.
2. Kristinsson SY, Björkholm M, Goldin LR, McMaster ML, Turesson I, Landgren O. Risk of lymphoproliferative disorders among first-degree relatives of lymphoplasmacytic lymphoma/Waldenstrom macroglobulinemia patients: a population-based study in Sweden. Blood. 2008;112(8):3052–6.
3. Wang H, Chen Y, Li F, Delasalle K, Wang J, Alexanian R, et al. Temporal and geographic variations of Waldenstrom macroglobulinemia incidence: a large population-based study. Cancer. 2012;118(15):3793–800.
4. Treon SP, Hunter ZR, Aggarwal A, Ewen EP, Masota S, Lee C, et al. Characterization of famil-

ial Waldenstrom's macroglobulinemia. Ann Oncol. 2006;17(3):488–94.
5. McMaster ML. Familial Waldenström macroglobulinemia: families informing populations. Hematol Oncol Clin North Am. 2018;32(5):787–809.
6. McMaster ML, Berndt SI, Zhang J, Slager SL, Li SA, Vajdic CM, et al. Two high-risk susceptibility loci at 6p25.3 and 14q32.13 for Waldenström macroglobulinemia. Nat Commun. 2018;9(1):4182.
7. Vajdic CM, Landgren O, McMaster ML, Slager SL, Brooks-Wilson A, Smith A, et al. Medical history, lifestyle, family history, and occupational risk factors for lymphoplasmacytic lymphoma/Waldenström's macroglobulinemia: the interlymph non-Hodgkin lymphoma subtypes project. J Natl Cancer Inst Monogr. 2014;2014(48):87–97.
8. Ögmundsdóttir HM, Steingrímsdóttir H, Haraldsdóttir V. Familial paraproteinemia: hyper-responsive B-cells as endophenotype. Clin Lymphoma Myeloma Leuk. 2011;11(1):82–4.
9. Varettoni M, Tedeschi A, Arcaini L, Pascutto C, Vismara E, Orlandi E, et al. Risk of second cancers in Waldenström macroglobulinemia. Ann Oncol. 2012;23(2):411–5.
10. Ojha RP, Thertulien R. Second malignancies among Waldenstrom macroglobulinemia patients: small samples and sparse data. Ann Oncol. 2012;23(2):542–3.
11. Castillo JJ, Olszewski AJ, Kanan S, Meid K, Hunter ZR, Treon SP. Survival outcomes of secondary cancers in patients with Waldenström macroglobulinemia: an analysis of the SEER database. Am J Hematol. 2015;90(8):696–701.
12. Kyle RA, Therneau TM, Rajkumar SV, Offord JR, Larson DR, Plevak MF, et al. A long-term study of prognosis in monoclonal gammopathy of undetermined significance. N Engl J Med. 2002;346(8):564–9.
13. Landgren O, Graubard BI, Katzmann JA, Kyle RA, Ahmadizadeh I, Clark R, et al. Racial disparities in the prevalence of monoclonal gammopathies: a population-based study of 12,482 persons from the National Health and Nutritional Examination Survey. Leukemia. 2014;28(7):1537–42.
14. Turesson I, Kovalchik SA, Pfeiffer RM, Kristinsson SY, Goldin LR, Drayson MT, et al. Monoclonal gammopathy of undetermined significance and risk of lymphoid and myeloid malignancies: 728 cases followed up to 30 years in Sweden. Blood. 2014;123(3):338–45.
15. Leleu X, O'Connor K, Ho AW, Santos DD, Manning R, Xu L, et al. Hepatitis C viral infection is not associated with Waldenström's macroglobulinemia. Am J Hematol. 2007;82(1):83–4.
16. Buske C, Sadullah S, Kastritis E, Tedeschi A, García-Sanz R, Bolkun L, et al. Treatment and outcome patterns in European patients with Waldenström's macroglobulinaemia: a large, observational, retrospective chart review. Lancet Haematol. 2018;5(7):e299–309.
17. Farhangi M, Merlini G. The clinical implications of monoclonal immunoglobulins. Semin Oncol. 1986;13(3):366–79.
18. Merlini G, Farhangi M, Osserman EF. Monoclonal immunoglobulins with antibody activity in myeloma, macroglobulinemia and related plasma cell dyscrasias. Semin Oncol. 1986;13(3):350–65.
19. Marmont AM, Merlini G. Monoclonal autoimmunity in hematology. Haematologica. 1991;76(6):449–59.
20. Stone MJ, Bogen SA. Evidence-based focused review of management of hyperviscosity syndrome. Blood. 2012;119(10):2205–8.
21. Stone MJ, Pascual V. Pathophysiology of Waldenström's macroglobulinemia. Haematologica. 2010;95(3):359–64.
22. Merlini G, Baldini L, Broglia C, Comelli M, Goldaniga M, Palladini G, et al. Prognostic factors in symptomatic Waldenstrom's macroglobulinemia. Semin Oncol. 2003;30(2):211–5.
23. Daoud MS, Lust JA, Kyle RA, Pittelkow MR. Monoclonal gammopathies and associated skin disorders. J Am Acad Dermatol. 1999;40(4):507–35; quiz 36–38.
24. Terrier B, Jaccard A, Harousseau J-L, Delarue R, Tournilhac O, Hunault-Berger M, et al. The clinical spectrum of IgM-related amyloidosis: a French nationwide retrospective study of 72 patients. Medicine (Baltimore). 2008;87(2):99–109.
25. Zanwar S, Abeykoon JP, Ansell SM, Gertz MA, Dispenzieri A, Muchtar E, et al. Primary systemic amyloidosis in patients with Waldenström macroglobulinemia. Leukemia. 2019;33(3):790–4.
26. Hivert B, Caron C, Petit S, Charpy C, Fankam-Siaka C, Lecocq S, et al. Clinical and prognostic implications of low or high level of von Willebrand factor in patients with Waldenstrom macroglobulinemia. Blood. 2012;120(16):3214–21.
27. Nobile-Orazio E, Marmiroli P, Baldini L, Spagnol G, Barbieri S, Moggio M, et al. Peripheral neuropathy in macroglobulinemia: incidence and antigen-specificity of M proteins. Neurology. 1987;37(9):1506–14.
28. Nemni R, Gerosa E, Piccolo G, Merlini G. Neuropathies associated with monoclonal gammapathies. Haematologica. 1994;79(6):557–66.
29. Chaudhry HM, Mauermann ML, Rajkumar SV. Monoclonal gammopathy-associated peripheral neuropathy: diagnosis and management. Mayo Clin Proc. 2017;92(5):838–50.
30. Weiss MD, Dalakas MC, Lauter CJ, Willison HJ, Quarles RH. Variability in the binding of anti-MAG and anti-SGPG antibodies to target antigens in demyelinating neuropathy and IgM paraproteinemia. J Neuroimmunol. 1999;95(1–2):174–84.
31. Svahn J, Petiot P, Antoine J-C, Vial C, Delmont E, Viala K, et al. Anti-MAG antibodies in 202 patients: clinicopathological and therapeutic features. J Neurol Neurosurg Psychiatry. 2018;89(5):499–505.

32. Garcia-Santibanez R, Zaidman CM, Sommerville RB, Lopate G, Weihl CC, Pestronk A, et al. CANOMAD and other chronic ataxic neuropathies with disialosyl antibodies (CANDA). J Neurol. 2018;265(6):1402–9.
33. Nobile-Orazio E, Gallia F. Multifocal motor neuropathy: current therapies and novel strategies. Drugs. 2013;73(5):397–406.
34. Löscher WN, Oberreiter E-M, Erdler M, Quasthoff S, Culea V, Berek K, et al. Multifocal motor neuropathy in Austria: a nationwide survey of clinical features and response to treatment. J Neurol. 2018;265(12):2834–40.
35. Viala K, Stojkovic T, Doncker A-V, Maisonobe T, Lenglet T, Bruneteau G, et al. Heterogeneous spectrum of neuropathies in Waldenström's macroglobulinemia: a diagnostic strategy to optimize their management. J Peripher Nerv Syst. 2012;17(1):90–101.
36. Briani C, Visentin A, Campagnolo M, Salvalaggio A, Ferrari S, Cavallaro T, et al. Peripheral nervous system involvement in lymphomas. J Peripher Nerv Syst. 2019;24(1):5–18.
37. D'Sa S, Kersten MJ, Castillo JJ, Dimopoulos M, Kastritis E, Laane E, et al. Investigation and management of IgM and Waldenström-associated peripheral neuropathies: recommendations from the IWWM-8 consensus panel. Br J Haematol. 2017;176(5): 728–42.
38. Berentsen S, Röth A, Randen U, Jilma B, Tjønnfjord GE. Cold agglutinin disease: current challenges and future prospects. J Blood Med. 2019;10:93–103.
39. Randen U, Trøen G, Tierens A, Steen C, Warsame A, Beiske K, et al. Primary cold agglutinin-associated lymphoproliferative disease: a B-cell lymphoma of the bone marrow distinct from lymphoplasmacytic lymphoma. Haematologica. 2014;99(3):497–504.
40. Mascaro JM, Montserrat E, Estrach T, Feliu E, Ferrando J, Castel T, et al. Specific cutaneous manifestations of Waldenström's macroglobulinaemia. A report of two cases. Br J Dermatol. 1982;106(2):217–22.
41. Rowczenio DM, Pathak S, Arostegui JI, Mensa-Vilaro A, Omoyinmi E, Brogan P, et al. Molecular genetic investigation, clinical features, and response to treatment in 21 patients with Schnitzler syndrome. Blood. 2018;131(9):974–81.
42. Ettl AR, Birbamer GG, Philipp W. Orbital involvement in Waldenström's macroglobulinemia: ultrasound, computed tomography and magnetic resonance findings. Ophthalmologica. 1992;205(1):40–5.
43. Simon L, Fitsiori A, Lemal R, Dupuis J, Carpentier B, Boudin L, et al. Bing-Neel syndrome, a rare complication of Waldenström macroglobulinemia: analysis of 44 cases and review of the literature. A study on behalf of the French innovative leukemia organization (FILO). Haematologica. 2015;100(12):1587–94.
44. Minnema MC, Kimby E, D'Sa S, Fornecker L-M, Poulain S, Snijders TJ, et al. Guideline for the diagnosis, treatment and response criteria for Bing-Neel syndrome. Haematologica. 2017;102(1):43–51.
45. Castillo JJ, Itchaki G, Paludo J, Varettoni M, Buske C, Eyre TA, et al. Ibrutinib for the treatment of Bing-Neel syndrome: a multicenter study. Blood. 2019;133(4):299–305.
46. Castillo JJ, Garcia-Sanz R, Hatjiharissi E, Kyle RA, Leleu X, McMaster M, et al. Recommendations for the diagnosis and initial evaluation of patients with Waldenström macroglobulinaemia: a task force from the 8th international workshop on Waldenström macroglobulinaemia. Br J Haematol. 2016;175(1):77–86.
47. Hunter ZR, Manning RJ, Hanzis C, Ciccarelli BT, Ioakimidis L, Patterson CJ, et al. IgA and IgG hypogammaglobulinemia in Waldenström's macroglobulinemia. Haematologica. 2010;95(3):470–5.
48. Nguyen-Khac F, Lambert J, Chapiro E, Grelier A, Mould S, Barin C, et al. Chromosomal aberrations and their prognostic value in a series of 174 untreated patients with Waldenström's macroglobulinemia. Haematologica. 2013;98(4):649–54.
49. Poulain S, Roumier C, Bertrand E, Renneville A, Caillault-Venet A, Doye E, et al. TP53 mutation and its prognostic significance in Waldenstrom's macroglobulinemia. Clin Cancer Res. 2017;23(20):6325–35.
50. Treon SP, Xu L, Yang G, Zhou Y, Liu X, Cao Y, et al. MYD88 L265P somatic mutation in Waldenström's macroglobulinemia. N Engl J Med. 2012;367(9):826–33.
51. Poulain S, Roumier C, Decambron A, Renneville A, Herbaux C, Bertrand E, et al. MYD88 L265P mutation in Waldenstrom macroglobulinemia. Blood. 2013;121(22):4504–11.
52. Treon SP, Xu L, Hunter Z. MYD88 mutations and response to ibrutinib in Waldenström's macroglobulinemia. N Engl J Med. 2015;373(6):584–6.
53. Treon SP, Cao Y, Xu L, Yang G, Liu X, Hunter ZR. Somatic mutations in MYD88 and CXCR4 are determinants of clinical presentation and overall survival in Waldenstrom macroglobulinemia. Blood. 2014;123(18):2791–6.
54. Hunter ZR, Yang G, Xu L, Liu X, Castillo JJ, Treon SP. Genomics, signaling, and treatment of Waldenström macroglobulinemia. J Clin Oncol. 2017;35(9):994–1001.
55. Roos-Weil D, Decaudin C, Armand M, Della-Valle V, MBK D, Ghamlouch H, et al. A recurrent activating missense mutation in Waldenström Macroglobulinemia affects the DNA binding of the ETS transcription factor SPI1 and enhances proliferation. Cancer Discov. 2019;9(6):796–811.
56. Bustoros M, Sklavenitis-Pistofidis R, Kapoor P, Liu C-J, Kastritis E, Zanwar S, et al. Progression risk stratification of asymptomatic Waldenström macroglobulinemia. J Clin Oncol. 2019;37(16):1403–11.
57. Morel P, Duhamel A. Comparison of prognostic scoring systems in primary myelofibrosis. Blood. 2010;115(3):745; author reply 6.
58. Morel P, Duhamel A, Gobbi P, Dimopoulos MA, Dhodapkar MV, McCoy J, et al. International prognostic scoring system for Waldenstrom macroglobulinemia. Blood. 2009;113(18):4163–70.
59. Kastritis E, Morel P, Duhamel A, Gavriatopoulou M, Kyrtsonis MC, Durot E, et al. A revised international

prognostic score system for Waldenstrom's macroglobulinemia. Leukemia. 2019;33(11):2654–61.
60. Dhodapkar MV, Jacobson JL, Gertz MA, Rivkin SE, Roodman GD, Tuscano JM, et al. Prognostic factors and response to fludarabine therapy in patients with Waldenström macroglobulinemia: results of United States intergroup trial (southwest oncology group S9003). Blood. 2001;98(1):41–8.
61. Gobbi PG, Bettini R, Montecucco C, Cavanna L, Morandi S, Pieresca C, et al. Study of prognosis in Waldenström's macroglobulinemia: a proposal for a simple binary classification with clinical and investigational utility. Blood. 1994;83(10):2939–45.
62. Kastritis E, Kyrtsonis M-C, Morel P, Gavriatopoulou M, Hatjiharissi E, Symeonidis AS, et al. Competing risk survival analysis in patients with symptomatic Waldenström macroglobulinemia: the impact of disease unrelated mortality and of rituximab-based primary therapy. Haematologica. 2015;100(11):e446–9.
63. Kastritis E, Kyrtsonis M-C, Hadjiharissi E, Symeonidis A, Michalis E, Repoussis P, et al. Validation of the international prognostic scoring system (IPSS) for Waldenstrom's macroglobulinemia (WM) and the importance of serum lactate dehydrogenase (LDH). Leuk Res. 2010;34(10):1340–3.
64. Dimopoulos MA, Gertz MA, Kastritis E, Garcia-Sanz R, Kimby EK, Leblond V, et al. Update on treatment recommendations from the fourth international workshop on Waldenstrom's macroglobulinemia. J Clin Oncol. 2009;27(1):120–6.
65. Kyle RA, Treon SP, Alexanian R, Barlogie B, Bjorkholm M, Dhodapkar M, et al. Prognostic markers and criteria to initiate therapy in Waldenstrom's macroglobulinemia: consensus panel recommendations from the second international workshop on Waldenstrom's macroglobulinemia. Semin Oncol. 2003;30(2):116–20.
66. Treon SP, Tripsas CK, Meid K, Warren D, Varma G, Green R, et al. Ibrutinib in previously treated Waldenstrom's macroglobulinemia. N Engl J Med. 2015;372(15):1430–40.
67. Kastritis E, Leblond V, Dimopoulos MA, Kimby E, Staber P, Kersten MJ, et al. Waldenstrom's macroglobulinaemia: ESMO clinical practice guidelines for diagnosis, treatment and follow-up. Ann Oncol. 2018;29(Suppl 4):iv41–50.
68. Dimopoulos MA, Anagnostopoulos A, Kyrtsonis MC, Zervas K, Tsatalas C, Kokkinis G, et al. Primary treatment of Waldenstrom macroglobulinemia with dexamethasone, rituximab, and cyclophosphamide. J Clin Oncol. 2007;25(22):3344–9.
69. Kastritis E, Gavriatopoulou M, Kyrtsonis MC, Roussou M, Hadjiharissi E, Symeonidis A, et al. Dexamethasone, rituximab, and cyclophosphamide as primary treatment of Waldenstrom macroglobulinemia: final analysis of a phase 2 study. Blood. 2015;126(11):1392–4.
70. Rummel MJ, Niederle N, Maschmeyer G, Banat GA, von Grunhagen U, Losem C, et al. Bendamustine plus rituximab versus CHOP plus rituximab as first-line treatment for patients with indolent and mantle-cell lymphomas: an open-label, multicentre, randomised, phase 3 non-inferiority trial. Lancet. 2013;381(9873):1203–10.
71. Treon SP, Hanzis C, Manning RJ, Ioakimidis L, Patterson CJ, Hunter ZR, et al. Maintenance rituximab is associated with improved clinical outcome in rituximab naive patients with Waldenstrom Macroglobulinaemia who respond to a rituximab-containing regimen. Br J Haematol. 2011;154(3):357–62.
72. Dimopoulos MA, Anagnostopoulos A, Kyrtsonis MC, Castritis E, Bitsaktsis A, Pangalis GA. Treatment of relapsed or refractory Waldenstrom's macroglobulinemia with bortezomib. Haematologica. 2005;90(12):1655–8.
73. Chen CI, Kouroukis CT, White D, Voralia M, Stadtmauer E, Stewart AK, et al. Bortezomib is active in patients with untreated or relapsed Waldenstrom's macroglobulinemia: a phase II study of the National Cancer Institute of Canada clinical trials group. J Clin Oncol. 2007;25(12):1570–5.
74. Ghobrial IM, Hong F, Padmanabhan S, Badros A, Rourke M, Leduc R, et al. Phase II trial of weekly bortezomib in combination with rituximab in relapsed or relapsed and refractory Waldenstrom macroglobulinemia. J Clin Oncol. 2010;28(8):1422–8.
75. Treon SP, Ioakimidis L, Soumerai JD, Patterson CJ, Sheehy P, Nelson M, et al. Primary therapy of Waldenstrom macroglobulinemia with bortezomib, dexamethasone, and rituximab: WMCTG clinical trial 05-180. J Clin Oncol. 2009;27(23):3830–5.
76. Sklavenitis-Pistofidis R, Capelletti M, Liu CJ, Reidy M, Zavidij O, Huynh D, et al. Bortezomib overcomes the negative impact of CXCR4 mutations on survival of Waldenstrom macroglobulinemia patients. Blood. 2018;132(24):2608–12.
77. Gertz MA, Rue M, Blood E, Kaminer LS, Vesole DH, Greipp PR. Multicenter phase 2 trial of rituximab for Waldenstrom macroglobulinemia (WM): an eastern cooperative oncology group study (E3A98). Leuk Lymphoma. 2004;45(10):2047–55.
78. Gustine JN, Meid K, Dubeau T, Hunter ZR, Xu L, Yang G, et al. Serum IgM level as predictor of symptomatic hyperviscosity in patients with Waldenström macroglobulinaemia. Br J Haematol. 2017;177(5):717–25.
79. Treon SP, Gustine J, Meid K, Yang G, Xu L, Liu X, et al. Ibrutinib monotherapy in symptomatic, treatment-naive patients with Waldenstrom macroglobulinemia. J Clin Oncol. 2018;36(27):2755–61.
80. Dimopoulos MA, Tedeschi A, Trotman J, Garcia-Sanz R, Macdonald D, Leblond V, et al. Phase 3 trial of Ibrutinib plus rituximab in Waldenstrom's macroglobulinemia. N Engl J Med. 2018;378(25):2399–410.

81. Dimopoulos MA, Trotman J, Tedeschi A, Matous JV, Macdonald D, Tam C, et al. Ibrutinib for patients with rituximab-refractory Waldenstrom's macroglobulinaemia (iNNOVATE): an open-label substudy of an international, multicentre, phase 3 trial. Lancet Oncol. 2017;18(2):241–50.
82. Owen RG, McCarthy H, Rule S, D'Sa S, Thomas SK, Tournilhac O, et al. Acalabrutinib monotherapy in patients with Waldenstrom macroglobulinemia: a single-arm, multicentre, phase 2 study. Lancet Haematol. 2020;7(2):e112–e21.
83. Tam CS, LeBlond V, Novotny W, Owen RG, Tedeschi A, Atwal S, et al. A head-to-head phase III study comparing zanubrutinib versus ibrutinib in patients with Waldenstrom macroglobulinemia. Future Oncol. 2018;14(22):2229–37.
84. Rummel MJ, Lerchenmüller C, Hensel M, Goerner M, Buske C, Schulz H, et al. Two years rituximab maintenance vs. observation after first line treatment with bendamustine plus rituximab (B-R) in patients with Waldenström's macroglobulinemia (MW): results of a prospective, randomized, multicenter phase 3 study (the StiL NHL7-2008 MAINTAIN trial). Blood. 2019;134(Suppl 1):343.
85. Kyriakou C, Canals C, Cornelissen JJ, Socie G, Willemze R, Ifrah N, et al. Allogeneic stem-cell transplantation in patients with Waldenstrom macroglobulinemia: report from the lymphoma working party of the European Group for Blood and marrow transplantation. J Clin Oncol. 2010;28(33):4926–34.
86. Kyriakou C, Canals C, Sibon D, Cahn JY, Kazmi M, Arcese W, et al. High-dose therapy and autologous stem-cell transplantation in Waldenstrom macroglobulinemia: the lymphoma working party of the European Group for Blood and marrow transplantation. J Clin Oncol. 2010;28(13):2227–32.

11 Mantle Cell Lymphoma

Elisabeth Silkenstedt, Martin Dreyling, and Simon Rule

Mantle cell lymphoma (MCL)

Clinical outline
Primarily a nodal disease of the adult and elderly. Frequently advanced stage with dissemination to bone marrow and other extranodal sites. The leukemic non nodal variant represents a clinic-biological subset, featuring a leukemic picture with splenomegaly and no nodal disease.

Cytology	Four main variants recognized: medium sized centrocytic (classical), CLL-like (small-cell) lymphoblast-like (blastoid) or large, like DLBCL (pleomorphic). Rare subtypes: Marginal-zone-like or lymphoplasmacytoid.	Mantle cell lymphoma, cytology	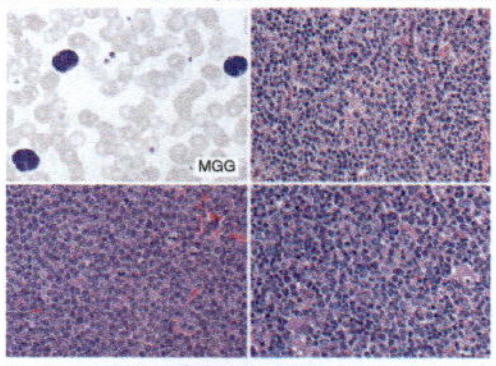
Histology	Variable growth pattern: mantle-zone with preserved GC, nodular and diffuse pattern.	Mantle cell lymphoma, hystology	

	CD20	CD5	CD23	CD10[1]	BCL6[1]	cyclin D1	CD103	FMC7	IgM	light chains
notes	[1]positive cases reported.									
other marker	Sox11 positive in most MCL, including cases negative for Cyclin D1 that carry translocations of cyclin D2 or D3. It is negative in the leukemic non-nodal MCL. Sox11 (see below) and in almost any other low grade B-cell lymphoma.									

▇ = majority of cases positive ▒ = variable fraction of cases positive ☐ = negative

Main differential diagnosis	CLL (should be CD23+, cyclin D1 negative and CD200+, the latter frequently used in flow cytometry). CD200+ in some leukemic non-nodal MCL.

M. Dreyling, M. Ladetto (eds.), *Indolent Lymphomas*, Hematologic Malignancies, https://doi.org/10.1007/978-3-030-55989-2_11

Key molecular features		
Cell cycle dysregulationand genomic instability due to altered DNA damage response. Frequent translocations: t(11;14)(q13;q32) in more than 95% of cases. Rarelytranslocations involving cyclin D2, *BCL6* or *MYC*. Frequent copy number alterations: gains of 3q26, 7p21, 8q24 (*MYC*), loss of 1p13-21, 6q23-27 (*TNFAIP3*), 9p21 (*CDKN2A*), 11q22-23 (*ATM*), 13q11-13, 13q14-34, 17p13 (*TP53*). Frequent mutations: *ATM, CCDD1, KMT2D, NOTCH1/2, TP53*		
Precursor lesions		
Circulating t(11;14)-positive lymphocytes in healthy donors; in situ mantle cell neoplasia.		
Progression		
Tendency to acquire genetic aberrations, higher proliferation and blastic morphology at relapse/progression. By definition such progression classified as MCL (and not as diffuse large B-cell lymphoma).		
Clinically relevant pathologic features	**Relevance**	**Evidence**
Proliferation	Prognostic: Ki67 is integrated in prognostic indexes (combined with MCL international prognostic index, MIPI)	**A**
TP53	Prognostic: unfavorable outcome (either defined by deletion and/or mutation or protein overexpression by immunohistochemistry)	**A**
Phenotypic markers	Prognostic: p53 overexpression (unfavorable)	**A**
	Prognostic: lack of SOX11 is common in the leukemic variant (favorable) but is also recurrent in MCL with aggressive cytology and/or with higher incidence of *TP53* anomaly (unfavorable)	**C**
Cytology	Prognostic: blastoid or pleomorphic cytology (unfavourable)	**B**
Leukemic non-nodal MCL	Blood, bone marrow and spleen involvement but no or little nodal disease. Clinical presentation associated with molecular features (lack of Sox11 expression, somatic IGHV hypermutation, low level genetic aberrations) and favourable outcome.	**B**
Legend: A = verified in multiple studies, randomized trials and/or integrated in guidelines; B = variable between studies/ needs definitive validation; C = preliminary/discrepant results.		

E. Silkenstedt · M. Dreyling (✉)
Department of Medicine III, LMU Hospital, München, Bayern, Germany
e-mail: elisabeth.hoering@med.uni-muenchen.de; martin.dreyling@med.uni-muenchen.de

S. Rule
Department of Haematology, Peninsula Medical School (Faculty of Health: Medicine, Dentistry and Human Sciences), Derriford Hospital, Plymouth, UK
e-mail: simon.rule@nhs.net

11.1 Definition and Epidemiology

Mantle cell lymphoma (MCL) was originally named centrocytic lymphoma. In 1992, the term mantle cell lymphoma was adopted for this entity because of morphologic and immunophenotypic similarities of the malignant cells to lymphocytes of the mantle zone of germinal centers [1].

Since the introduction of the Revised European-American Classification of the International Lymphoma Study Group (R.E.A.L. classification) in 1994, mantle cell lymphoma is regarded as a distinctive lymphoma subtype in the nowadays renowned World Health Organization classification of malignant lymphoid disorders [2].

MCL occurs with an incidence of 1–2 per 100,000 people per year and accounts for 5–7% of malignant lymphomas in Western Europe. The median age is around 65 years with a male to female ratio of about 3:1 [3].

11.2 Histology and Immunophenotype

The affected lymph node shows effacement of the nodal architecture with an infiltrative process with pathological features that may include diffuse, vaguely nodular, mantle zone, or rarely follicular patterns, or a combination of these. A prominent meshwork of follicular dendritic cells is usually present [4]. A mantle zone pattern may represent an earlier phase of the disease [5].

The cytologic features in classical MCL cases consist of small- to intermediate-size cells with irregular, cleaved nuclei, dense chromatin, and indistinct nucleoli. Centroblasts and immunoblasts are typically absent, thus facilitating differentiation to other lymphoma subtypes, especially follicular lymphoma [2, 4].

A leukemic non-nodal variant, resembling chronic lymphocytic leukemia (CLL), usually missing SOX11 expression, is associated with a more indolent course [6]. In contrast, the blastoid variant, characterized by neoplastic cells resembling lymphoblasts, with dispersed chromatin, prominent nucleoli, and high mitotic figures and often featuring high proliferation rates, displays a more aggressive clinical course, whereby a Ki-67 $\geq$ 30% can be considered prognostically relevant [2, 4, 7].

Immunophenotypically, the cells resemble the lymphocytes in the mantle zone of normal germinal follicles with co-expression of B-cell antigens at variable intensities (CD19, CD20, CD79a, secretory immunoglobulin sIgM, sIgD) accompanied by diagnostically relevant aberrant expression of the T-cell–associated marker CD5+. Based on their predominantly pregerminal center origin, MCL cells stain strongly for the antiapoptotic protein BCL-2 but are negative for germinal center markers like CD10 and BCL-6 [2].

In contrast to CLL, FMC7 and CD38 are commonly positive, whereas expression of CD23 is absent [4]. Because of the morphologic heterogeneity of MCL, detection of MCL genetic hallmark, either by immunohistochemistry (cyclin D1 overexpression) or fluorescence in situ hybridization (chromosomal translocation t(11;14) (q13;q32)), is crucial to confirm the diagnosis. In rare cases that are negative for cyclin D1, cyclin D2 or cyclin D3 may be overexpressed [2]. Furthermore, staining for SOX11, a transcription factor specifically expressed in more than 90% of MCL cases, may help to establish the diagnosis [8]. In analogy to follicular lymphoma, an "in situ" mantle cell lymphoma has to be distinguished from the diagnosis of a manifest classical MCL. In these cases, the lymphoma involvement is limited to the inner mantle zone, and lymphoma cells express cyclin D1 (BCL-1) and CD5 and are weakly BCL2+ [4].

11.3 Pathogenesis, Cytogenetics, and Molecular Genetics

The chromosomal t(11;14)(q13;q32) translocation is the genetic hallmark of MCL and considered the primary oncogenic event in the pathogenesis leading to overexpression of cyclin D1 and dysregulation of cell cycle at the G1–S phase transition [9, 10]. Furthermore, the constitutive activation of the B-cell receptor (BCR) and its downstream signaling pathways plays an important role in the development of the disease [11–13].

Additionally, genomic profiling revealed a high number of secondary genetic alterations and recurrent mutations affecting, for example, regulation of cell cycle, DNA damage response, and apoptosis pathways that contribute to the pathogenesis and aggressiveness of MCL [11]. Mutation of the ataxia-telangiectasia mutant (ATM) gene facilitates genomic instability in lymphoma cells through impaired response to DNA damage. Phosphoinositide 3′-kinase (PI3K) and mammalian target of rapamycin (mTOR) are important downstream targets of this signaling pathway. MCL has one of the highest levels of genomic instability among the malignant lymphoid neoplasms. These genetic abnormalities include losses in chromosomes 1p13–p31, 2q13, 6q23–27, 8p21, 9p21, 10p14–15, 11q22–23, 13q11–13, 13q14–34, 17p13, and 22q12; gains in chromosomes 3q25, 4p12–13, 7p21–22, 8q21, 9q22, 10p11–12, 12q13, and 18q11q23; and high-copy-number amplifications of certain chromosomal regions.

Recurrent somatic mutations have been, among others, detected in *CCND1* (~7–35%), *WHSC1* (~10%), *KMT2D/MLL2* (~14–15%), *BIRC3*, *MEF2B*, and *NOTCH1/2* (all <10%) [14, 15]. Yet, prognostic and functional relevance remains unclear for most of the mutations and is currently under further investigation. Genetic mutations that have been described to be associated with a poor clinical outcome affect *TP53* and *NOTCH1/2* [14, 16–18].

11.4 Prognostic Factors

Important clinical and serological factors, associated with a worse clinical outcome, include age, poor general condition, advanced stage of disease (Ann Arbor stage III or IV), splenomegaly and anemia, the serum level of β2-microglobulin and LDH, blastoid cytology, extranodal presentation, and constitutional symptoms. A prognostic score that has been confirmed in numerous series, the MIPI (MCL International Prognostic Index), was established implementing four independent prognostic factors: age, performance status, LDH, and leukocyte count (Fig. 11.1) [19, 20].

Yet, the most important prognostic marker independent of clinical features is the proliferation rate and the expression of genes related to proliferation, respectively. A cell proliferation gene signature that distinguishes patient subsets that differ by more than 5 years in median survival has been identified [21, 22]. In the clinical setting, immunohistochemical determination of Ki-67 expression, a cell cycle–related protein, has been prospectively confirmed as a reliable prognostic marker and is, in combination with the MIPI (MIPI-c), a highly recommended tool to estimate individual risk profile and to identify high-risk patients (Ki-67 > 30%) who may qual-

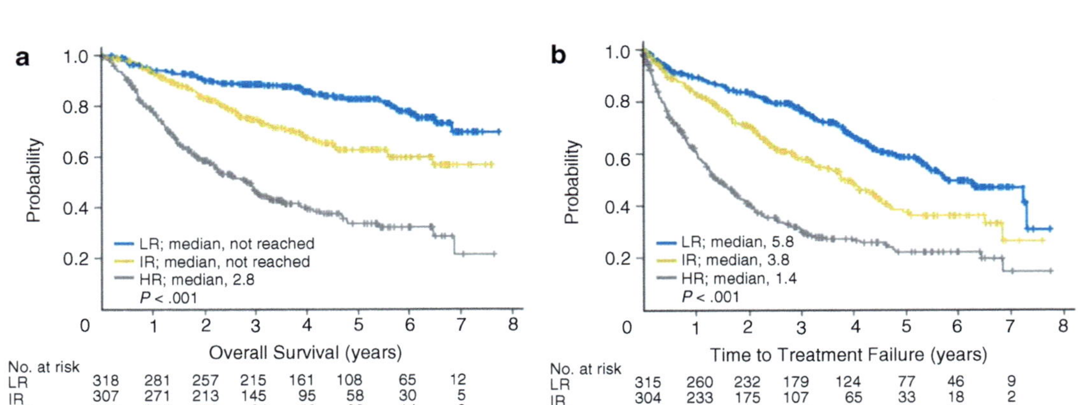

Fig. 11.1 Overall survival (**a**) and time-to-treatment failure (**b**) depending on MIPI risk group (low risk (LR), intermediate risk (IR), high risk (HR)) [19]

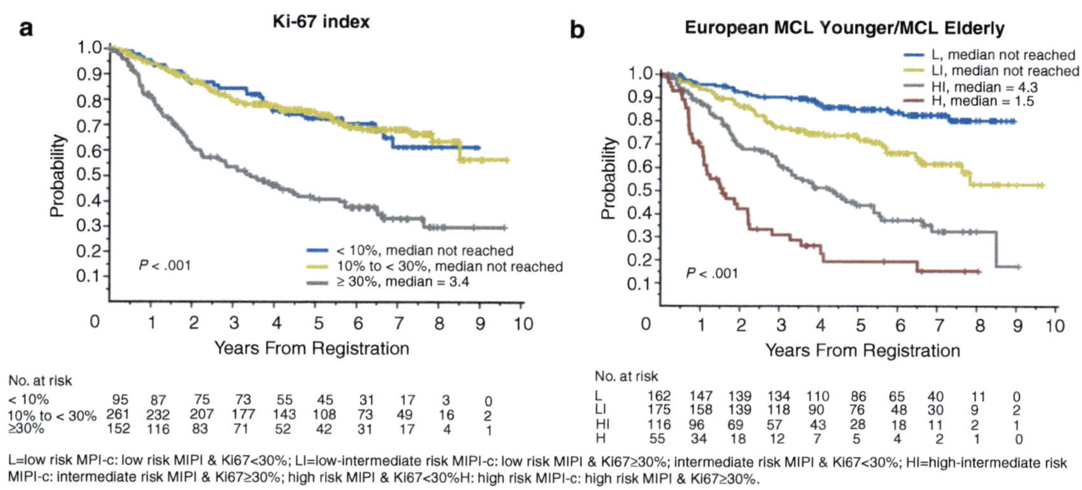

Fig. 11.2 Overall survival depending on cell proliferation (Ki-67) alone and in combination with MIPI [7]

ify for more aggressive therapeutic approaches [7, 23, 24] (Fig. 11.2).

11.5 Clinical Presentation

MCL typically presents with lymphadenopathy of several sites; most of the patients are diagnosed with advanced-stage disease (Ann Arbor stage III, IV). Extranodal manifestations occur in 90% of patients, including infiltration of bone marrow (53–82%), blood (50%), liver (25%), and the gastrointestinal tract (20–60%), presenting as *polyposis coli* [3, 25]. The spleen is enlarged in 40% of patients [3]. In some cases, leukemic manifestation in combination with massive splenomegaly is clinically prominent. These nonnodal, leukemic cases are often characterized by a more indolent clinical course, sometimes characterized by a very low Ki-67 index and missing SOX11 expression [6].

The patient may be asymptomatic, but some experience fever, night sweats, or weight loss.

The frequency of CNS disease is low at first diagnosis but increases with subsequent relapses and correlates with elevated lactate dehydrogenase (LDH), blastoid cytology, and cell proliferation (Ki-67) [26].

11.6 Diagnosis and Differential Diagnosis

Tissue diagnostic, preferentially lymph node excision, is crucial for diagnosis of MCL. Immunohistochemical workup of expression pattern of B- and T-cell antigens and immunoglobulins and cytogenetic analysis or FISH diagnostic to identify the t(11;14) translocation are usually sufficient for diagnosis finding. In the rare cases of cyclin D negativity, expression of SOX11 may be helpful to support the diagnosis of MCL. The clinical presentation of MCL may resemble CLL or other indolent nodal lymphomas. Therefore, immunohistochemical differentiation from other entities is of great importance. There are overlapping cytologic features between CLL/SLL and MCL. Also, the vaguely nodular patterns in MCL and the pseudo-follicles in CLL/SLL may resemble one another. The immunophenotype of CLL is also similar, with co-expression of immunoglobulin IgM and IgD and of the B-cell–associated antigens CD19 and CD20 and aberrant expression of the T-cell antigen CD5. In contrast to MCL cells, however, CD23 is typically highly expressed in CLL, and unlike CLL, MCL cells express FMC7, CD79a, and BCL-1 nuclear protein. The vague nodular pattern in MCL may mimic follicular pattern in FL, and like FL, MCL is positive for CD20 and BCL-2, but in contrast to FL, the neoplastic cells of MCL lack centroblasts and immunoblasts and do not express CD10 and BCL6. However, as these expression patterns vary, analysis of cyclin D1 overexpression or t(11;14) remains crucial to confirm or exclude the diagnosis of MCL [4].

To define the clinical stage, a CT scan of the neck, chest, and abdomen is recommended. Extranodal manifestations occur in >90% of patients; further interventional diagnostic such as endoscopic evaluation is only recommended for symptomatic patients and, because of the therapeutic consequence, to confirm (rare) early stages [3]. If CNS involvement is clinically suspected, liquor diagnostic should be supplemented. Diagnostic recommendations are summarized in Table 11.1.

11.7 Therapy

The clinical course of MCL is characterized by generally high initial response rates; however, early relapses are frequent, and most patients follow an aggressive clinical course. Nevertheless, 10–15% of patients present with a more indolent subtype. These cases are commonly characterized by a leukemic, non-nodal lymphoma manifestation or a very low Ki-67 index (<10%). In these cases, watchful waiting under close monitoring is considered an appropriate strategy [27]. Yet, the majority of cases require an early treatment initiation even though advanced-stage disease (stage III/IV) is still considered incurable.

11.7.1 Localized Stage

In the (rare) early stages I and II with low tumor burden, long-term remissions after involved-field radiotherapy (30–36 Gy) have been reported [28]. In contrast, in a randomized trial, frequent early relapses after radiotherapy alone were observed [29]. Therefore, in these localized cases, a shortened immunochemotherapy followed by a consolidating radiotherapy is considered most appropriate.

11.7.2 Advanced Stage

11.7.2.1 Conventional Chemotherapy

Due to the characteristic aggressive clinical course of MCL, an anthracycline-containing chemotherapy regimen is considered the standard chemotherapy backbone in the treatment of MCL [3], even though a small randomized trial did not confirm a major clinical benefit [30].

Table 11.1 Diagnostic recommendations

Laboratory workup	• Blood and differential count.
	• Serologic diagnostic including LDH, uric acid, liver and renal function, electrophoresis.
	• Optional: ß2-microglobulin, immune fixation.
	• FACS (in >20% of cases detection of circulating MCL cells).
	• In the case of clinical suspicion: liquor diagnostic (cell count, cytology, immunohistochemistry).
	• Hepatitis B/C and HIV serology.
Tissue diagnostic	• Preferably excisional lymph node biopsy (cytology, immunohistochemistry, cytogenetic/FISH). • Bone marrow aspiration and biopsy (cytology, immunohistochemistry, cytogenetic/FISH).
Imaging	• CT neck, chest, abdomen, pelvis.
	• Abdominal ultrasound .
	• MRI only in selected locations (CNS).
	• If clinically symptomatic or in early stages: gastroscopy, colonoscopy.
	• PET-CT prior to radiation in early stages.
Toxicity scans	• Creatinine clearance.
	• Electrocardiogram.
	• Cardiac ultrasound.
	• Pulmonary function (before ASCT).

Table 11.2 Conventional immunochemotherapy in newly diagnosed MCL

Author (year)	Phase	Number of patients	Regimen	ORR (CR) %	Median PFS (months)	Median OS %
Howard [33] (2002)	II	40	R-CHOP	96 (48)	17	95 (3 years)
Herold [34] (2015)	III	90	MCP R-MCP	63 (15) 71 (32)	34.9 93.4	55.9 (8 years) 76.1 (8 years)
Rummel [35] (2013)	III	94	R-CHOP BR	91 (30) 93 (40)	21 35	No difference
Kluin-Nelemans [36] (2012)	III	560	R-CHOP R-FC	86 (34) 78 (40)	28 (TTF) 26 (TTF)	62 (4 years) 47 (4 years)
Flinn [37] 2019	III	447	B R-CHOP/R-CVP	97 91	65.5% (5 years) 55.8% (5 years)	No difference

ORR overall response rate, *CR* complete response, *PFS* progression-free survival, *OS* overall survival, *R* rituximab, *CHOP* cyclophosphamide/doxorubicin/vincristine/prednisone, *MCP* mitoxantrone/chlorambucil/prednisone, *BR* bendamustine/rituximab, *R-FC* rituximab/fludarabine/cyclophosphamide

11.7.2.2 Combined Immunochemotherapy

Monotherapy with the anti-CD20 antibody rituximab showed only limited effectivity with response rates of approximately 25% [31] and should therefore be used only in medically unfit patients who are not able to tolerate cytotoxic therapy. However, addition of rituximab to conventional chemotherapy improved complete response rates, overall response rates, and overall survival. In a randomized trial, combination of rituximab and CHOP resulted in a significant improvement of response rates (94% vs. 75%) and time-to-treatment failure (21 vs. 14 months) [32]. Different trials confirmed superior response rates and improved overall survival (Table 11.2) [33–37], making immunochemotherapy the standard of care in both first-line and relapsed settings for patients with advanced-stage MCL.

In several phase 3 trials, different immunotherapy regimens were compared: A bendamustine-based combination resulted in similar response rates (93% vs. 91%) and was even superior in progression-free survival (PFS) (35 vs. 21 months). Most importantly, a more favorable toxicity profile was observed, particularly with regard to alopecia and peripheral neuropathy, making the bendamustine and rituximab (BR) regimen a useful alternative and currently the most favored regimen especially in elderly patients [35]. In contrast, a combination of rituximab with cyclophosphamide, vincristine, and prednisone (R-CVP) resulted in significantly inferior response rates and PFS [37]. Similarly, fludarabine-based combinations (R-FC: rituximab with fludarabine and cyclophosphamide) reached significantly worse overall survival rates (46% vs. 62% at 4 years) to those achieved with R-CHOP and resulted in prolonged cytopenias [36]. Therefore, this regimen cannot be recommended for first-line therapy of patients with MCL.

11.7.2.3 Therapy in Patients ≤65 years

In young and fit patients (≤65 years), a dose-intensified concept containing an immunochemotherapy induction followed by a high-dose consolidation regimen and autologous stem cell transplantation (ASCT) constitutes the current standard of care [3]. In several studies, either intensified up-front therapy or the addition of high-dose consolidation followed by ASCT resulted in impressive survival rates (Table 11.3) [38–41].

Induction: Dose-Intensified, Cytarabine-Containing Regimen

Promising results were achieved by sequential application of R-CHOP and the cytarabine-containing R-DHAP regimen (rituximab, dexamethasone, high-dose cytarabine, cisplatin): four cycles of R-DHAP following four cycles of R-CHOP improved CR rates from 12% to 57% [38]. Similarly, the rituximab plus hyperfractionated cyclophosphamide, vincristine, doxorubicin,

Table 11.3 Dose-intensified regimens in newly diagnosed MCL

Author (year)	Number of patients	Induction regimen	Consolidation regimen	ORR (CR) %	Median PFS (years)	Median OS% (years)
Delarue [38] 2013	60	R-CHOP/R-DHAP	ASCT	100 (96)	6.9	75% (5 years)
Chihara [39] 2016	97	R-hyper-CVAD/MA	–	90 (87)	4.8	10.7 years
Hermine [40] 2016	455	R-CHOP	ASCT	90 (63)	4.3	69% (5 years)
		R-CHOP/R-DHAP	ASCT	94 (61)	9.1	76% (5 years)
Le Gouill [41] 2017	299	R-DHAP	ASCT + R-maintenance	89 (after induction)	79% (4 years)	89% (4 years)
		R-DHAP	ASCT + observation		61% (4 years)	80% (4 years)
Eskelund [42] 2016	159	R-CHOP/R-high-dose cytarabine	ASCT		12.7	8,5

Dose-intensified therapy in newly diagnosed MCL. *ORR* overall response rate, *CR* complete response, *PFS* progression-free survival, *OS* overall survival, *R* rituximab, *CHOP* cyclophosphamide/doxorubicin/vincristine/prednisone, *DHAP* dexamethasone/high-dose cytarabine/cisplatin/dexamethasone, *hyper-CVAD* cyclophosphamide/doxorubicin/vincristine/dexamethasone, *MA* high-dose methotrexate/high-dose cytarabine

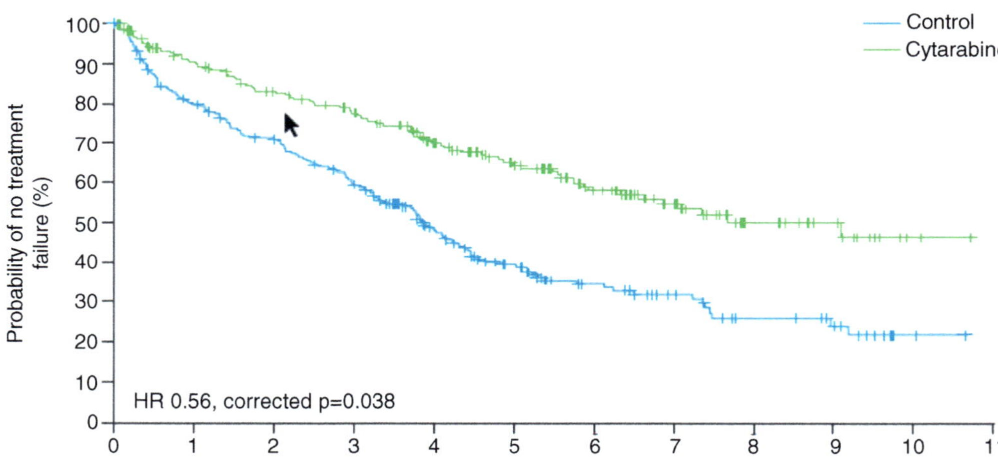

Number at risk

	0	1	2	3	4	5	6	7	8	9	10	11
Control	234	177	154	126	87	61	41	29	18	13	3	0
Cytarabine	232	290	170	151	119	92	67	41	22	14	2	0

Fig. 11.3 Time-to-treatment failure (TTF) after cytarabine-containing induction therapy (alternating R-CHOP/R-DHAP) followed by ASCT compared to R-CHOP alone [40]

and dexamethasone (R-hyper-CVAD) regimen achieved high complete response rates and long-term remissions [39]. However, this regimen is hampered by significant therapy-associated toxicity, including secondary malignancies, and should only be considered in young, fit patients [43, 44]. In a large, randomized European trial, the administration of the R-CHOP/DHAP regimen compared to administration of R-CHOP alone prior to myeloablative consolidation with ASCT more than doubled time-to-treatment failure (TTF) (109 vs. 47 months) [40] (Fig. 11.3).

Consolidation: Autologous Stem Cell Transplantation

In several studies, the addition of high-dose consolidation followed by autologous stem cell transplantation (ASCT) resulted in impressive survival rates [38, 40, 41]. A large randomized trial proved that consolidation by myeloablative radiochemo-

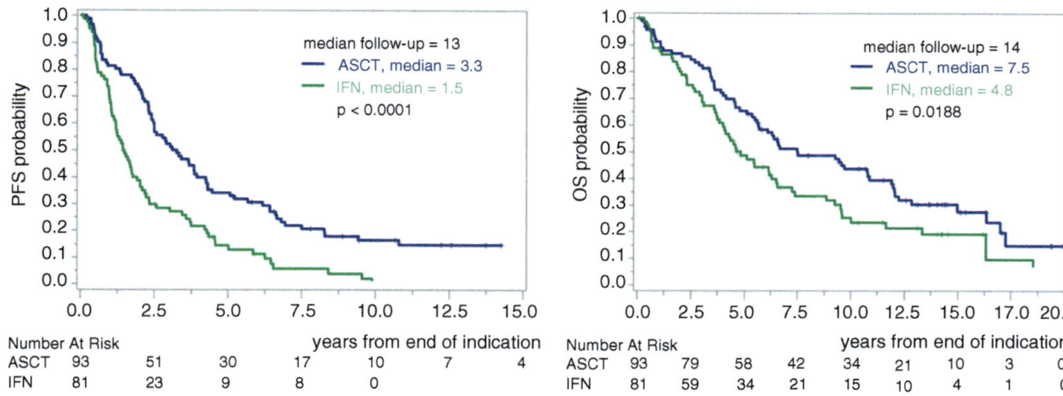

Fig. 11.4 Progressions-free survival and overall survival after ASCT compared to maintenance with Interferon (IFN) [46]

therapy followed by ASCT in first remission significantly prolonged PFS (3.3 vs. 1.5 years) (Fig. 11.4) and OS [45, 46] independently of the addition of rituximab. A retrospective comparison of different trials showed a benefit of a total-body irradiation (TBI)–containing high-dose consolidation only in patients having achieved partial remission after induction, whereas the addition of conventionally dosed radioimmunotherapy did not result in this benefit [47].

Unfortunately, even after such intensive consolidation regimens, a majority of patients relapses. This might be due to contamination of stem cell products with circulating MCL cells. Promising results were achieved by "in vivo purging" with a rituximab-containing induction regimen before apheresis, showing further improvement of long-term survival.

Maintenance

Rituximab maintenance after ASCT is currently considered standard of care for younger patients with MCL based on the results of a large phase III trial showing a significant optimization of PFS (83% vs. 64% after 4 years) and OS (89% vs. 80% after 4 years) after 3 years of rituximab maintenance compared to observation only [41].

Recently, another phase III trial revealed a benefit from a lenalidomide maintenance after autologous transplantation with improved PFS (80% vs. 64% after 3 years) compared to observation [48]. However, due to the elevated toxicity profile (especially hematotoxicity), lenalidomide maintenance should be only considered in patients not suitable to receive rituximab.

Radioimmunotherapy

Radioimmunotherapy as another alternative for treatment optimization has been evaluated in several studies. Applied to relapsed/refractory mantle cell lymphoma patients, radioimmunotherapy has achieved long-term remissions in some patients, although efficacy as a single approach is limited, with a median time to progression of only 5 months [49, 50]. Radioimmunotherapy consolidation after a shortened R-CHOP induction resulted in a 10-year overall survival of 56% (younger patients) and 33% (older patients), respectively, thereby proving as an active regimen for initial treatment of MCL [51].

11.7.2.4 Therapy in Patients >65 Years

Induction

The group of the over 65-year-olds ineligible for transplantation presents very heterogeneous regarding physical and cognitive performance. Fit patients >65 years should receive conventional immunochemotherapy followed by rituximab maintenance [36]. A combination of bortezomib, rituximab, cyclophosphamide, doxorubicin, and prednisone (VR-CAP) represents the new standard induction therapy for this group of patients based on a recently published international phase III trial comparing R-CHOP with VR-CAP. In this trial, VR-CAP doubled overall survival (OS) after 82 months compared to R-CHOP (90.7 vs. 45.7 months). However, hematologic toxicity (especially grade ≥3 thrombocytopenia) was significantly increased in the experimental arm (57% vs. 6%) [52].

The combination of rituximab, bendamustine, and cytarabine (R-BAC) offers another useful option [53]. Yet, this regimen was accompanied by severe hematotoxicities and should therefore only be administered to very fit older patients with high-risk features (e.g., blastoid variant, high LDH count).

Alternatively, for patients not qualifying for such intensive therapy regimens, R-bendamustine offers an appropriate alternative. This combination resulted in similar response rates (93% vs. 91%) compared to R-CHOP and was even superior in progression-free survival (PFS) (35 vs. 21 months) with a more favorable toxicity profile observed [35]. In frail patients, choice of therapy should mainly be aimed at control of symptoms.

Taken together, VR-CAP and BR represent the current standard approaches in older patients, who represent the majority of MCL patients. Based on clinical presentation, BR may be preferable especially in patients with a more indolent CLL-like presentation or in patients not qualifying for aggressive regimens, whereas VR-BAC seems to be appropriate in the more aggressive cases. Especially in blastoid variants, one might consider cytarabine-containing regimens based on the improved results in younger patients [40].

Maintenance

A large, randomized, European phase III trial confirmed that rituximab maintenance compared to interferon maintenance clearly improved PFS and OS after induction therapy with R-CHOP (5-year PFS R vs. IFN 51% vs. 22%, 5-year OS R vs. IFN 79% vs. 59%) [54] so that rituximab maintenance is now generally recommended.

11.7.3 Recurrent and Refractory Disease

Relapsed disease is often characterized by an even more aggressive clinical course. Resistance of MCL to conventional doses of chemotherapy becomes especially apparent in these relapsed cases. Conventional immunochemotherapy options, some of them highly effective in first-line treatment, achieve only short-term remissions in relapsed disease [55–59].

11.7.3.1 Allogenic Transplantation

For younger patients, the option of allogeneic transplantation as a curative approach should be discussed early, based on the observed graft-versus-lymphoma activity in MCL. Reduced-intensity conditioning may be applicable also in patients older than age 60 years. Yet, transplantation-associated severe acute and delayed toxicities, including chronic graft-versus-host disease and 20–25% treatment-related mortality, are frequent [60–63]. Therefore, allogeneic transplantation is not recommended in the first-line setting and should only be discussed in relapsed disease [3, 60–63]. Recently, the high efficacy of CAR T-cell therapy has been also confirmed in relapsed MCL even in the patient subset with high-risk features and may become the preferred alternative based on the more favorable toxicity profile [64].

11.7.3.2 Molecular Targeted Therapies

For patients not eligible for allogeneic transplantation, salvage immunochemotherapies or molecular targeted therapies should be applied. Yet, chemotherapy alone has only short-term activity in relapsed disease. Several targeted therapy approaches have been investigated in different studies as single agents or in combination with immunochemotherapies or other targeted therapies (Table 11.4).

Targeting the *B-cell receptor pathway* with the *Bruton's tyrosine kinase* (BTK) inhibitor ibrutinib resulted in remarkable response rates leading to its approval in relapsed MCL. In a large international phase II study, response rates of 68% were achieved with ibrutinib in patients with relapsed disease. The combination with rituximab was effective in all cases with low Ki-67, whereas in highly proliferating disease, only half of the patients responded to this approach [13]. A pooled analysis of the results of three different trials testing ibrutinib as monotherapy revealed overall response rates of 66% with median PFS and OS of 12.8 and 25 months,

Table 11.4 Molecular targeted therapies in MCL

Regimen	Phase	Number of patients	ORR (CR) %	Median PFS (years)	Author (year)
Bortezomib	Phase II	141	33 (8)	6.7 (TTP)	Goy [65]
Bortezomib + R-HAD	Retrospective	8	50 (25)	5	Weigert [66]
CHOP vs. bortezomib + CHOP	Phase II	46	48 (22) 83(35)	17 8	Furtado [67]
Temsirolimus 175/75 mg vs. temsirolimus 175/25 mg vs. chemotherapy	Phase III	162	22 (2) 6 (0) 2 (2)	4.8 3.4 1.9	Hess [68]
Temsirolimus + BR	Phase I/II	32	87 (8)	18	Hess [69]
R + temsirolimus	Phase II	69	59 (19)	9.7	Ansell [70]
Lenalidomide	Phase II	134	28 (88)	4	Goy [71]
Lenalidomide	Phase II	57	35 (12)	8.8	Zinzani [72]
Lenalidomide vs. monochemotherapy	Phase II	170 84	46 (11) 23 (8)	8.7 5.2	Trneny [73]
Lenalidomide + rituximab	Phase II	44	57 (36)	11.1	Wang [74]
Lenalidomide + rituximab	Phase II	38	92 (64)	64% (after 5 years)	Ruan [75]
Ibrutinib	Phase II	111	68 (21)	13.9	Wang [13]
Ibrutinib vs. temsirolimus	Phase III	280	72 (19) 40 (1)	14.6 6.2	Dreyling [76]
Ibrutinib + rituximab	Phase II	50	88 (44)		Wang [77]
Ibrutinib + bortezomib	Phase II				Novak [78]
Ibrutinib + lenalidomide + rituximab	Phase II	50	76	16	Jerkeman [79]
Idelalisib	Phase I	16	62	3.0	Kahl [80]
Abt-199 (venetoclax)	Phase I	28	75 (21)	14	Davids [81]
Abt-199 (venetoclax) + ibrutinib	Phase II	24	71	NA	Tam [82]
Acalabrutinib	Phase II	124	81	NA	Wang [83]

Molecular targeted therapies in MCL. *ORR* overall response rate, *CR* complete response, *PFS* progression-free survival, *OS* overall survival, *R* rituximab, *CHOP* cyclophosphamide/doxorubicin/vincristine/prednisone, *HAD* high-dose cytarabine/dexamethasone

respectively [84]. The compound is very well tolerated with only slight immunosuppression, bleeding, and atrial fibrillation being the predominant side effects. Yet, in patients with mutations in the *P53* gene, median PFS was significantly worse [84]. Furthermore, patients suffering early relapses after ibrutinib therapy demonstrated very aggressive clinical courses [85]. For this patient cohort, a monotherapy with the *B-cell-lymphoma 2 (bcl2) inhibitor* Abt-199 (venetoclax) might be a promising alternative, as a phase I trial showed response rates of 75% in patients with relapsed MCL [81] and 60% in patients having received prior ibrutinib therapy [86].

Second-generation BTK inhibitors such as acalabrutinib are currently being tested in different trials with promising results especially regarding tolerability [83]. Furthermore, BTK inhibitors combined with immunochemotherapy or other targeted therapies are under investigation. Recently, the combination of ibrutinib and venetoclax proved to be highly effective in a small study cohort [82].

Immunomodulatory drugs represent another molecular therapeutic approach. Various studies confirmed a benefit of the orally available lenalidomide in relapsed MCL, with response rates of 35–50% [71–74]. In a randomized phase II trial, this approach was superior to monochemotherapy (response rate 46% vs. 23%) [73]. Based on an in vitro synergism, lenalidomide in combination with rituximab resulted in long-lasting remissions in first-line therapy of a rather low-risk patient cohort [75].

Bortezomib, a first-generation *proteasome inhibitor*, has shown response rates of 30–40% in relapsed disease, with a median PFS of approximately 6 months, leading to the first Food and Drug Administration approval of a targeted drug in relapsed MCL [65]. Based on the encouraging results achieved with a combination of bortezomib and different immuno- and chemotherapeutic regimens [66, 87, 88], a large phase III trial combining bortezomib with rituximab, cyclophosphamide, doxorubicin, and prednisone (VR-CAP) as first-line therapy resulted in an almost doubling of PFS and significantly improved overall survival compared with R-CHOP [52].

Mammalian target of rapamycin inhibitor temsirolimus has been approved for relapsed disease based on the results of a large randomized trial proving it to be superior compared to monotherapy in a highly refractory patient population (response rate, 22% vs. 2%) [68]. Convincing response rates have also been observed in combination with bendamustine [69].

11.8 Outlook

The prospects of patients have significantly improved over the last decades due to optimization of chemotherapy regimens and addition of rituximab leading to improved overall survival. Yet, MCL remains an incurable disease with often aggressive clinical courses and early relapses despite initial response to therapy.

The implementation of targeted therapies, especially the BTK inhibitor ibrutinib, has already proven to be an effective strategy in the treatment of relapsed or refractory disease. Combined approaches for first-line therapy are now required to achieve prolonged remission durations. An overview of therapeutic recommendations is depicted in Fig. 11.5.

Improved clinical (MIPI), immunohistochemical (Ki-67, SOX11), and molecular genetic (*P53*) diagnostic tools have already paved the way to better estimate individual risk profiles and accordingly choose a therapeutic strategy.

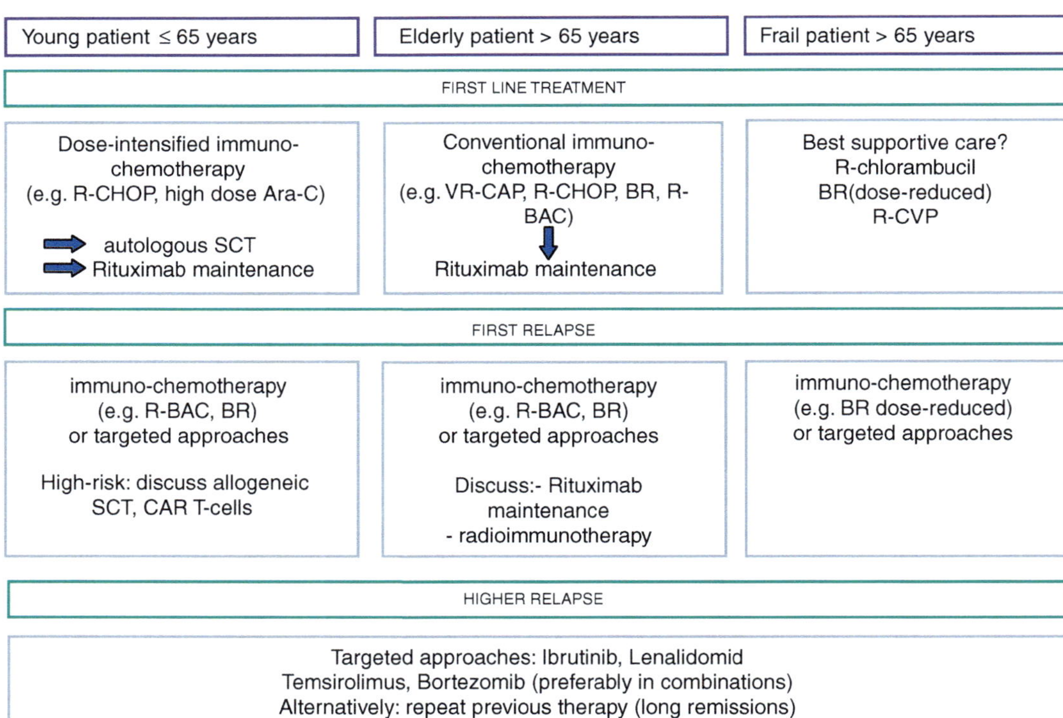

Fig. 11.5 Therapeutic recommendations in MCL

Nevertheless, the impact of prognostic and functional relevance of other recurrently mutated genes in MCL is still unclear and requires further investigation to individualize treatment strategies and allow patients to achieve optimal outcomes.

References

1. Banks PM, Chan J, Cleary ML, et al. Mantle cell lymphoma. A proposal for unification of morphologic, immunologic, and molecular data. Am J Surg Pathol. 1992;16(7):637–40.
2. Swerdlow SH, Campo E, Harris NL, et al. WHO classification of tumours of haematopoietic and lymphoid tissues. In: Bosman FT, Jaffe ES, Lakhani SR, Ohgaki H, editors. World Health Organization classification of tumours. Revised 4th Edition, Volume 2.2. Lyon: IARC; 2017.
3. Dreyling M, Campo E, Hermine O, et al. Newly diagnosed and relapsed mantle cell lymphoma: ESMO Clinical Practice Guidelines for diagnosis, treatment and follow-up. Ann Oncol. 2017;28(Suppl_4):iv62–71.
4. Naeim F. Atlas of hematopathology. Morphology, immunophenotype, cytogenetics and molecular approaches. 1st ed. New York: Academic Press; 2012. p. 411–25.
5. Tiemann M, Schrader C, Klapper W, et al. Histopathology, cell proliferation indices and clinical outcome in 304 patients with mantle cell lymphoma (MCL): a clinicopathological study from the European MCL Network. Br J Haematol. 2005;131(1):29–38.
6. Fernandez V, Salamero O, Espinet B, et al. Genomic and gene expression profiling defines indolent forms of mantle cell lymphoma. Cancer Res. 2010;70(4):1408–18.
7. Hoster E, Rosenwald A, Berger F, et al. Prognostic value of Ki-67 index, cytology, and growth pattern in mantle-cell lymphoma: results from randomized trials of the European Mantle Cell Lymphoma Network. J Clin Oncol. 2016;34(12):1386–94.
8. Fu K, Weisenburger DD, Greiner TC, et al. Cyclin D1-negative mantle cell lymphoma: a clinicopathologic study based on gene expression profiling. Blood. 2005;106(13):4315–21.
9. Jares P, Colomer D, Campo E. Genetic and molecular pathogenesis of mantle cell lymphoma: perspectives for new targeted therapeutics. Nat Rev Cancer. 2007;7(10):750–62.
10. Fernandez V, Hartmann E, Ott G, et al. Pathogenesis of mantle-cell lymphoma: all oncogenic roads lead to dysregulation of cell cycle and DNA damage response pathways. J Clin Oncol. 2005;23(26):6364–9.
11. Jares P, Colomer D, Campo E. Molecular pathogenesis of mantle cell lymphoma. J Clin Invest. 2012;122(10):3416–23.
12. Young RM, Staudt LM. Targeting pathological B cell receptor signalling in lymphoid malignancies. Nat Rev Drug Discov. 2013;12(3):229–43.
13. Wang ML, Rule S, Martin P, et al. Targeting BTK with ibrutinib in relapsed or refractory mantle-cell lymphoma. N Engl J Med. 2013;369(6):507–16.
14. Bea S, Valdes-Mas R, Navarro A, et al. Landscape of somatic mutations and clonal evolution in mantle cell lymphoma. Proc Natl Acad Sci U S A. 2013;110(45):18250–5.
15. Zhang J, Jima D, Moffitt AB, et al. The genomic landscape of mantle cell lymphoma is related to the epigenetically determined chromatin state of normal B cells. Blood. 2014;123(19):2988–96.
16. Yang P, Zhang W, Wang J, et al. Genomic landscape and prognostic analysis of mantle cell lymphoma. Cancer Gene Ther. 2018;25(5–6):129–40.
17. Eskelund CW, Dahl C, Hansen JW, et al. TP53 mutations identify younger mantle cell lymphoma patients who do not benefit from intensive chemoimmunotherapy. Blood. 2017;130(17):1903–10.
18. Aukema SM, Hoster E, Rosenwald A, et al. Expression of TP53 is associated with the outcome of MCL independent of MIPI and Ki-67 in trials of the European MCL Network. Blood. 2018;131(4):417–20.
19. Hoster E, Klapper W, Hermine O, et al. Confirmation of the mantle-cell lymphoma international prognostic index in randomized trials of the European Mantle-Cell Lymphoma Network. J Clin Oncol. 2014;32(13):1338–46.
20. Hoster E, Dreyling M, Klapper W, et al. A new prognostic index (MIPI) for patients with advanced-stage mantle cell lymphoma. Blood. 2008;111(2):558–65.
21. Wang ML, Lee H, Chuang H, et al. Ibrutinib in combination with rituximab in relapsed or refractory mantle cell lymphoma: a single-centre, open-label, phase 2 trial. Lancet Oncol. 2016;17(1):48–56.
22. Rauert-Wunderlich H, Mottok A, Scott DW, et al. Validation of the MCL35 gene expression proliferation assay in randomized trials of the European Mantle Cell Lymphoma Network. Br J Haematol. 2019;184(4):616–24.
23. Scott DW, Abrisqueta P, Wright GW, et al. New molecular assay for the proliferation signature in mantle cell lymphoma applicable to formalin-fixed paraffin-embedded biopsies. J Clin Oncol. 2017;35(15):1668–77.
24. Clot G, Jares P, Gine E, et al. A gene signature that distinguishes conventional and leukemic nonnodal mantle cell lymphoma helps predict outcome. Blood. 2018;132(4):413–22.
25. Romaguera JE, Medeiros LJ, Hagemeister FB, et al. Frequency of gastrointestinal involvement and its clinical significance in mantle cell lymphoma. Cancer. 2003;97(3):586–91.
26. Cheah CY, George A, Gine E, et al. Central nervous system involvement in mantle cell lymphoma: clinical features, prognostic factors and outcomes from the European Mantle Cell Lymphoma Network. Ann Oncol. 2013;24(8):2119–23.

27. Martin P, Chadburn A, Christos P, et al. Outcome of deferred initial therapy in mantle-cell lymphoma. J Clin Oncol. 2009;27(8):1209–13.
28. Dabaja BS, Zelenetz AD, Ng AK, et al. Early-stage mantle cell lymphoma: a retrospective analysis from the International Lymphoma Radiation Oncology Group (ILROG). Ann Oncol. 2017;28(9):2185–90.
29. Engelhard M, Unterhalt M, Hansmann M, et al. Follicular lymphoma, immunocytoma, and mantle cell lymphoma: randomized evaluation of curative radiotherapy in limited stage nodal disease. Ann Oncol. 2008;19(Suppl 4):418.
30. Meusers P, Engelhard M, Bartels H, et al. Multicentre randomized therapeutic trial for advanced centrocytic lymphoma: anthracycline does not improve the prognosis. Hematol Oncol. 1989;7(5):365–80.
31. Ghielmini M, Schmitz SF, Cogliatti S, et al. Effect of single-agent rituximab given at the standard schedule or as prolonged treatment in patients with mantle cell lymphoma: a study of the Swiss Group for Clinical Cancer Research (SAKK). J Clin Oncol. 2005;23(4):705–11.
32. Lenz G, Dreyling M, Hoster E, et al. Immunochemotherapy with rituximab and cyclophosphamide, doxorubicin, vincristine, and prednisone significantly improves response and time to treatment failure, but not long-term outcome in patients with previously untreated mantle cell lymphoma: results of a prospective randomized trial of the German Low Grade Lymphoma Study Group (GLSG). J Clin Oncol. 2005;23(9):1984–92.
33. Howard OM, Gribben JG, Neuberg DS, et al. Rituximab and CHOP induction therapy for newly diagnosed mantle-cell lymphoma: molecular complete responses are not predictive of progression-free survival. J Clin Oncol. 2002;20(5):1288–94.
34. Herold M, Scholz CW, Rothmann F, et al. Long-term follow-up of rituximab plus first-line mitoxantrone, chlorambucil, prednisolone and interferon-alpha as maintenance therapy in follicular lymphoma. J Cancer Res Clin Oncol. 2015;141(9):1689–95.
35. Rummel MJ, Niederle N, Maschmeyer G, et al. Bendamustine plus rituximab versus CHOP plus rituximab as first-line treatment for patients with indolent and mantle-cell lymphomas: an open-label, multicentre, randomised, phase 3 non-inferiority trial. Lancet. 2013;381(9873):1203–10.
36. Kluin-Nelemans HC, Hoster E, Hermine O, et al. Treatment of older patients with mantle-cell lymphoma. N Engl J Med. 2012;367(6):520–31.
37. Flinn IW, van der Jagt R, Kahl B, et al. First-line treatment of patients with indolent non-Hodgkin lymphoma or mantle-cell lymphoma with bendamustine plus rituximab versus R-CHOP or R-CVP: results of the BRIGHT 5-year follow-up study. J Clin Oncol. 2019;37(12):984–91.
38. Delarue R, Haioun C, Ribrag V, et al. CHOP and DHAP plus rituximab followed by autologous stem cell transplantation in mantle cell lymphoma: a phase 2 study from the Groupe d'Etude des Lymphomes de l'Adulte. Blood. 2013;121(1):48–53.
39. Chihara D, Cheah CY, Westin JR, et al. Rituximab plus hyper-CVAD alternating with MTX/Ara-C in patients with newly diagnosed mantle cell lymphoma: 15-year follow-up of a phase II study from the MD Anderson Cancer Center. Br J Haematol. 2016;172(1):80–8.
40. Hermine O, Hoster E, Walewski J, et al. Addition of high-dose cytarabine to immunochemotherapy before autologous stem-cell transplantation in patients aged 65 years or younger with mantle cell lymphoma (MCL younger): a randomised, open-label, phase 3 trial of the European Mantle Cell Lymphoma Network. Lancet. 2016;388(10044):565–75.
41. Le Gouill S, Thieblemont C, Oberic L, et al. Rituximab after autologous stem-cell transplantation in mantle-cell lymphoma. N Engl J Med. 2017;377(13):1250–60.
42. Eskelund CW, Kolstad A, Jerkeman M, et al. 15-year follow-up of the Second Nordic Mantle Cell Lymphoma trial (MCL2): prolonged remissions without survival plateau. Br J Haematol. 2016;175(3):410–8.
43. Merli F, Luminari S, Ilariucci F, et al. Rituximab plus HyperCVAD alternating with high dose cytarabine and methotrexate for the initial treatment of patients with mantle cell lymphoma, a multicentre trial from Gruppo Italiano Studio Linfomi. Br J Haematol. 2012;156(3):346–53.
44. Bernstein SH, Epner E, Unger JM, et al. A phase II multicenter trial of hyperCVAD MTX/Ara-C and rituximab in patients with previously untreated mantle cell lymphoma; SWOG 0213. Ann Oncol. 2013;24(6):1587–93.
45. Dreyling M, Lenz G, Hoster E, et al. Early consolidation by myeloablative radiochemotherapy followed by autologous stem cell transplantation in first remission significantly prolongs progression-free survival in mantle-cell lymphoma: results of a prospective randomized trial of the European MCL Network. Blood. 2005;105(7):2677–84.
46. Zoellner A-K, et al. Autologous stem cell transplantation in first remission significantly prolongs progression-free and overall survival in mantle cell lymphoma. In: International conference on malignant lymphoma, Lugano; 2019.
47. Hoster E, Geisler CH, Doorduijn J, et al. Total body irradiation after high-dose cytarabine in mantle cell lymphoma: a comparison of Nordic MCL2, HOVON-45, and European MCL Younger trials. Leukemia. 2016;30(6):1428–30.
48. Ladetto M, Cortelazzo S, Ferrero S, et al. Lenalidomide maintenance after autologous stem cell transplantation in mantle cell lymphoma: results of a multicentre randomised phase III trial. Lancet Oncology (in press).
49. Ferrero S, Pastore A, Scholz CW, et al. Radioimmunotherapy in relapsed/refractory mantle cell lymphoma patients: final results of a

European MCL Network Phase II Trial. Leukemia. 2016;30(4):984–7.
50. Wang M, Oki Y, Pro B, et al. Phase II study of yttrium-90-ibritumomab tiuxetan in patients with relapsed or refractory mantle cell lymphoma. J Clin Oncol. 2009;27(31):5213–8.
51. Smith MR, Hong F, Li H, et al. Mantle cell lymphoma initial therapy with abbreviated R-CHOP followed by (90)Y-ibritumomab tiuxetan: 10-year follow-up of the phase 2 ECOG-ACRIN study E1499. Leukemia. 2017;31(2):517–9.
52. Robak T, Jin J, Pylypenko H, et al. Frontline bortezomib, rituximab, cyclophosphamide, doxorubicin, and prednisone (VR-CAP) versus rituximab, cyclophosphamide, doxorubicin, vincristine, and prednisone (R-CHOP) in transplantation-ineligible patients with newly diagnosed mantle cell lymphoma: final overall survival results of a randomised, open-label, phase 3 study. Lancet Oncol. 2018;19(11):1449–58.
53. Visco C, Chiappella A, Nassi L, et al. Rituximab, bendamustine, and low-dose cytarabine as induction therapy in elderly patients with mantle cell lymphoma: a multicentre, phase 2 trial from Fondazione Italiana Linfomi. Lancet Haematol. 2017;4(1):e15–23.
54. Kluin-Nelemans H, Hoster E, Hermine O, et al. Treatment of older patients with mantle cell lymphoma: long-term follow-up of the randomized European MCL elderly trial. J Clin Oncol. 2020;38(3):248–56.
55. Forstpointner R, Dreyling M, Repp R, et al. The addition of rituximab to a combination of fludarabine, cyclophosphamide, mitoxantrone (FCM) significantly increases the response rate and prolongs survival as compared with FCM alone in patients with relapsed and refractory follicular and mantle cell lymphomas: results of a prospective randomized study of the German Low-Grade Lymphoma Study Group. Blood. 2004;104(10):3064–71.
56. Rummel MJ, Al-Batran SE, Kim SZ, et al. Bendamustine plus rituximab is effective and has a favorable toxicity profile in the treatment of mantle cell and low-grade non-Hodgkin's lymphoma. J Clin Oncol. 2005;23(15):3383–9.
57. Robinson KS, Williams ME, van der Jagt RH, et al. Phase II multicenter study of bendamustine plus rituximab in patients with relapsed indolent B-cell and mantle cell non-Hodgkin's lymphoma. J Clin Oncol. 2008;26(27):4473–9.
58. Weide R, Hess G, Koppler H, et al. High anti-lymphoma activity of bendamustine/mitoxantrone/rituximab in rituximab pretreated relapsed or refractory indolent lymphomas and mantle cell lymphomas. A multicenter phase II study of the German Low Grade Lymphoma Study Group (GLSG). Leuk Lymphoma. 2007;48(7):1299–306.
59. Dreyling M, Aurer I, Cortelazzo S, et al. Treatment for patients with relapsed/refractory mantle cell lymphoma: European-based recommendations. Leuk Lymphoma. 2018;59(8):1814–28.
60. Tam CS, Bassett R, Ledesma C, et al. Mature results of the M. D. Anderson Cancer Center risk-adapted transplantation strategy in mantle cell lymphoma. Blood. 2009;113(18):4144–52.
61. Le Gouill S, Kroger N, Dhedin N, et al. Reduced-intensity conditioning allogeneic stem cell transplantation for relapsed/refractory mantle cell lymphoma: a multicenter experience. Ann Oncol. 2012;23(10):2695–703.
62. Hamadani M, Saber W, Ahn KW, et al. Allogeneic hematopoietic cell transplantation for chemotherapy-unresponsive mantle cell lymphoma: a cohort analysis from the center for international blood and marrow transplant research. Biol Blood Marrow Transplant. 2013;19(4):625–31.
63. Zoellner AK, Fritsch S, Prevalsek D, et al. Sequential therapy combining clofarabine and T-cell-replete HLA-haploidentical haematopoietic SCT is feasible and shows efficacy in the treatment of refractory or relapsed aggressive lymphoma. Bone Marrow Transplant. 2015;50(5):679–84.
64. Wang M, Munoz J, Goy A, et al. KTE-X19 car T-cell therapy in relapsed or refractory mantle-cell lymphoma. N Engl J Med. 2020;382(14):1331–42.
65. Goy A, Bernstein SH, Kahl BS, et al. Bortezomib in patients with relapsed or refractory mantle cell lymphoma: updated time-to-event analyses of the multicenter phase 2 PINNACLE study. Ann Oncol. 2009;20(3):520–5.
66. Weigert O, Weidmann E, Mueck R, et al. A novel regimen combining high dose cytarabine and bortezomib has activity in multiply relapsed and refractory mantle cell lymphoma - long-term results of a multicenter observation study. Leuk Lymphoma. 2009;50(5):716–22.
67. Furtado M, Johnson R, Kruger A, et al. Addition of bortezomib to standard dose chop chemotherapy improves response and survival in relapsed mantle cell lymphoma. Br J Haematol. 2015;168(1):55–62.
68. Hess G, Herbrecht R, Romaguera J, et al. Phase III study to evaluate temsirolimus compared with investigator's choice therapy for the treatment of relapsed or refractory mantle cell lymphoma. J Clin Oncol. 2009;27(23):3822–9.
69. Hess G, Keller U, Scholz CW, et al. Safety and efficacy of Temsirolimus in combination with bendamustine and rituximab in relapsed mantle cell and follicular lymphoma. Leukemia. 2015;29(8):1695–701.
70. Ansell SM, Tang H, Kurtin PJ, et al. Temsirolimus and rituximab in patients with relapsed or refractory mantle cell lymphoma: a phase 2 study. Lancet Oncol. 2011;12(4):361–8.
71. Goy A, Sinha R, Williams ME, et al. Single-agent lenalidomide in patients with mantle-cell lymphoma who relapsed or progressed after or were refractory to bortezomib: phase II MCL-001 (EMERGE) study. J Clin Oncol. 2013;31(29):3688–95.
72. Zinzani PL, Vose JM, Czuczman MS, et al. Long-term follow-up of lenalidomide in relapsed/refractory

mantle cell lymphoma: subset analysis of the NHL-003 study. Ann Oncol. 2013;24(11):2892–7.
73. Trneny M, Lamy T, Walewski J, et al. Lenalidomide versus investigator's choice in relapsed or refractory mantle cell lymphoma (MCL-002; SPRINT): a phase 2, randomised, multicentre trial. Lancet Oncol. 2016;17(3):319–31.
74. Wang M, Fayad L, Wagner-Bartak N, et al. Lenalidomide in combination with rituximab for patients with relapsed or refractory mantle-cell lymphoma: a phase 1/2 clinical trial. Lancet Oncol. 2012;13(7):716–23.
75. Ruan J, Martin P, Christos P, et al. Five-year follow-up of lenalidomide plus rituximab as initial treatment of mantle cell lymphoma. Blood. 2018;132(19):2016–25.
76. Dreyling M, Jurczak W, Jerkeman M, et al. Ibrutinib versus temsirolimus in patients with relapsed or refractory mantle-cell lymphoma: an international, randomised, open-label, phase 3 study. Lancet. 2016;387(10020):770–8.
77. Wang ML, Lee H, Chuang H, et al. Ibrutinib in combination with rituximab in relapsed or refractory mantle cell lymphoma: a single-centre, open-label, phase 2 trial. Lancet Oncol. 2016;17(1):48–56.
78. Novak U, Fehr M, Zander T, et al. SAKK 36/13–Ibrutinib and bortezomib followed by ibrutinib maintenance in patients with relapsed and refractory mantle cell lymphoma: phase I report of a phase I/II trial. In: Supplement: 14th international conference on malignant lymphoma Palazzo dei Congressi (Lugano, Switzerland), 14–17 June, 2017; 2017;35(S2). p. 207.
79. Jerkeman M, Eskelund CW, Hutchings M, et al. Ibrutinib, lenalidomide, and rituximab in relapsed or refractory mantle cell lymphoma (PHILEMON): a multicentre, open-label, single-arm, phase 2 trial. Lancet Haematol. 2018;5(3):e109–e16.
80. Kahl BS, Spurgeon SE, Furman RR, et al. A phase 1 study of the PI3Kdelta inhibitor idelalisib in patients with relapsed/refractory mantle cell lymphoma (MCL). Blood. 2014;123(22):3398–405.
81. Davids MS, Roberts AW, Seymour JF, et al. Phase I first-in-human study of venetoclax in patients with relapsed or refractory non-Hodgkin lymphoma. J Clin Oncol. 2017;35(8):826–33.
82. Tam CS, Anderson MA, Pott C, et al. Ibrutinib plus venetoclax for the treatment of mantle-cell lymphoma. N Engl J Med. 2018;378(13):1211–23.
83. Wang M, Rule S, Zinzani PL, et al. Acalabrutinib in relapsed or refractory mantle cell lymphoma (ACE-LY-004): a single-arm, multicentre, phase 2 trial. Lancet. 2018;391(10121):659–67.
84. Rule S, Dreyling M, Goy A, et al. Ibrutinib for the treatment of relapsed/refractory mantle cell lymphoma: extended 3.5-year follow up from a pooled analysis. Haematologica. 2019;104(5):e211–e4.
85. Martin P, Maddocks K, Leonard JP, et al. Postibrutinib outcomes in patients with mantle cell lymphoma. Blood. 2016;127(12):1559–63.
86. Jiang H, Lwin T, Zhao X, et al. Venetoclax as a single agent and in combination with PI3K-MTOR1/2 kinase inhibitors against ibrutinib sensitive and resistant mantle cell lymphoma. Br J Haematol. 2019;184(2):298–302.
87. Baiocchi RA, Alinari L, Lustberg ME, et al. Phase 2 trial of rituximab and bortezomib in patients with relapsed or refractory mantle cell and follicular lymphoma. Cancer. 2011;117(11):2442–51.
88. Lamm W, Kaufmann H, Raderer M, et al. Bortezomib combined with rituximab and dexamethasone is an active regimen for patients with relapsed and chemotherapy-refractory mantle cell lymphoma. Haematologica. 2011;96(7):1008–14.

12 Hairy Cell Leukemia

Tadeusz Robak and Sascha Dietrich

Hairy cell leukemia (HCL)

Clinical outline Adult patients with symptoms mainly related to bone marrow (BM) infiltration and splenomegaly; circulating neoplastic cells are few. Rarely mass forming, nodal or other extranodal. Granulopenia frequent.

Cytology	"Hairy cells", i.e. small to medium sized cells with oval to indented nucleus and circumferential cytoplasmic projections.	Hairy cell leukemia, cytology	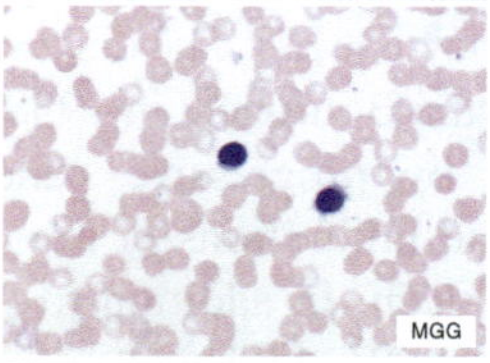
Histology	Frequent punctio sicca. BM biopsy with maturation arrest and decrease of granulopoiesis. Interstitial cells with "fried egg" appearance with accompanying reticulin fibrosis. Diagnosis may be challenging due to relative low infiltration grade. Diffuse expansion in red pulp of spleen.	Hairy cell leukemia, hystology	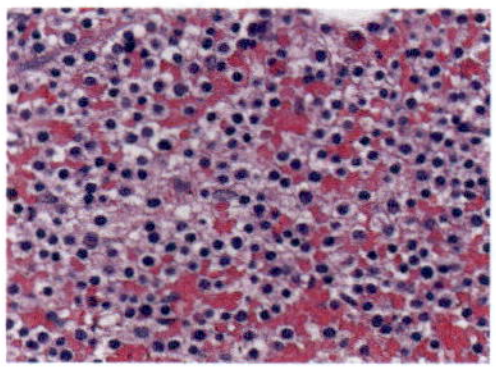

	CD20	CD5	CD23	CD10[1]	BCL6	cyclin D1[2]	CD103	FMC7	IgM	light chains
notes	[1]few positive cases reported. [2]faint staining but no translocation of cyclin D1,									
other marker	"HCL-phenotype" on flow cytometry: FMC7+, CD11c+, CD103+, CD123+, CD25+, CD200+ Histology markers: BRAF-V600E +, Annexin-A +, DBA44 +, T-BET+									

= majority of cases positive   = variable fraction of cases positive   = negative

Main differential diagnosis	Splenic marginal zone lymphoma (should be CD103 and BRAF-V600E negative), Hairy cell leukemia variant (should be CD103 positive, BRAF-V600E negative and show distinct cytology),

M. Dreyling, M. Ladetto (eds.), *Indolent Lymphomas*, Hematologic Malignancies,
https://doi.org/10.1007/978-3-030-55989-2_12

Key molecular features
IGH genes are rearranged, somatic hypermutation and IGHV usage bias. BRAF-V600E in vast majority. Few cases without BRAF-V600E mutation but MAP2K1 mutations (relation to HCL or Hairy cell leukemia variant uncertain so far)
Frequent translocations: none reported.
Precursor lesions
Not known.
Progression
Transformation rare (only sporadic cases reported).
Clinically relevant pathologic features
Clinically relevant subtypes not identified. BRAF-V600E mutation negative variants may be a predictive subgroup but relation to hairy cell leukemia variant still uncertain.

12.1 Introduction

Hairy cell leukemia (HCL) is a rare type of chronic lymphoid leukemia originated from a mature B lymphocyte [1, 2]. The disease was first described by Bertha Bouroncle in 1958 [3]. HCL is characterized by progressive pancytopenia, splenomegaly, and infiltrations of the bone marrow, liver, and spleen. In addition to the classic form of HCL, the World Health Organization (WHO) now recognizes HCL variant (HCL-V) as a provisional entity distinct from classic HCL; it is regarded as an unclassifiable splenic B-cell leukemia/lymphoma, together with splenic diffuse red pulp small B-cell lymphoma (SDRPL) [4, 5]. However, the relationship between SDRPL and HCL-V remains unclear. HCL-V was first described in 1980 by Cawley et al. [6]. The disease is characterized by splenomegaly, lymphocytosis, and hypercellular bone marrow. In comparison to classic HCL, patients with HCL-V are often older, present with lymphocytosis, and are resistant to purine nucleoside analogs. Biologically, HCL-V is more closely related to splenic lymphomas and shares several overlapping clinical and morphological features with other disorders characterized by villous circulating cells. In the last three decades, tremendous progress in the biology and treatment of classic HCL and HCL-V has been made, which has resulted in an improvement in overall life expectancy and quality of life, mainly due to the introduction of purine nucleoside analogs, cladribine and pentostatin, as well as supportive care regimens. Thanks to the use of these drugs, classic HCL has evolved from a disease with poor prognosis to a highly treatable disorder and affords near-normal survival [7]. HCL-V has usually poorer prognosis than classic HCL.

12.2 Epidemiology

Hairy cell leukemia (HCL) is a rare mature B-cell malignancy with an incidence of 0.3 cases per 100,000 individuals and is four times more common in men than women [8]. It predominantly occurs in elderly patients with a median age of 49–51 years at initial diagnosis, but younger patients are also affected. These young patients with HCL have shorter responses to treatment and require more lines of therapy to maintain disease control while attaining similar long-term survival [9]. HCL-V is estimated to be 0.2 cases per 100,000 and the disease comprises 2% of all leukemias [8].

T. Robak (✉)
Department of Hematology, Medical University of Lodz, Lodz, Poland
e-mail: robaktad@csk.umed.lodz.pl

S. Dietrich
Department of Medicine V, University of Heidelberg, Heidelberg, Germany
e-mail: sascha.dietrich@embl.de

12.3 Molecular Biology and Pathogenesis

During recent years, many new discoveries have revolutionized the molecular understanding of HCL [10]. In 2011, Tiacci et al. discovered that classical HCL is characterized by a gain-of-function mutation of the BRAF serine/threonine protein kinase (V600E) [11, 12]. In the initial validation series, all HCL patients showed this particular mutation; however, a set of 195 B-cell lymphomas and leukemias did not harbor a mutated *BRAF* gene. The vast majority of *BRAF*-V600E mutations in HCL are heterozygous, but while homozygous mutations are rare, they have been suggested to be associated with a more aggressive disease course [13]. Recurrent deletions of the *BRAF* gene locus on chromosome 7q34 have been described in HCL and lead to loss of heterozygosity [14]. BRAF mutations, different from V600E, seem to be extremely rare in HCL and have been described in only two patients so far [15]. The incidence of BRAF mutations in nearly 100% HCL cases at diagnosis, i.e., encompassing the whole disease spectrum, their somatic nature, and presence in the entire tumor clone, as well as their high stability at relapse, strongly suggests that the pathogenesis of HCL critically depends on constitutively activated BRAF [11, 12, 16].

Chung et al. report that *BRAF*-V600E mutations are already present in hematopoietic stem cells (HSCs) or B-cell lymphoid progenitors of HCL patients and that these patients exhibit marked alterations in hematopoietic stem/progenitor cell (HSPC) frequencies [17]. Transplantation of *BRAF*-V600E-mutant HSCs from an HCL patient into immunodeficient mice resulted in stable engraftment of *BRAF*-V600E-mutant human hematopoietic cells, highlighting the functional self-renewal capacity of HCL HSCs. However, none of the transplanted mice developed a typical HCL, strongly suggesting that the development of a full HCL phenotype may require a permissive epigenetic background, likely restricted to a particular stage of B-cell differentiation, and/or the acquirement of further genetic lesions.

The *BRAF*-V600E mutation constitutively activates BRAF providing oncogenic signaling through the MEK-ERK cascade [11]. Both in vitro and in vivo studies have demonstrated that BRAF-dependent phospho-ERK activation is a critical signaling event in HCL. Moreover, in vitro treatment of primary purified HCL cells with BRAF and MEK inhibitors has resulted in the marked dephosphorylation of MEK/ERK, silencing of the RAF-MEK-ERK pathway transcriptional output, loss of the specific HCL gene expression profile signature, change of the characteristic morphology of the leukemic cells (from "hairy" to "smooth"), and eventual apoptosis [18].

Aberrant expression of cell cycle-related proteins such as cyclin D1 have been shown to be reversible using inhibitors of activated BRAF signaling, suggesting that expression is not a constitutive disease trait but elicited by MEK/ERK signaling and oncogenic BRAF mutations, respectively. This concept may have important consequences for minimal residual disease (MRD) assessment in the context of inhibitor treatment, as the marker profile (cyclin D1) could be dynamic, as well as for targeted drug treatment, which may be curtailed by the on-target effect of inhibitors.

In addition to the *BRAF*-V600E mutation, the most common genetic alteration in classical HCL was a loss in copy number for chromosome 7q. The minimally deleted region of this copy number alteration includes the wild-type locus of *BRAF*. This genetic lesion subdivides classical HCL into those with hemizygous versus those with heterozygous mutations of *BRAF* [12]. Whole exome sequencing study of relapsed and refractory HCL patients revealed known cancer-associated genes such as *EZH2* and *ARID1A*, as well as novel inactivating mutations of the cell cycle inhibitor *CDKN1B* (p27). In a cohort of 81 mostly untreated HCL patients, the incidence of *CDKN1B* mutations was 16% [19]. While a clinical impact of *CDKN1B* mutations was not found, *CDKN1B* was found to be the second most commonly mutated gene in HCL. *CDKN1B* is a critical element in cell cycle control and a known tumor suppressor in different solid cancers [20].

CDKN1B prevents the activation of cyclin E-CDK2 or cyclin D-CDK4 complexes and therefore regulates cell cycle progression in the G1 phase. Interestingly, BRAF-induced senescence in premalignant nevi is circumvented by deletion or mutation of *CDKN2A* in invasive melanoma. In *BRAF*-mutated hairy cell leukemia, *CDKN1B* loss may serve as a mechanism to escape oncogene-induced senescence [21]. In addition to *CDKN1B*, mutations cooperating with *BRAF*-V600E, recurrent, inactivating mutations in *KMT2C* (*MLL3*) were identified in 15% and 13% of classical HCL and HCL variant, respectively [12]. Another study described somatic mutations or deletions of the *Krüppel-like factor 2* (*KLF2*) in 4 of 24 (16%) HCL patients examined, but *KLF2* mutations are more frequent in other B-cell malignancies, such as SMZL (31%), and diffuse large B-cell lymphoma (26%). Although better descriptions of the genetic landscape of HCL have been obtained during recent years, the function of mutations cooperating with *BRAF*-V600E remains to be elucidated.

12.4 Differential Diagnosis

Historically, there were two different forms of HCL, the more common classical HCL (90%) and the less frequent HCL-V (10%). HCL-V is characterized by a more aggressive disease course and a poor response to purine analogs [22]. Most importantly, HCL-V cases are commonly negative for *BRAF*-V600E mutation. A small subset of patients with bona fide classical HCL but who also do not harbor any *BRAF* mutation has been reported but only in a single study [23]. However, these cases are often characterized by an *IGHV4-34* immunoglobulin rearrangement, which is generally absent in classic HCL, and it is associated with a similar poor prognosis as HCL-V.

Almost 50% of HCL-V and IGHV4-34-expressing HCL cases were found to harbor activating mutations in the *MAP2K1* gene encoding MEK1. All but one of the identified mutations (n = 15) have been described and are known to strongly increase phospho-ERK levels and, consequently, cell proliferation [24]. These findings underline the importance of constitutive MEK-ERK signaling even in this HCL-like disorder.

HCL cells typically show a distinctive immunophenotype coexpressing CD19, CD20, CD11c, CD25, CD103, and CD123. In contrast, HCL-V cells lack the expression of CD25 and CD123 [25]. Moreover, HCL cells strongly express CD200, which can also be used as another distinctive marker to differentiate HCL [26]. *BRAF*-V600E is now regarded as a specific oncogenic mutation occurring only in HCL [27]. Another distinctive feature of HCL is the expression of annexin A1, which is easily accessible by immunohistochemical staining [28]. In addition to HCL-V, the 2016 revision of the WHO classification of lymphoid neoplasms recognizes two provisional entities resembling HCL: splenic marginal zone lymphoma (SMZL), usually associated with *NOTCH2* mutations, and splenic diffuse red pulp small B-cell lymphoma (SDRPBCL) whose genomic landscape has not been yet clarified. Table 12.1 summarizes the most important differential diagnosis of HCL and their characteristic markers.

Testing for *BRAF*-V600E mutation can be helpful as an additional marker in routine clinical practice if there is any diagnostic uncertainty. For relapsed and refractory patients, we strongly recommend evaluating *BRAF* mutation status, since this may serve as therapeutic target. The limited number of HCL cells present in the peripheral blood requires highly sensitive molecular assays to detect *BRAF* mutations (e.g., allele-specific polymerase chain reaction). Alternatively, *BRAF*-V600E mutation-specific antibodies can be used for immunohistochemical staining in bone marrow biopsies [5]. However, further validation of the diagnostic utility of these reagents in a larger number of cases is required.

12.5 Prognosis

Hairy cell leukemia belongs to the group of indolent lymphoid malignancies. Standard treatment with purine analogs induces complete remission in more than 80% of patients with classical hairy cell leukemia. If complete remission is achieved,

Table 12.1 Differential diagnosis of HCL and the characteristic features of related entities

	HCL	HCL variant	SMZL	SDRPBCL
Frequency	0.3/100,000	0.03/100,000	0.13/100,000	N.a.
Ratio m:f	4:1 (m:w)	1–2:1 (m:w)	1:3 (m:w)	1–2:1 (m:w)
Median age	50–55	>70	65–70	65–75
Lymphocytosis	≤10%	≥90%	≥50%	≥50%
Immunophenotype	CD11c+ CD103+ CD25+ CD200+ CD23− CD5−	CD11c+ CD103+/− CD25− CD200− CD23− CD5−	CD11c− CD103−/+ CD5−/+ CD200+ CD23+/− CD5−/+	CD11c+ CD103− CD25−/+ – CD23− CD5−/+
Immunohistochemistry	DBA.44+ Cyclin D1+ Annexin A1+	DBA.44+ Cyclin D1+/− Annexin A1−	DBA.44+ Cyclin D1− Annexin A1−	DBA.44+ Cyclin D1− Annexin A1−
Genotype	*BRAF*-V600E Mutation	*BRAF* wt ≈50% *MEK1* mutations, ≈50% IGHV4-34 rearrangement	*BRAF* wild-type Frequent Notch2 mutations	*BRAF* wild-type

the median time to next treatment is more than 10 years [29]. In case of a partial remission, patients have a significantly shorter treatment-free interval of only 3 years. If retreatment is necessary, and a subsequent complete remission can be achieved, patients with classical hairy cell leukemia enjoy again a very long treatment-free interval of more than 10 years [29]. However, the proportion of patients who achieve a CR decreases with each treatment round. Altogether, it has been shown that many classical hairy cell leukemia patients have an overall survival which is comparable with the normal population. Even younger patients with hairy cell leukemia, who tend to have shorter treatment-free intervals, seem to have a very good long-term outcome [9]. It is important to note that in contrast to classical HCL, it has been found that HCL-V and HCL with *VH4-34* gene usage have a considerably poorer response and long-term outcome [30].

12.6 Treatment Response Evaluation and Disease Progression

Treatment response criteria are defined according the consensus guidelines and ESMO guidelines [1, 2]. Complete remission (CR) required morphologic absence of hairy cells on peripheral blood (PB) and bone marrow (BM) aspiration or biopsy specimens and normalization of organomegaly and peripheral blood counts. Patients in CR should have near normalization of peripheral blood counts including hemoglobin >11 g/dL, platelets >100,000/μL, and an absolute neutrophil count >1500/μL. It is recommended that an assessment for CR following cladribine should be performed 4–6 months after treatment, and at this time a BM biopsy should be performed to document a CR. A partial response (PR) is described as normalization of PB counts, with at least 50% reduction in organomegaly and bone marrow hairy cells and below 5% of circulating hairy cells. All other outcomes are considered as nonresponse. Patients with a CR demonstrate longer remission duration and longer survival than those achieving a PR [31]. Relapse is defined as deterioration in blood counts related to the detection of hairy cells in PB and/or BM and/or increasing splenomegaly. Progressive disease is defined by a 25% decrease in PB hematologic parameters that lasts for 2 months or more or an increase in the hairy cell infiltration of the BM [1]. In addition, 25% increase in either the size of the spleen or the liver based on the nadir measurements achieved following therapy is consistent with disease progression.

The evaluation of minimal residual disease (MRD) in HCL remains controversial and is generally not recommended in routine clinical practice. Preliminary studies indicate that the extent of MRD may predict the duration of remission. For quantitative evaluation of MRD, immunohistochemical staining of the BM core biopsy for CD20, DBA.44, VE-1, or CD79a may be useful. However, the level of disease involvement for MRD negativity is not yet established. Some authors indicate that risk of relapse is low if immunohistochemical staining reveals an MRD level below 1% and high if MRD is greater than 5% positive cells in the BM [32]. In another study, the PB-MRD panel consisted of 2 four-color tubes, including CD19, CD11c, CD25, CD22, and CD103 antigens, or 2 six-color tubes with the addition of CD123 and CD200 [33]. The sensitivity of this test was established as 0.01% and remained constant over the entire period of observation. This study has confirmed that patients with PB-MRD negativity at 6 months (0.01% cutoff) have a low probability of disease relapse. However, further studies are needed to establish the predictive value of PB flow cytometric monitoring for MRD relapse.

12.7 Treatment of Newly Diagnosed Patients with Classic HCL

Similarly to other indolent lymphoid malignancies, a "watch and wait" strategy is recommended in HCL patients asymptomatic at diagnosis. Approximately 10% of HCL patients do not require immediate therapy after diagnosis, and they should be monitored until treatment is indicated. Treatment should be initiated if symptomatic and/or progressive disease is recognized, especially cytopenia and/or symptomatic organomegaly [1]. According to current consensus guidelines, treatment should be initiated if one or more of the following hematologic parameters are met: hemoglobin less than 11 g/dL, platelet count less than $100 \times 10^3/\mu L$, or absolute neutrophil count less than 1000/μL [1, 2]. Symptomatic splenomegaly with or without cytopenias is also an indication for treatment.

Cladribine and pentostatin are the drugs of choice in the treatment of HCL [1, 2]. These agents have significantly improved the prognosis of patients with HCL as they typically induce very long-lasting remissions. Pentostatin was first used by Spiers et al. in 1984 for the treatment of two men with advanced but previously untreated HCL [34]. Quick clearance of hairy cells from the blood and regression of splenomegaly and lymphadenopathy were observed in both patients, as was correction of anemia, thrombocytopenia, and granulocytopenia. In 1990, the Piro group from Scripps Clinic, San Diego, reported 12 patients with HCL treated with cladribine (2-CDA, 2-chlorodeoxyadenosine) at a dose of 0.1 mg per kilogram of body weight per day, by continuous infusion for 7 days [35]. Eleven patients had CR with the normalization of PB and BM with disappearance of leukemic cells. The median duration of response was 15.5 months with the longest remission being 3.8 years and no relapse at the time of publication. Further studies confirmed these early reports. Both agents induce durable and unmaintained CR in more than 70% of patients, and the relapse rates were about 30–40% after 5–10 years of follow-up (Table 12.2) [29, 36–46].

Cladribine is most commonly administered as a continuous i.v. infusion at a dose of 0.09 mg/kg over a 5- to 7-day period or as a 2-h i.v. infusion at a dose of 0.12–0.14 mg/kg for 5–7 days [37, 47]. Administration of cladribine can result in severe neutropenia that can last weeks or longer. Cladribine is also not recommended for patients presenting with active infection requiring therapy for the underlying leukemia. Cladribine can be also given at a dose of 0.12–0.15 mg/kg in a 2-h infusion once a week for six doses. Weekly and daily administration induces similar OR and CR rates. In addition, randomized trials indicate no difference in the occurrence of adverse events, including infections and hematological toxicity, between the weekly and daily schedule [38, 48]. Cladribine given subcutaneously is as equally effective as the intravenous formulation but more convenient for patients [49].

Table 12.2 Larger clinical trials with purine analogs in treating classic hairy cell leukemia

Study	Treatment	No. of pts	CR rate	Duration of CR (time to relapse)
Saven et al. 1998 [36]	2-CDA 0.087 or 0.1 mg/kg/day c.i. × 7 days	349	91%	96% survival at 48 months
Goodman et al. 2003 [31]	2-CDA 0.1 mg/kg/day c.i. × 7 days	207	95%	Median duration of CR—98 monts
Cheson et al. 1998 [37]	2-CDA 0.1 mg/kg/day c.i. × 7 days	861	50%	Median duration of CR not reached
Robak et al. 1999 [39]	2-CDA 0.12 mg/kg/day in 2 h i.v. infusion/5 days	97	77.3%	Median duration of CRc—37.4 months
Robak et al. 2007 [38]	2-CDA 0.12 mg/kg/day in 2 h i.v. infusion/5 days vs. once a week for 6 weeks	116	76% vs. 72%	Median duration of CRc—4.3 years vs. 5.1 years
Grever et al. 1995 [40]	Pentostatin 2–4 mg/m² i.v. biweekly	154	76%	67% estimated DFS at 10 years; 18.5% relapse at 111 months
Maloisel et al. 2003 [42]	Pentostatin 4 mg/m² i.v. biweekly	230	79%	68.8% estimated DFS at 10 years
Flinn et al. 2000 [42]	Pentostatin 4 mg/m² i.v. biweekly	241	76%	67% estimated RFS at 10 years
Else et al. 2005, 2009 [29]	Pentostatin 4 mg/m² i.v. every 1 or 2 weeks	185	81%	Median time to relapse—15 years; 24% of relapse at 5 years, 42% at 10 years
Zinzani et al. 2010 [44]	2-CDA 0.14 mg/kg/day i.v. for 5 days or once a week for five cycles	121	77%	Median time to relapse—2.7 years
Inbar et al. 2018 [45]	2-CDA i.v. (62%) or s.c. (38%) as a daily injection for 5 consecutive days	159	NR	Median time to next treatment after first-line therapy—9.3 (0–15.5) years.
Forconi et al. 2010 [46]	2-CDA s.c. 0.5–0.7 mg/kg as a single course	148	68.2%	After a median follow-up of 37.5 months (range 12–67), 5-year TFS, 67%; RFS, 71%; and OS, 94%

2-CDA 2-chlorodeoxiadenosine, cladribine, *CR* complete response, *DFS* disease-free survival, *OS* overall survival, *RFS* relapse-free survival, *TFS* treatment free survival

Pentostatin is usually administered at a dose of 4 mg/m² i.v. every second week, until CR with one or two consolidating injections [29, 40, 42, 43]. Pentostatin is more effective than interferon-α (IFN-α) in HCL patients, as confirmed in a large, multicenter, randomized trial [40]. Purine nucleoside analogs dramatically improved the prognosis for patients with HCL. Durable and unmaintained remission is observed in 76–98% of patients, with relapse rates of about 30–40% after 5–10 years of observation, and in many patients, overall OS is longer than 20 years [29, 43, 50].

Although no direct comparison between pentostatin and cladribine has been performed in any randomized trial, no significant difference has been found between the two with regard to their efficacy or safety. Both agents can be used as frontline treatment of HCL. Cladribine is most commonly used due to its simpler administration and its lower renal toxicity [51, 52]. However, pentostatin has been successfully administered to patients with an active infection due to the gradual administration of titrated doses of this drug. In addition, cladribine can induce remissions in patients resistant to pentostatin [53–56]. A summary description of larger clinical trials with purine analogs in classic HCL is given in Table 12.2.

Whether rituximab should be administered concurrently or sequentially with cladribine to obtain the maximum benefit in previously untreated patients remains unclear [57]. In a recent phase 2 study, cladribine 5.6 mg/m² was given intravenously daily for 5 days, followed approximately 1 month later with rituximab 375 mg/m^2 i.v. weekly for 8 weeks. In 59 patients with untreated HCL, the CR rate was 100%. With a median follow-up of 60 months, 5-year failure-free survival (FFS) was 95%. In addition, 94% of the patients achieved negative MRD. However, the combination of rituximab with a purine nucleoside analog as up-front therapy for classic HCL has not been prospectively compared to purine analog therapy alone.

IFN-α may still have a place in front-line treatment of HCL, but its use is currently limited. It can be used in pregnancy and in patients presenting with neutropenia below 0.2/μL, when the risk of infection due to nucleoside analog therapy is high [58, 59].

The indications for splenectomy are limited in the era of currently available drugs. Splenectomy can be considered in pregnancy when INF-α treatment fails [60, 61]. Moreover, splenectomy can be effective for patients with splenic rupture and in patients with disease refractory to available therapeutic agents.

12.8 Treatment of Relapsed and Refractory Patients with Classic HCL

Despite the high efficacy of purine analogs, several patients will relapse during the course of their disease. However, similarly to previously untreated patients, relapsed patients do not always require treatment at the time of diagnosis, and indications for subsequent lines of therapy are similar to those made at diagnosis. In relapsed patients, re-induction with cladribine or pentostatin again induces remissions. However, in many patients treated with purine analogs as a single agent, responses are usually shorter and some patients develop refractory disease. Patients who relapse within 2–3 years after the first course of treatment have worse prognosis and a lower likelihood of achieving second durable CR; in addition, some patients have disease refractory to purine analog therapy. The median duration of response to second-line cladribine monotherapy is around 3 years [42, 44].

In early relapse (before 12–18 months), rituximab may be given at a dose of 375 mg/m^2 for four to eight doses as weekly IV infusions [62]. Response is seen usually in more than 50% of patients with refractory to or relapsing disease. Longer responses are achievable with sequential cladribine followed by rituximab [43, 57, 62]. In one study of the use of cladribine followed by rituximab for relapsed disease, the CR rate was found to be 100%, and the 5-year FFS and OS 100% among 14 participating patients [57]. Of this group, the median duration of response was found to be longer among the 12 patients who had received prior cladribine monotherapy, i.e., as second-line treatment with cladribine followed by rituximab, than two treatment-naïve patients, who received this course as first-line cladribine monotherapy (P = 0.004). Alternatively, rituximab can be administered concurrently with purine analogs; this combination is more active than rituximab alone but is also more toxic than sequential treatment.

Few treatment options are available for patients who progress following first-line therapy with a purine analog and/or rituximab. Interferon-α (IFN-α) may be an effective treatment option for selected patients with relapsed HCL. However, only PRs can be achieved in the majority of patients, and prolonged treatment is necessary to maintain remission [63–65]. Although IFN-α eliminates leukemic cells from the blood and reduces bone marrow fibrosis, continuous therapy is less convenient to the patient and decreases quality of life due to flu-like symptoms and fatigue. Patients experiencing side effects may lower their dose or temporarily discontinue the treatment (drug holiday) and resume IFN-α at the time of relapse.

The use of fludarabine or bendamustine combined with rituximab could be also considered in relapsed patients. Fludarabine given at a dose of 40 mg/m^2 p.o. on 5 consecutive days in combination with an intravenous injection of rituximab 375 mg/m^2 on day 1, every 28 days for 4 cycles, may be a therapeutic option in relapsed or refractory patients previously treated with cladribine [66]. After a median follow-up of 35 months, 5-year PFS was found to be 89% and OS 83%.

The combination of bendamustine and rituximab has also activity in multiply relapsed/refractory HCL. Burotto et al. treated 12 patients with HCL with two or more prior therapies requiring treatment with rituximab 375 mg/m^2 on days 1 and 15 and bendamustine 70–90 mg/m^2 on days 1 and 2, for 6 cycles at 4-week intervals [67]. The overall response rate was 100%, including CR in seven patients. MRD was absent in six patients with CR, who remained in CR for 30–35 months of follow-up. The most common adverse events (AEs) were thrombocytopenia (83%), lymphopenia (75%), leukopenia (58%), and neutropenia (42%).

The anti-CD22 recombinant immunotoxin moxetumomab pasudotox (LUMOXITI™, Astra Zeneca) is now an important drug for the treatment of HCL, especially in patients where conventional therapies produce limited responses or treatment failure. Moxetumomab pasudotox is composed of the Fv fragment of an anti-CD22 monoclonal antibody fused to a 38-kDa fragment of *Pseudomonas* exotoxin A, PE38. The drug was investigated in a phase 1 trial in 26 patients with refractory/relapsed HCL [68]. Nineteen patients (73.1%) responded with a CR rate of 34.6% and a PR rate of 38.5%. Moxetumomab pasudotox produced inferior responses in splenectomized patients and in patients with massive splenomegaly. In an extension study, the combined 33-patient cohort displayed 88% OR, including 64% CR [69]. Importantly, CR duration was longer (42.1 months) in 11 MRD-negative patients than in 9 MRD-positive patients (13.5 months) ($P < 0.001$). Among MRD-negative CRs, ten patients had ongoing CR and nine were without MRD at the end of the study. Moxetumomab pasudotox is so far the only nonchemotherapy treatment that can eliminate MRD in a significant percentage of HCL patients. The results from the phase 1 study have been confirmed recently in a pivotal, multicenter, open-label trial performed in 80 relapsed/refractory patients [70]. The objective response rate was 75% and durable CR rate was 41%. Among patients who achieved a CR, 27 (85%) achieved MRD negativity as evaluated by immunohistochemistry. The most frequent AEs included peripheral edema (39%), nausea (35%), fatigue (34%), and headache (33%). Hemolytic uremic syndrome (7.5%) and capillary leak syndrome (5%) were also observed, but they were reversible and generally manageable with supportive care and treatment discontinuation. In 2018, moxetumomab pasudotox received FDA approval for the treatment of patients with relapsed or refractory HCL who had received at least two prior systemic therapies, including treatment with a purine nucleoside analog [71]. Patients refractory to purine analog therapy and moxetumomab pasudotox should be enrolled on clinical trials that use new agents whenever possible.

Splenectomy may be indicated in patients who have resistant massive symptomatic splenomegaly (>10 cm below the costal margin) and accompanying low-level bone marrow infiltration [52]. Another indication for splenectomy is progressive HCL refractory to nucleoside analogs and IFN-α. Chemotherapy should not be given until at least 6 months after splenectomy.

Allogeneic stem cell transplantation should be considered in heavily pretreated younger patients who have had multiple relapses and are refractory to purine analogs and rituximab [72–74].

12.9 Treatment of Hairy Cell Leukemia Variant

Potential treatment options for HCL-V patients include splenectomy, purine nucleoside analogs (cladribine, pentostatin), IFN-α, monoclonal antibodies and immunotoxins, and immunochemotherapy [24, 75]. The results of cladribine monotherapy in HCL-V are inferior to those achieved with cladribine in classic HCL, with a response rate of less than 55% and few examples of CR being reported [39, 76, 77]. However, some reports indicate that HCL-V patients had shorter time to next treatment than those with classical HCL but demonstrated similar OS [78]. Rituximab combined with cladribine is more effective in treating HCL-V than cladribine alone or rituximab alone. In a study performed by Kreitman et al., cladribine was given at a dose of 0.15 mg/kg on days 1–5, with eight weekly doses of 375 mg/m^2 rituximab, beginning on day 1 [79].

Of 10 patients, 9 achieved a CR, including 8 (88%) with MRD negativity at 12–48 (median 27) months of follow-up. In other study, the efficacy of cladribine followed by four weekly doses of rituximab was also evaluated in seven patients with HCL-V [57]. CR rate was 86%, 5-year FFS 64%, and OS 51.4%. Cladribine followed by immediate rituximab seems also to be an effective first-line treatment in HCL-V. Visentin et al. reported three previously untreated elderly patients who were effectively treated with four cycles of this combination [80]. All patients achieved a CR with no evidence of MRD. After a median follow-up of 19 months, all three patients were still in CR. Similar results were recently reported by Letendre and Doll [81]. Complete responses were also observed in relapsed patients treated with moxetumomab pasudotox [70]. Novel agents like ibrutinib and trametinib are also considered for the treatment of this disease [82, 83]. Splenectomy is recommended in some patients as it may induce clinical responses, correct cytopenias, remove the bulk of the tumor, and improve responses to chemo- or immunochemotherapy. In addition, autologous and allogenic hematopoietic stem cell transplantation can be taken into account in relapsed/refractory cases.

12.10 Novel Agents

Recently, new targeted drugs are investigated in HCL, including vemurafenib and ibrutinib (Table 12.3). Vemurafenib (Zelboraf™, Roche) is the oral BRAF V600 inhibitor that has remarkable activity in multiply relapsed and refractory HCL patients with rapidly decreased splenomegaly, increased platelet counts, and normalization of hemoglobin and granulocyte counts [13, 84–87]. The safety and activity of vemurafenib were assessed in relapsed and refractory patients with classic HCL in two phase 2, multicenter studies in Italy and in the USA [86]. Vemurafenib was administered at a dose of 960 mg twice daily for a median of 16 weeks in the Italian study and 18 weeks in the US study, resulting in OR rates of 96% (CR 35%) in the Italian study and 100% (CR 42%) in the US study. Among the patients with CR, the median relapse-free survival (RFS) was 19 months, and the median treatment-free survival (TFS) was 25 months. Among those with PR, PFS was 6 months and TFS 18 months. Rash and arthralgia or arthritis were the most frequent AEs, and secondary cutaneous tumors was observed in 7 of 50 patients. Lower doses of vemurafenib are also effective in HCL. Dietrich et al. treated 21 heavily pretreated patients with vemurafenib starting at 240 mg BID and escalating to 720 or 960 mg in four patients [87]. CR was achieved in 40% (6/15) of evaluable patients, and median event-free survival (EFS) was 17 months. The response rate and kinetics of response were independent of vemurafenib dosage, and no significant difference in CR rate was found between lower and higher doses of vemurafenib. Vemurafenib is usually better tolerated than purine nucleoside analogs, and the risk of myelosuppression is relatively low. In addition, vemurafenib administration is associated with improvement in peripheral blood counts in infected patients. However, profound cytopenias and severe infections were also observed in HCL patients [88]. Other side effects noted with BRAF inhibitors include skeletal pain, photosensitivity, skin tumors, and renal toxicity. Secondary diffuse large B-cell lymphoma and well-differentiated squamous cell carcinoma were also observed in HCL patients treated with vemurafenib [89].

Vemurafenib combined with anti-CD20 monoclonal antibodies is even more effective than vemurafenib alone [90]. A phase 2 study by Tiaci et al. evaluated 31 patients who were either relapsed or refractory to purine analogs. Vemurafenib was administered at a dose of 960 mg twice daily for 8 weeks and rituximab at a dose of 375 mg/m^2 on days 1 and 15. In addition, four doses of rituximab were given every 2 weeks after vemurafenib dosing. CRs were achieved in all 27 patients evaluable for efficacy. In addition, about two-thirds of the patients were found to be MRD negative in the BM by immunohistochemistry and flow cytometry. In the median follow-up period of 1.5 years, only 1 of 27 evaluable patients progressed. This chemotherapy-free regimen produces deep and durable responses in heavily pretreated patients

Table 12.3 Larger clinical trials with novel agents in classic hairy cell leukemia

Study	Treatment regimen	Patient characteristics	*N*	Clinical activity	Side effects
Phase 2 Kreitman et al. 2009 [96]	BL22: 40 μg/kg i.v. every other day for three doses on cycle 1. Patients without HR retreated at 30 μg/kg every other day for three doses every 4 weeks	Relapsed/refractory HCL, needed treatment	36	CR—61% + PR – 19% CR—86% for doses 40–50 μg/kg every other day for three doses; median CR duration not reached at 22+ months (range: 5 to 46+)	Most common—gr 1 to 2 hypoalbuminemia, AST/ALT elevation, edema, myalgia, proteinuria, fatigue, nausea, and fever; HUS, 8%; neutralizing Antibodies, 11%
Phase 1 Kreitman et al. 2012; 2018 [68, 69]	Moxetumomab pasudotox: 5–50 μg/kg every other day for three doses (QOD × 3), up to 16 cycles repeating at ≥4-week intervals	Relapsed/refractory HCL after ≥2 prior therapies	33	OR—88%; CR—64%; 11 MRD-negative CRs; median CR duration—42.4 months	Dose-limiting toxicity not observed; grade 1–2 hypoalbuminemia, aminotransferase elevations, edema, headache, hypotension, nausea, fatigue; grade 2 HUS—2 pts
Phase 3 Kreitman et al. 2018 [70]	Moxetumomab pasudotox 40 μg/kg i.v. on days 1, 3, and 5 every 28 days for ≤6 cycles	Two or more prior systemic therapies, including two courses of a purine nucleoside analog or one course of rituximab or a *BRAF* inhibitor following a single prior purine nucleoside analog course	80	OR—80%; CR—41%; among CR, 27 (85%) MRD negative	AE—peripheral edema (39%), nausea (35%), fatigue (34%), headache (33%). Treatment-related serious AE—HUS (7.5%) and CLS (5%)
Phase 2 Tiaci et al. 2015 [86]	Vemurafenib 960 mg twice daily for 16 (*N* = 26, Italian study) or 18 (*N* = 24, US study) weeks	Primary refractory to PNA, early relapsed and/or repeatedly relapsed after PNA	50	Italian study: OR, 96% and 100%; CR, 34.6% (9/26); median RFS, 19 months; TFS 25 months in CR and RFS 6; and TFS 18 months PR; US study: OR, 100%; CR, 41.7% (10/24); 1-year PFS, 73%; 1-year OS, 91%	Skin toxicities (especially rash and photosensitivity), arthralgias/arthritis, pyrexia, and bilirubin increase
Phase II Dietrich et al. 2016 [87]	Vemurafenib started dose of 240 mg bid in 18 pts.; in 4 pts. doses escalated to 720 or 960 mg; retreatment—6 pts.	Previously treated (19) or untreated (2), median prior treatment lines—3 (range: 0–12)	21	CR, 40% (6/15); median EFS 17 months. Similar response in retreatment	Arthralgia ($n = 4$), reversible elevation of liver enzymes ($n = 4$), phototoxicity ($n = 4$)
Phase II Jones et al. 2015 [94]	Ibrutinib 420–840 mg daily in 28-day cycles for a median of 16 weeks	Previously treated with classic HCL (11), untreated (1), HCL-v (1); median prior therapies—4 (range: 1–11)	13	OR, 46%, at median follow-up of 14.5 months, 9 pts. (69%) remain on treatment and progression-free	Gr 3/4 AE—hypophosphatemia (30%), neutropenia (23%), infections (23%) Gr 1/2 AE—myalgias (61%), headache (38%), dizziness (38%), diarrhea (38%), arthralgias (30%), rash (30%), fatigue (30%)

AE adverse event, *CLS* capillary leak syndrome, *CR* complete response, *EFS* event-free survival, *HUS* hemolytic uremic syndrome, *RFS* relapse-free survival, *TFS* treatment-free survival, *PFS* progression-free survival, *OR* overall response, *OS* overall survival, *PNA* purine nucleoside analogs, *RFS* relapse-free survival with HCL and is superior to monotherapy with either vemurafenib or rituximab in the previous trials.

Dabrafenib, another BRAF inhibitor, is also promising and merits further evaluation in larger clinical trials [91, 92]. Combination therapy with BRAF and MEK inhibitors can be also more effective than vemurafenib alone and overcome vemurafenib resistance. A recent report presented interim analysis results of treatment with the combination of BRAF inhibitor dabrafenib and MEK inhibitor trametinib [93]. Treatment was used in 43 patients with heavily pretreated *BRAF*-V600E-mutated HCL that was refractory to first-line treatment with a purine analog or relapsed after two or more prior lines of treatment. This drug combination was well tolerated and demonstrated a high rate of durable responses. OR rate was 78% including 49% CR and 15% CR without MRD. Sixteen (50%) responses lasted 18 months or longer and 97.6% PFS and OS rates at 12 months.

Finally, Bruton's tyrosine kinase pathway inhibitor ibrutinib is also being tested in patients with HCL and can induce a stable disease in most patients, including those with HCL-V [82, 94]. Consequently, multicenter phase 2 trials evaluating the role of ibrutinib in patients with relapsed HCL have been initiated (NCT01981512, NCT01841723). In the coming years, new agents will assist standard therapy for patients with HCL who may currently have suboptimal results after treatment with purine nucleoside analogs [95].

12.11 Treatment Complications and Supportive Care

Chemotherapy with purine analogs commonly leads to immune suppression and myelosuppression with cytopenias, as well as high risk of infections and bleeding, leading to hospitalization. In patients with febrile neutropenia, investigation for opportunistic, fungal, and viral infections is indicated, and treatment with broad-spectrum antibiotics and antifungal and antiviral drugs is recommended [2]. Patients treated with purine nucleoside analogs should receive prophylaxis for herpes simplex virus and varicella zoster virus, as well as prophylaxis against *Pneumocystis jirovecii* [2]. In patients with lymphopenia treated with cladribine or pentostatin, co-trimoxazole (960 mg three times per week) and aciclovir (200 mg three times per day) are recommended 1 week after purine analog administration. This prophylaxis should be given until the lymphocyte count increases to $>1 \times 10^9$/L [2].

Granulocyte colony-stimulating factor may be considered for patients with severe neutropenia and life-threatening infection, but their role has not been proven. Annual influenza immunizations are also indicated as well as immunizations against *Streptococcus pneumoniae*. However, live viral vaccines are contraindicated. Transfused blood products should be irradiated to prevent transfusion-associated graft-versus-host disease.

12.12 Conclusions

Hairy cell leukemia is characterized by progressive pancytopenia, splenomegaly, and leukemic infiltrations of the bone marrow, liver, and spleen, The recent WHO classification distinguishes classic form of HCL and its HCL variant (HCL-V) as two distinct entities. Hairy cell leukemia usually has an indolent disease course. Most cases with classic HCL are *BRAF*-V600E-positive, but no cases of *BRAF*-V600E mutation have been described in HCL-V. The purine nucleoside analogs cladribine and pentostatin are effective drugs in the treatment of HCL; however, the disease mostly remains incurable, and new treatment options are needed for patients resistant to purine analog therapy. Rituximab is an active drug in HCL. The combination of rituximab with purine nucleoside analogs increases the occurrence and duration of response rates. Recently, the immunotoxin moxetumomab pasudotox received approval in the USA for the treatment of relapsed or refractory HCL patients who received at least two prior systemic therapies,

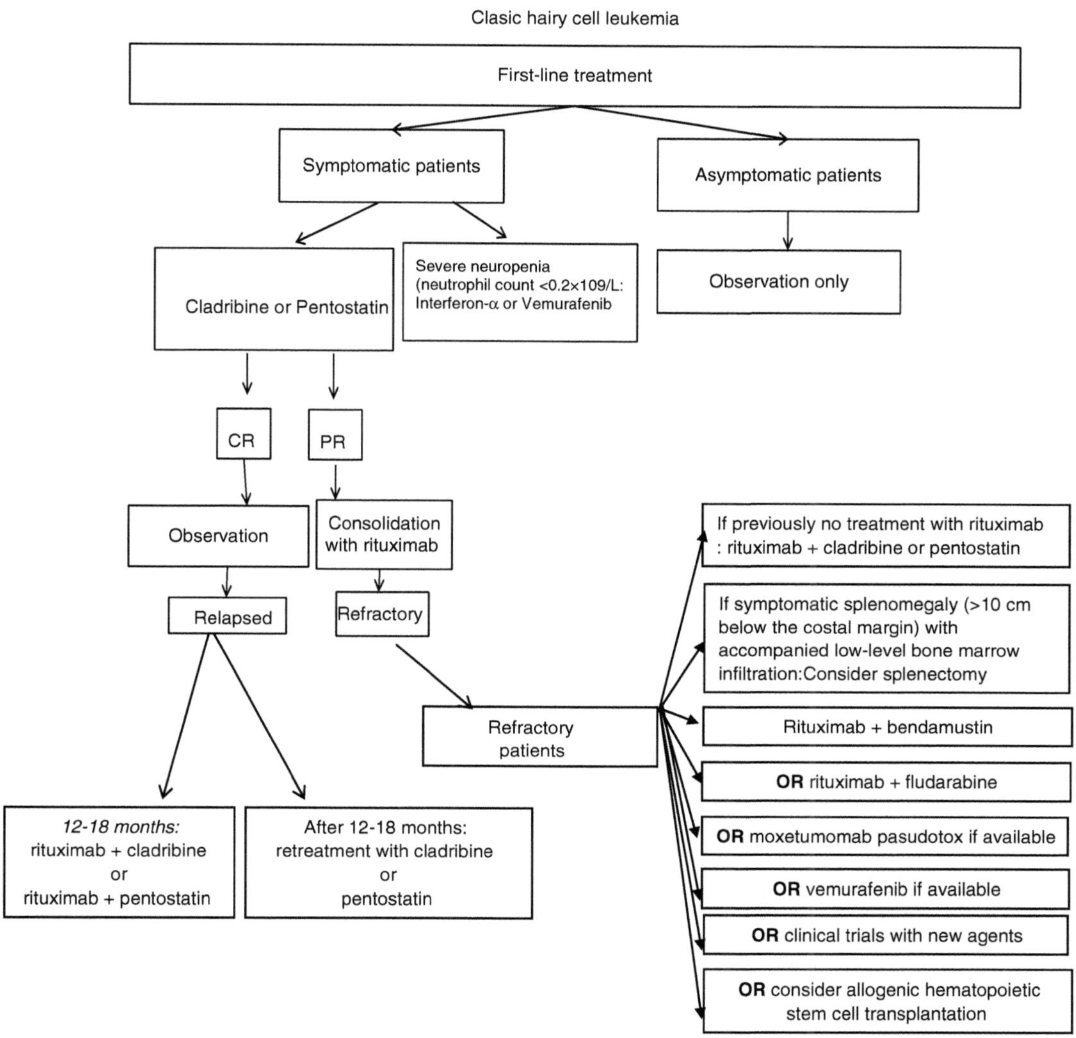

Fig. 12.1 Therapeutic algorithm for the treatment of patients with classic hairy cell leukemia

including treatment with a purine nucleoside analog. Vemurafenib, an ATP-competitive BRAF inhibitor, is an active and well-tolerated drug in refractory or relapsed patients with classic HCL but not with HCL-V. Ibrutinib, an inhibitor of Bruton's tyrosine kinase, has been shown to demonstrate antitumor activity in HCL patients, including HCL-V. The therapeutic algorithm for the treatment of patients with classic HCL is presented in Fig. 12.1.

Conflicts of Interest No potential conflicts of interest were disclosed.

References

1. Grever MR, Abdel-Wahab O, Andritsos LA, et al. Consensus guidelines for the diagnosis and management of patients with classic hairy cell leukemia. Blood. 2017;129:553–60.
2. Robak T, Matutes E, Catovsky D, Zinzani PL, Buske C, ESMO Guidelines Committee. Hairy cell leukaemia: ESMO clinical practice guidelines for diagnosis, treatment and follow-up. Ann Oncol. 2015;26(Suppl 5):v100–7.
3. Bouroncle BA, Wiseman BK, Doan CA. Leukemic reticuloendotheliosis. Blood. 1958;13:609–30.
4. Wang X, Spielberger R, Huang Q. Hairy cell leukemia variant, a new entity of the WHO 2008. J Clin Oncol. 2011;29(36):e864–6.

5. Swerdlow SH, Campo E, Pileri SA, et al. The 2016 revision of the World Health Organization classification of lymphoid neoplasms. Blood. 2016;127:2375–90.
6. Cawley JC, Burns GF, Hayhoe FG. A chronic lymphoproliferative disorder with distinctive features: a distinct variant of hairy-cell leukaemia. Leuk Res. 1980;4:547–59.
7. Chandran R, Gardiner SK, Smith SD, Spurgeon SE. Improved survival in hairy cell leukaemia over three decades: a SEER database analysis of prognostic factors. Br J Haematol. 2013;163:407–9.
8. Teras LR, DeSantis CE, Cerhan JR, Morton LM, Jemal A, Flowers CR. 2016 US lymphoid malignancy statistics by World Health Organization subtypes. CA Cancer J Clin. 2016;66:443. https://doi.org/10.3322/caac.21357.
9. Getta BM, Woo KM, Devlin S, et al. Treatment outcomes and secondary cancer incidence in young patients with hairy cell leukaemia. Br J Haematol. 2016;175:402–9.
10. Roider T, Falini B, Dietrich S. Recent advances in understanding and managing hairy cell leukemia. F1000 Res. 2018;7. pii: F1000 Faculty Rev-509.
11. Tiacci E, Schiavoni G, Forconi F, et al. Simple genetic diagnosis of hairy cell leukemia by sensitive detection of the BRAF-V600E mutation. Blood. 2012;119:192–5.
12. Tiacci E, Trifonov V, Schiavoni G, et al. BRAF mutations in hairy-cell leukemia. N Engl J Med. 2011;364:2305–15.
13. Samuel J, Macip S, Dyer MJ. Efficacy of vemurafenib in hairy-cell leukemia. N Engl J Med. 2014;370:286–8.
14. Durham BH, Getta B, Dietrich S, et al. Genomic analysis of hairy cell leukemia identifies novel recurrent genetic alterations. Blood. 2017;130:1644–8.
15. Tschernitz S, Flossbach L, Bonengel M, Roth S, Rosenwald A, Geissinger E. Alternative BRAF mutations in BRAF V600E-negative hairy cell leukaemias. Br J Haematol. 2014;165:529–33.
16. Tiacci E, Pettirossi V, Schiavoni G, Falini B. Genomics of hairy cell leukemia. J Clin Oncol. 2017;35:1002–10.
17. Chung SS, Kim E, Park JH, et al. Hematopoietic stem cell origin of BRAFV600E mutations in hairy cell leukemia. Sci Transl Med. 2014;6:238ra71.
18. Falini B, Martelli MP, Tiacci E. BRAF V600E mutation in hairy cell leukemia: from bench to bedside. Blood. 2016;128:1918–27.
19. Andrulis M, Penzel R, Weichert W, von Deimling A, Capper D. Application of a BRAF V600E mutation-specific antibody for the diagnosis of hairy cell leukemia. Am J Surg Pathol. 2012;36:1796–800.
20. Uppal G, Ly V, Wang ZX, et al. The utility of BRAF V600E mutation-specific antibody VE1 for the diagnosis of hairy cell leukemia. Am J Clin Pathol. 2015;143:120–5.
21. Dietrich S, Hüllein J, Lee SC, et al. Recurrent CDKN1B (p27) mutations in hairy cell leukemia. Blood. 2015;126:1005–8.
22. Tiacci E, Schiavoni G, Martelli MP, et al. Constant activation of the RAF-MEK-ERK pathway as a diagnostic and therapeutic target in hairy cell leukemia. Haematologica. 2013;98:635–9.
23. Pettirossi V, Santi A, Imperi E, et al. BRAF inhibitors reverse the unique molecular signature and phenotype of hairy cell leukemia and exert potent antileukemic activity. Blood. 2015;125:1207–16.
24. Robak T. Hairy-cell leukemia variant: recent view on diagnosis, biology and treatment. Cancer Treat Rev. 2011;37:3–10.
25. Xi L, Arons E, Navarro W, et al. Both variant and IGHV4-34-expressing hairy cell leukemia lack the BRAF V600E mutation. Blood. 2012;119:3330–2.
26. Waterfall JJ, Arons E, Walker RL, et al. High prevalence of MAP2K1 mutations in variant and IGHV4-34-expressing hairy-cell leukemias. Nat Genet. 2014;46:8–10.
27. Sandes AF, de Lourdes Chauffaille M, Oliveira CR, et al. CD200 has an important role in the differential diagnosis of mature B-cell neoplasms by multiparameter flow cytometry. Cytometry B Clin Cytom. 2014;86:98–105.
28. Pillai V, Pozdnyakova O, Charest K, Li B, Shahsafaei A, Dorfman DM. CD200 flow cytometric assessment and semiquantitative immunohistochemical staining distinguishes hairy cell leukemia from hairy cell leukemia-variant and other B-cell lymphoproliferative disorders. Am J Clin Pathol. 2013;140:536–43.
29. Else M, Dearden CE, Matutes E, et al. Long-term follow-up of 233 patients with hairy cell leukaemia, treated initially with pentostatin or cladribine, at a median of 16 years from diagnosis. Br J Haematol. 2009;145:733–40.
30. Arons E, Suntum T, Stetler-Stevenson M, Kreitman RJ. VH4-34+ hairy cell leukemia, a new variant with poor prognosis despite standard therapy. Blood. 2009;114:4687–95.
31. Goodman GR, Burian C, Koziol JA, Saven A. Extended follow-up of patients with hairy cell leukemia after treatment with cladribine. J Clin Oncol. 2003;21:891–6.
32. Mhawech-Fauceglia P, Oberholzer M, Aschenafi S, et al. Potential predictive patterns of minimal residual disease detected by immunohistochemistry on bone marrow biopsy specimens during a long-term follow-up in patients treated with cladribine for hairy cell leukemia. Arch Pathol Lab Med. 2006;130:374–7.
33. Ortiz-Maldonado V, Villamor N, Baumann T, et al. Is there a role for minimal residual disease monitoring in the management of patients with hairy-cell leukaemia? Br J Haematol. 2018;183:127–9.
34. Spiers AS, Parekh SL, Bishop MB. Hairy cell leukaemia: induction of complete remission with pentostatin (2′-deoxycoformycin). J Clin Oncol. 1984;2:1336–42.

35. Piro LD, Carrera CJ, Carson DA, Beutler E. Lasting remissions in hairy cell leukemia induced by a single infusion of 2-chlorodeoxyadenosine. N Engl J Med. 1990;322:1117–21.
36. Saven A, Burian C, Kozioł JA, Piro LD. Long-term follow-up of patients with hairy cell leukemia after cladribine treatment. Blood. 1998;92:1918–26.
37. Cheson BD, Sorensen JM, Vena DA. Treatment of hairy cell leukemia with 2-chlorodeoxyadenosine via the group protocol mechanism of the National Cancer Institute: a report of 979 patients. J Clin Oncol. 1998;16:3007–15.
38. Robak T, Jamroziak K, Gora-Tybor J, et al. Cladribine in a weekly versus daily schedule for untreated active hairy cell leukemia: final report from the Polish Adult Leukemia Group (PALG) of a prospective, randomized, multicenter trial. Blood. 2007;109:3672–5.
39. Robak T, Błasińska-Morawiec M, Błoński J, et al. 2-chlorodeoxyadenosine: (cladribine) in the treatment of hairy cell leukemia and hairy cell leukemia variant 7-year experience in Poland. Eur J Haematol. 1999;62:49–56.
40. Grever M, Kopecky K, Foucar MK, et al. Randomized comparison of pentostatin versus interferon alfa-2a in previously untreated patients with hairy cell leukemia: an intergroup study. J Clin Oncol. 1995;13:974–82.
41. Maloisel F, Benboubker L, Gardembas M, et al. Long-term outcome with pentostatin treatment in hairy cell leukemia patients. A French retrospective study of 238 patients. Leukemia. 2003;17:45–51.
42. Flinn IW, Kopecky KJ, Foucar MK, et al. Long-term follow-up of remission duration, mortality and second malignancies in hairy cell leukemia patients treated with pentostatin. Blood. 2000;96:2981–6.
43. Else M, Dearden CE, Catovsky D. Long-term follow-up after purine analogue therapy in hairy cell leukaemia. Best Pract Res Clin Haematol. 2015;28:217–29.
44. Zinzani PL, Pellegrini C, Stefoni V, et al. Hairy cell leukemia: evaluation of the long-term outcome in 121 patients. Cancer. 2010;116:4788–92.
45. Inbar M, Herishanu Y, Goldschmidt N, et al. Hairy cell leukemia: retrospective analysis of demographic data and outcome of 203 patients from 12 medical centers in Israel. Anticancer Res. 2018;38:6423–9.
46. Forconi F, Cencini E, Zaja F, et al. Analysis of toxicity and efficacy of subcutaneous cladribine at reduced or standard doses (five versus seven consecutive days) in patients with hairy cell leukemia (HCL) in the ICGHCL2004 protocol by the Italian Cooperative Group on HCL. Blood. 2010;116:Abstravt 701.
47. Robak T, Blasinska-Morawiec M, Krykowski E, et al. 2-chlorodeoxyadenosine (2-CdA) in 2-hour versus 24-hour intravenous infusion in the treatment of patients with hairy cell leukemia. Leuk Lymphoma. 1996;22:107–11.
48. Zenhäusern R, Schmitz SF, Solenthaler M, et al. Randomized trial of daily versus weekly administration of 2-chlorodeoxyadenosine in patients with hairy cell leukemia: a multicenter phase III trial (SAKK 32/98). Leuk Lymphoma. 2009;50:1501–11.
49. von Rohr A, Schmitz SF, Tichelli A, et al. Treatment of hairy cell leukemia with cladribine (2-chlorodeoxyadenosine) by subcutaneous bolus injection: a phase II study. Ann Oncol. 2002;13:1641–9.
50. Sigal DS, Sharpe R, Burian C, Saven A. Very long-term eradication of minimal residual disease in patients with hairy cell leukemia after a single course of cladribine. Blood. 2010;115:1893–6.
51. Cornet E, Delmer A, Feugier P, et al. Recommendations of the SFH (French Society of Haematology) for the diagnosis, treatment and follow-up of hairy cell leukaemia. Ann Hematol. 2014;93:1977–83.
52. Jones G, Parry-Jones N, Wilkins B, Else M, Catovsky D. Revised guidelines for the diagnosis and management of hairy cell leukaemia and hairy cell leukaemia variant. Br J Haematol. 2012;156:186–95.
53. Piro LD, Ellison DJ, Saven A. The Scripps clinic experience with 2-chlorodeoxyadenosine in the treatment of hairy cell leukemia. Leuk Lymphoma. 1994;14(Suppl 1):121–5.
54. Saven A, Piro LD. Complete remissions in hairy cell leukemia with 2-chlorodeoxyadenosine after failure with 2′-deoxycoformycin. Ann Intern Med. 1993;119:278–83.
55. Dearden CE, Matutes E, Hilditch BL, Swansbury GJ, Catovsky D. Long-term follow-up of patients with hairy cell leukaemia after treatment with pentostatin or cladribine. Br J Haematol. 1999;106:515–9.
56. Estey EH, Kurzrock R, Kantarjian HM, et al. Treatment of hairy cell leukemia with 2-chlorodeoxyadenosine (2-CdA). Blood. 1992;79:882–7.
57. Chihara D, Kantarjian H, O'Brien S, et al. Long-term durable remission by cladribine followed by rituximab in patients with hairy cell leukaemia: update of a phase II trial. Br J Haematol. 2016;174:760–6.
58. Baer MR, Ozer H, Foon KA. Interferon-alpha therapy during pregnancy in chronic myelogenous leukaemia and hairy cell leukaemia. Br J Haematol. 1992;81:167–9.
59. Habermann TM, Rai K. Historical treatments of in hairy cell leukemia, splenectomy and interferon: past and current uses. Leuk Lymphoma. 2011;52:18–20.
60. Adeniji BA, Fallas M, Incerpi M, et al. Laparoscopic splenectomy for hairy cell leukemia in pregnancy. Case Report Med. 2010;2010. pii: 136823.
61. Stiles GM, Stanco LM, Saven A, et al. Splenectomy for hairy cell leukemia in pregnancy. J Perinatol. 1998;18:200–1.
62. Leclerc M, Suarez F, Noël MP, et al. Rituximab therapy for hairy cell leukemia: a retrospective study of 41 cases. Ann Hematol. 2015;94:89–95.
63. Seymour JF, Estey EH, Keating MJ, Kurzrock R. Response to interferon-α in patients with hairy cell leukemia relapsing after treatment with 2-chlorodeoxyadenosine. Leukemia. 1995;9:929–32.
64. Hoffman MA. Interferon-alpha is a very effective salvage therapy for patients with hairy cell leukemia relapsing after cladribine: a report of three cases. Med Oncol. 2011;28:1537–41.

65. Silva WFD, Teixeira LLC, Rocha V, Buccheri V. Current role of interferon in hairy cell leukemia therapy: a timely decision. Hematol Transfus Cell Ther. 2019;41:88–90.
66. Gerrie AS, Zypchen LN, Connors JM. Fludarabine and rituximab for relapsed or refractory hairy cell leukemia. Blood. 2012;119:1988–91.
67. Burotto M, Stetler-Stevenson M, Arons E, et al. Bendamustine and rituximab in relapsed and refractory hairy cell leukemia. Clin Cancer Res. 2013;19:6313–21.
68. Kreitman RJ, Tallman MS, Robak T, et al. Phase I trial of anti-CD22 recombinant immunotoxin moxetumomab pasudotox (CAT-8015 or HA22) in patients with hairy cell leukemia. J Clin Oncol. 2012;30:1822–8.
69. Kreitman RJ, Tallman MS, Robak T, et al. Minimal residual hairy cell leukemia eradication with moxetumomab pasudotox: phase 1 results and long-term follow-up. Blood. 2018;131:2331–4.
70. Kreitman RJ, Dearden C, Zinzani PL, et al. Moxetumomab pasudotox in relapsed/refractory hairy cell leukemia. Leukemia. 2018;32:1768–77.
71. Dhillon S. Moxetumomab pasudotox: first global approval. Drugs. 2018;78:1763–7.
72. Cheever MA, Fefer A, Greenberg PD, et al. Treatment of hairy-cell leukemia with chemoradiotherapy and identical-twin bone-marrow transplantation. N Engl J Med. 1982;307:479–81.
73. Zinzani PL, Bonifazi F, Pellegrini C, et al. Hairy cell leukemia: allogeneic transplantation could be an optimal option in selected patients. Clin Lymphoma Myeloma Leuk. 2012;12:287–9.
74. Kiyasu J, Shiratsuchi M, Ohtsuka R, et al. Achievement of complete remission of refractory hairy cell leukemia by rituximab progressing after allogeneic hematopoietic stem cell transplantation. Int J Hematol. 2009;89:403–5.
75. Robak T. Management of hairy cell leukemia variant. Leuk Lymphoma. 2011;52(Suppl 2):53–6.
76. Matutes E, Wotherspoon A, Catovsky D. The variant form of hairy-cell leukaemia. Best Pract Res Clin Haematol. 2003;16:41–56.
77. Tetreault SA, Robbins BA, Saven A. Treatment of hairy cell leukemia-variant with cladribine. Leuk Lymphoma. 1999;35:347–54.
78. Getta B, Woo KM, Devlin S, et al. Hairy cell leukemia variant has similar survival to classical disease despite poorer responses to initial therapy: a 30-year experience from Memorial Sloan Kettering Cancer Center. Blood. 2015;126:Abstract 1476.
79. Kreitman RJ, Wilson W, Calvo KR, et al. Cladribine with immediate rituximab for the treatment of patients with variant hairy cell leukemia. Clin Cancer Res. 2013;19:6873–81.
80. Visentin A, Imbergamo S, Frezzato F, et al. Bendamustine plus rituximab is an effective first-line treatment in hairy cell leukemia variant: a report of three cases. Oncotarget. 2017;8:110727–31.
81. Letendre P, Doll D. Novel therapeutics in the treatment of hairy cell leukemia variant. Leuk Res. 2018;75:58–60.
82. Bohn JP, Wanner D, Steurer M. Ibrutinib for relapsed refractory hairy cell leukemia variant. Leuk Lymphoma. 2017;58:1224–6.
83. Andritsos LA, Grieselhuber NR, Anghelina M, et al. Trametinib for the treatment of IGHV4-34, MAP2K1-mutant variant hairy cell leukemia. Leuk Lymphoma. 2018;59:1008–11.
84. Dietrich S, Zenz T. BRAF inhibitor therapy in HCL. Best Pract Res Clin Haematol. 2015;28:246–52.
85. Dietrich S, Glimm H, Andrulis M, et al. BRAF inhibition in refractory hairy-cell leukemia. N Engl J Med. 2012;366:2038–40.
86. Tiacci E, Park JH, De Carolis L, et al. Targeting mutant BRAF in relapsed or refractory hairy-cell leukemia. N Engl J Med. 2015;373:1733–47.
87. Dietrich S, Pircher A, Endris V, et al. BRAF inhibition in hairy cell leukemia with low-dose vemurafenib. Blood. 2016;127:2847–55.
88. Shenoi DP, Andritsos LA, Blachly JS, et al. Classic hairy cell leukemia complicated by pancytopenia and severe infection: a report of 3 cases treated with vemurafenib. Blood Adv. 2019;3:116–8.
89. Bhangoo MS, Saven A. Secondary malignancies after treatment with single-agent vemurafenib in two patients with refractory hairy cell leukemia. Leuk Lymphoma. 2018;15:1–3. https://doi.org/10.1080/10428194.2018.1519809.
90. Tiacci E, Carolis LD, Zaja F, et al. The chemotherapy-free combination of vemurafenib and rituximab produces deep and durable responses in relapsed or refractory hairy cell leukemia (HCL) patients. Blood. 2017;130:Abstract 409.
91. Blachly JS, Lozanski G, Lucas DM, Grever MR, Kendra K, Andritsos LA. Cotreatment of hairy cell leukemia and melanoma with the BRAF inhibitor dabrafenib. J Natl Compr Cancer Netw. 2015;13:9–13.
92. Vergote V, Dierickx D, Janssens A, et al. Rapid and complete hematological response of refractory hairy cell leukemia to the BRAF inhibitor dabrafenib. Ann Hematol. 2014;93:2087–9.
93. Kreitman RJ, Moreau P, Hutchings M, et al. Treatment with combination of dabrafenib and trametinib in patients with recurrent/refractory BRAF V600E-mutated hairy cell leukemia (HCL). Blood. 2018;132:Abstract 391.
94. Jones JA, Andritsos LA, Lucas DM. Preliminary safety and efficacy of the Bruton's tyrosine kinase (BTK) inhibitor ibrutinib (IBR) in patients (pts) with hairy cell leukemia (HCL). J Clin Oncol. 2014;32(15 Suppl):Abstract 7063.
95. Robak T, Wolska A, Robak P. Potential breakthroughs with investigational drugs for hairy cell leukemia. Expert Opin Investig Drugs. 2015;24:1419–31.
96. Kreitman RJ, Stetler-Stevenson M, Margulies I, et al. Phase II trial of recombinant immunotoxin RFB4(dsFv)-PE38 (BL22) in patients with hairy cell leukemia. J Clin Oncol. 2009;27:2983–90.

Treatment of Chronic Lymphocytic Leukemia

13

Nisha De Silva and Barbara Eichhorst

Chronic lymphocytic leukemia / small lymphocytic lymphoma (CLL/SLL)

Clinical outline
leukemic in most patients (≥ 5000 cells/µl, see section "precursor lesion"); non-leukemic presentation in SLL. Frequent involvement of spleen, lymph nodes and bone marrow. All tissues can be involved, frequently as incidental findings.

Cytology	Small cells rsembling lymphocytes with narrow rim of cytoplasm. Variable number of prolymphocytes.	CLL, cytology	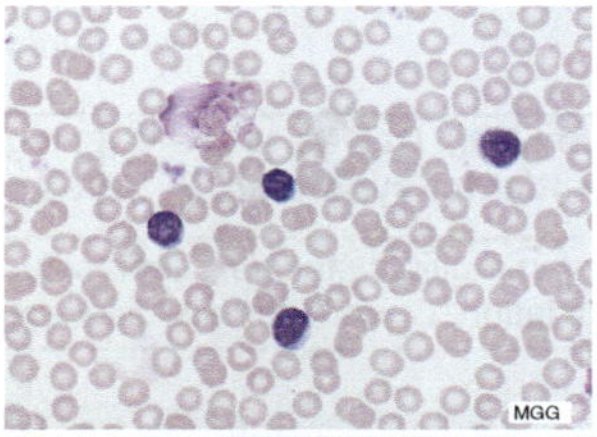
Histology	Diffuse infiltration of tissues with variable amount of larger cells (prolymphocytes and paraimmunoblasts) in pseudofollicles (proliferation centers). Some cases harbor features of plasmacytic differentiation.	CLL, hystology	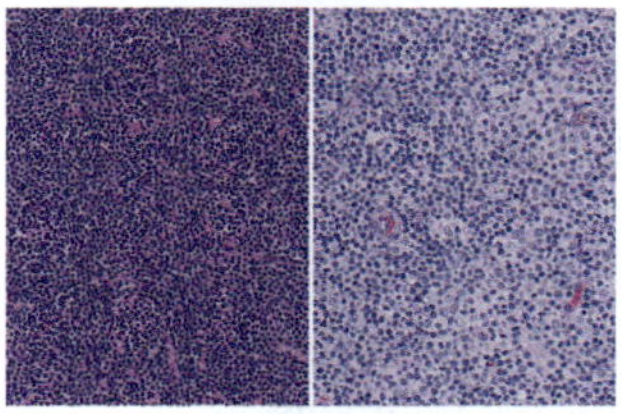

	CD20[1]	CD5	CD23[2]	CD10	BCL6	cyclin D1[3]	CD103	FMC7	IgM	light chains
notes	[1]typically weak expression, [2]stronger on larger cells, [3]some positivity in proliferation centers									
other marker	Ki67 low (higher rates in proliferation centers and in progression and transformation LEF1 positive (transcription factor negative in normal B-cells and low in other small B-cell lymphomas)									

■ = majority of cases positive   ▒ = variable fraction of cases positive   □ = negative

Main differential diagnosis	MCL (should be cyclin D1+ and CD23-); SMZL (should be CD5-)

M. Dreyling, M. Ladetto (eds.), *Indolent Lymphomas*, Hematologic Malignancies,
https://doi.org/10.1007/978-3-030-55989-2_13

Key molecular features
Two main subsets subdivided upon presence vs absence of IGHV mutation. 30% of cases have B-cell receptor stereotypy . Frequent copy number alterations: del13q14.3 (miR-16-1, miR-15a), trisomy 12, del 11q22-23 (*ATM*, *BIRC3*), del17p (TP53). Frequent mutations: NOTCH1, SF3B1, TP53, BIRC3, POT1, MYD88. Frequent translocations: -
Precursor lesions
Monoclonal B-cell lymphocytosis of the CLL type (defined as clonal cells with CLL phenotype of <5000/µl)
Progression
Prolymphocytoid transformation; diffuse large B-cell lymphoma (clonally related or unrelated) or classical Hodgkin lymphoma (mostly clonally unrelated), both defined as "Richter-syndrome".

Clinically relevant pathologic features	Relevance	Evidence
IGHV mutation status	prognostic (unmutated, unfavourable) predictive (estimation of treatment response)	A
***TP53* anomaly (17p deletion, *TP53* mutation)**	prognostic (unfavourable) predictive (subtype-specific protocols available)	A
Complex karyotype, 11q deletion	prognostic (unfavourable) predictive (subtype-specific protocols available)	B
Increase in large cells and / or proliferative index; expanded proliferation center.	prognostic (unfavourable)	C
Phenotypic markers	prognostic (p53, CD38 and ZAP70 expression, unfavourable),predictive (BCL2 inhibitors)	C
Clonal relationship of the DLBCL to the underlying CLL in Richter syndrome	prognostic (clonally identical cases have shorter OS as compared to unrelated (de novo) DLBCL	C
Legend: A = verified in multiple studies, randomized trials and/or integrated in guidelines; B = variable between studies/ needs definitive validation; C = preliminary/discrepant results.		

13.1 Treatment

This chapter summarizes current treatment options including chemoimmunotherapy as well as chemotherapy-free regimens.

13.1.1 Indication for Treatment Initiation

In general, newly diagnosed patients with asymptomatic early stage disease (Rai 0, Binet A) should be monitored unless they develop symptoms of active and/or progressive disease, as defined by the IWCLL guidelines [1]. Treatment should be initiated in patients with advanced stage disease (Rai III and IV or Binet C) due to hematopoietic insufficiency. Patients with intermediate stage (Rai I and II or Binet B) can be monitored until they have symptoms of progression and/or symptomatic disease.

N. De Silva · B. Eichhorst (✉)
Department I for Internal Medicine, Center for Integrated Oncology Aachen-Bonn-Cologne-Duesseldorf, University of Cologne, Cologne, Germany
e-mail: nisha.de-silva@uk-koeln.de; Barbara.Eichhorst@uk-koeln.de

13.1.2 General Considerations for the Choice of Therapy

For the treatment decision in this disease of mostly elderly people, a number of factors should be considered for the choice of initial as well as later therapies:

- *Genetic risk of the leukemia*: FISH and molecular testing for deletion of the short arm of chromosome 17 [del(17p)], or mutation of the *TP53* gene, which is associated with a poor prognosis and resistance to chemotherapeutic agents [2, 3]. Because of the possibility of genetic evolution [4, 5], testing for specific genetic markers should be repeated before treatment initiation if the previous testing was done more than 6 months ago or at any stage if the clinical course has become more aggressive.

- *Fitness and comorbidity burden including renal function* [6, 7].
- *Co-medication*: Consider patient compliance and potential interactions with co-medication.

13.2 Frontline Treatment

13.2.1 Treatment of Fit Patients

Treatment with chemoimmunotherapy is still a considerable treatment option in frontline of CLL but should be done only in patients with favorable genetic profile including mutated immunoglobulin heavy-chain variable region (IGHV) status and exclusion of *TP53* mutation/deletion. Combinations of anti-CD20 antibodies with fludarabine-based chemotherapeutic backbone are the most intensive chemoimmunotherapeutic options in CLL resulting in high rates of MRD negativity. The CLL8 trial of the German CLL study group (GCLLSG), with 817 patients, demonstrated the superiority of fludarabine, cyclophosphamide, and rituximab (FCR) over fludarabine and cyclophosphamide (FC) with high rates of undetectable minimal residual disease (MRD) (63% vs. 35% $p < 0.001$) [8] resulting in a significantly improved progression-free survival (PFS) and overall survival (Table 13.1) [9]. In addition, after more than 5 years' observation time, median PFS is still not reached in the FCR-treated patients with mutated IGHV status [10].

The combination of the alkylating agent bendamustine with rituximab (BR) showed promising activity in a phase II trial [11]. BR was compared with FCR in the phase III trial of the GCLLSG (CLL10) trial, showing that patients treated with FCR achieved a longer median PFS (55.2 vs. 41.7 months, HR = 1.643, 95% CI 1.308–2.064, $p = 0.0003$) than with BR, but no difference in OS was observed. Of note, significantly more common toxicity criteria (CTC) grade three and four neutropenias and infections occurred with FCR particularly in patients >65 years old [12]. Based on these results, the BR combination is used commonly in fit, elderly patients (recommended cutoff at 65 years).

Randomized trials have shown that targeted agents inhibiting kinases downstream of the B-cell receptor, which play a major role in the pathogenesis of CLL, are superior to chemoimmunotherapy, particularly in patients with less favorable genetic profile. Ibrutinib is a first-in-class orally available inhibitor of Bruton's tyrosine kinase (BTK). This substance is given continuously and is only discontinued in the event of intolerable side effects or progression of CLL.

In the frontline setting, the phase III RESONATE II trial showed the advantage of ibrutinib over chlorambucil in 269 elderly, untreated CLL patients with regard to overall response rate (ORR) (86% vs. 35%), median PFS (not reached vs. 18.9 months), and 2-year OS (98% vs. 85%) (85) (Table 13.2) [13]. Based on this, ibrutinib was approved for therapy of treatment-naïve as well as pretreated CLL patients, including patients with 17p deletion.

The phase III ECOG-ACRIN E1912 frontline trial demonstrated superiority of six cycles of ibrutinib and rituximab (IR) (after a single cycle of ibrutinib monotherapy) followed by ibrutinib monotherapy until disease progression in 354 patients over six cycles of FCR treatment in 175 patients [14]. The PFS advantage of the ibrutinib-containing arm was 89.4% vs. 72.9% at 3 years and OS advantage 98.8% vs. 91.5% at 3 years. The significantly superior PFS of the IR arm over the FCR arm were only demonstrated in patients without the immunoglobulin heavy-chain variable region (IGHV) mutation (90.7% vs. 62.5%) at 3 years, unlike those with mutated IGHV status (87.7% vs. 88.0%).

Other currently ongoing trials as the FLAIR trial of the UK-CLL study group or the GAIA/CLL13 trial of the GCLLSG are currently evaluating other combination therapies, such as fixed duration of venetoclax plus obinutuzumab or a

Table 13.1 Efficacy of selected chemoimmunotherapies in frontline of CLL

Reference and study design	No. patients	Treatment regimen	Clinical response		Progression-free survival	Overall survival
			CR	CR + PR		
Fit/young patients						
Fludarabine, cyclophosphamide + rituximab full dosed (FCR)						
Keating et al., JCO 2005 [55, 56] Phase II	224	F 25 mg/m² d1–3 iv q 28 d × 6 C 250 mg/m² d1–3 iv q 28d × 6 R 375 mg/m² d1 C1 and R 500 mg/m² d1 C2–6	70%	95%	Median 6.4 years	Median 12.7 years
Hallek et al., Lancet 2010 (GCLLSG CLL8) [9, 10] Phase III	408	F 25 mg/m² d1–3 iv q 28 d × 6 C 250 mg/m² d1–3 iv q 28 d × 6 R 375 mg/m² d1 C1 and R 500 mg/m² d1 C2–6	44%	93%	Median 57 mo	79% at 5 years
Bendamustine + rituximab (BR)						
Fischer et al., JCO 2012 Phase II [11]	117	B 90 mg/m² d1 + 2 q 28 × 6 R 375 mg/m² d1 C1 and R 500 mg/m² d1 C2–6	23%	88%	Median 34 mo (event-free survival)	At 2 years 90%
Eichhorst et al., Lancet Oncol 2016 [12] Phase III	279	B 90 mg/m² d1 + 2 q 28 × 6 R 375 mg/m² d1 C1 and R 500 mg/m² d1 C2–6	31%	98%	Median 42 mo	At 3 years 92%
Chlorambucil + obinutuzumab (ClbO)						
Goede et al. NEJM 2014 [15] Phase III randomized	333	Clb 0.5 mg/kg BW d1 + 15 q28 × 6 O 1000 mg d1,8,15 C1 and 1000 mg d1 C2–6	22%	77%	Median 26.7 mo	Median not reached
Bendamustine + rituximab (BR)						
Michallet et al., Haematol 2018 [16] Phase IIIb	121	B 90 mg/m² d1 + 2 q 28 × 6 R 375 mg/m² d1 C1 and R 500 mg/m² d1 C2–6	24%	91%	Median 40 mo	n.a.

All agents were given intravenously unless otherwise specified
F fludarabine, *CYC* cyclophosphamide, *R* rituximab, *B* bendamustine, *Clb* chlorambucil, *O* obinutuzumab, *d* day, *C* cycle, *mo* months, *n.a.* not available

triple combination (venetoclax plus ibrutinib plus obinutuzumab) or the oral combination of ibrutinib plus venetoclax alone (see below).

13.2.2 Treatment of Less Fit Patients

Single agent chlorambucil (Clb) has been widely used in this patient group and in combination treatment. The phase III CLL11 of the GCLLSG trial with 781 patients demonstrated superior PFS of Clb plus obinutuzumab over rituximab plus chlorambucil (ClbR) or single agent Clb (26.7 vs. 16.3 vs. 11.1 months $p < 0.0001$), respectively [15]. An updated analysis showed that OS in the ClbO arm was also significantly improved in comparison to Clb alone (HR 0.47, 95% CI 0.29–0.76, $p = 0.0014$) (Table 13.1).

The randomized phase IIIb MABLE study of BR in comparison to ClbR in 241 elderly patients ineligible for frontline therapy with FCR as well as 116 patients at second-line therapy showed a significantly extended median PFS in the BR arm, in comparison to the ClbR group (40 vs. 30 months;

Table 13.2 Efficacy of novel agents alone or in combination in frontline CLL

Reference and study design	No. patients	Treatment regimen	Clinical response CR	CR + PR	Progression-free survival	Overall survival
Ibrutinib						
Burger et al., NEJM 2015 [13] Phase III randomized	269	Ibrutinib 420 mg daily until progression	4%	86%	Median not reached	At 2 years: 98%
Shanafelt et al., NEJM 2019 [14] Phase III randomized	529	Ibrutinib 420 mg daily until progression R 50 mg/m² d1 c1 R 375 mg/m² d2 c2 and R 500 mg/m² d1 c3–7	17.2%	95.8%	89.4% at 33.6 months	At 3 years: 98.8%
Woyach et al., NEJM 2018 [17] Phase III randomized	547	Ibrutinib 420 mg daily until progression or ibrutinib 420 mg daily until progression + R 375 mg/m² C1 d1 d8 d14 d21 d1 c2–6	7%		Not reached	At 2 years: 90%
			12%		Not reached	At 2 years: 94%
Moreno et al., Lancet Onc 2018 [18] Phase III randomized	229	Ibrutinib 420 mg daily until progression Obinutuzumab 1000 mg d1,8,15 C1 and 1000 mg d1 C2-C6	19%	88%	Not reached	At 30 months: 86%
Venetoclax						
Fischer et al., NEJM 2019 [26] Phase III randomized	432	Venetoclax c1 d22 (ramp up) Venetoclax 400 mg daily c2–12) Obinutuzumab 1000 mg d1,8,15 C1 and 1000 mg d1 C2-C6	49.5%	84.7%	88.2% at 24 months	Not yet reached

$p = 0.003$) [16]. No difference in OS was observed. A greater number of SAEs due to infections were observed with BR (19% versus 8%).

Also in elderly patients, newer targeted agents have been investigated and showed an improved PFS, but not OS in comparison to chemoimmunotherapies. In the phase III ALLIANCE trial for patients >65 years, ibrutinib monotherapy and ibrutinib with rituximab were compared to bendamustine and rituximab (BR) treatment, with 182 patients in each of the three arms [17]. PFS has not yet been reached in either ibrutinib-containing arm but was 41 months in the BR arm. No significant survival difference has yet been demonstrated between any of the three arms, providing possible reassurance that ibrutinib monotherapy is equally efficacious as IR.

The phase III frontline ILLUMINATE trial of 229 patients aged >65 years or ≤65 with coexisting conditions demonstrated a longer PFS with ibrutinib plus obinutuzumab over chlorambucil plus obinutuzumab (not reached vs. 19.0 months at a median follow-up of 31.3 months, independent of high-risk features) [18].

However, besides the improvement of response and response duration, the continuous administration of BTK inhibitors is associated with additional morbidity, particularly cardiovascular morbidity. Severe atrial fibrillation was reported in 6% of patients [17], and more than threefold increased risk was described during ibrutinib therapy [19]. The development of new or worsening of preexisting arterial hypertension was reported in up to 78% of the patients during the course of ibrutinib intake [20]. Other BTK inhibitors as acalabrutinib or zanubrutinib may have a more favorable toxicity profile, but head-head comparisons between those substances are still missing [21–23]. However, results from a randomized phase III trial in elderly CLL patients comparing acalabrutinib alone or in combination with obinutuzumab versus chlorambucil plus obinutuzumab demonstrated superiority of both BTK inhibitor-containing treatment arms versus chemoimmunotherapy [21].

Venetoclax, an oral *BCL2* inhibitor, shows promising data with regard to deep responses, including high rates of MRD negativity [24, 25]. The phase III frontline CLL14 trial including 432 patients compared fixed duration venetoclax and obinutuzumab with chlorambucil and obinutuzumab in less fit patients and those with a CIRS score >6 or calculated creatinine clearance <70 mL/min. The 2-year PFS was significantly higher in the venetoclax and obinutuzumab arm (88.2% vs. 64.1%) with this advantage also seen in patients with a *TP53* deletion and/or mutation and unmutated IGHV status. MRD negativity was also higher in this patient group, in peripheral blood (75.5% vs. 35.2%) and in bone marrow (56.9% vs. 17.1%). Toxicities, which were mainly hematologic toxicities as well as infections and infusion-related reactions, and mortality are thus far statistically similar between the two arms [26].

Randomized trials comparing the two principles of chemotherapy-free treatment – continuous administration of BCR inhibitor versus time-limited therapy of bcl2-inhibiotr plus anit-CD20 antibody, have just started. Before these results are available with each patient individually, the choice of therapy has to be discussed based on consideration of comorbidity, co-medication, genetic profile, and ability to come to the physician's office.

13.3 Conclusion

Though FCR remains a treatment option in physically fit patients up to the age 65 years and with a mutated IGHV status, targeted therapies are the treatment of choice particularly in patients with unmutated IGHV status or *TP53* mutation or deletion. In fit patients, overall survival was longer for ibrutinib versus FCR within a randomized trial without crossover. Other trials in elderly or less fit evaluating the BTK inhibitors ibrutinib or acalabrutinib or the time-limited therapy of the bcl2 inhibitor venetoclax plus obinutuzumab versus chemoimmunotherapy demonstrated superiority with respect to PFS. In comparison to the less intensive chemoimmunotherapy with chlorambucil and obinutuzumab, ibrutinib and venetoclax demonstrated superiority in both subgroups, patients with mutated and unmutated IGHV. Data with respect to the combination of venetoclax plus obinutuzumab in fit patients are still pending.

13.4 Relapse Treatment

According to the *IWCLL* guidelines, relapsed patients are defined as those who have previously achieved a complete response (CR) or partial response (PR) but demonstrated evidence of disease progression after a period of 6 or more months [1]. Treatment-refractory CLL is defined as disease without PR or CR or disease progression within 6 months following the last antileukemic therapy.

The response to subsequent or second-line treatment depends on a variety of factors including clinical stage, adverse biological prognostic factors, and numbers of prior therapies. Patients refractory to previous therapy including BCR inhibitors and those with a del(17p)/*TP53* mutation have particularly poor prognosis [27–30]. In clinical studies, del(17p) has been identified in around 7% of previously untreated patients and as many as 50% with relapsed/refractory disease. Disease progression within 2 years of the initiation of frontline chemoimmunotherapy is an independent negative predictor of survival [31]. However, also progression of CLL on continuous treatment with targeted agents is associated with genetic evolution resulting in resistance mutations and poor outcome [29, 30, 32].

Therapy for relapsed and refractory patients after time-limited frontline therapy should be planned according to:

- Clinical stage of disease.
- Response to the previous treatment.
- Genetic results.
- Fitness of the patients.
- Laboratory parameters such as renal function.
- Bone marrow reserve.

If progression occurs on continuous therapy with targeted agents, treatment should not be stopped before an alternate treatment plan exists, because progression of CLL might accelerate immediately [33]. Repeat FISH testing and molecular testing for *TP53* mutation at the time of relapse is important to optimize treatment for high-risk patients. Testing for *BTK* mutations or other mutations in genes coding for targeted kinases is not yet performed in routine.

13.4.1 Management of Late Relapsed Patients After Chemoimmunotherapy

The European Society for Medical Oncology (ESMO) recommendations indicate that frontline treatment with chemoimmunotherapy may be repeated if the relapse or progression occurred within 24–36 months or longer after initial therapy [2]. However, in the era of new drugs, only a small proportion of relapsed patients are retreated with previous chemoimmunotherapies. Though patients may still show remarkable response rates, response duration is rather short in this situation and significant myelotoxicity may occur [34]. Because of more favorable side effect and efficacy profile, targeted drugs are the treatment of choice in the majority of relapsed patients.

13.4.2 Inhibitors of the B-Cell Receptor Pathway to Treat r/r Patients

Ibrutinib was compared with ofatumumab in a large, multicenter, phase III study (RESONATE I), performed in 391 patients with relapsed or refractory CLL (Table 13.3) [35]. The median PFS was not reached in the ibrutinib group but was 8.1 months in the ofatumumab group ($p < 0.001$). Ibrutinib administration also significantly improved the OR and the OS rates. In February 2014, the FDA approved ibrutinib for CLL in patients who had received at least one previous therapy and subsequently to patients with 17p deletion.

Ibrutinib can be also used after CLL relapse following allogeneic hematopoietic cell transplant (allo-HCT). *In a study* of 27 patients with relapsed CLL following allo-HCT who subsequently received ibrutinib salvage therapy, an 87.5% OR rate was observed with only three progressions after the 24-month observation [36].

Idelalisib is a phosphoinositide 3-kinase (PI3K)γ target, causing downstream inhibition of the B-cell receptor. The substance showed remarkable efficacy in comparison to rituximab in a heavily pretreated elderly patient population (Table 13.3) [37]. Significant toxicities observed in several trials as severe diarrhea, pneumonitis including *Pneumocystis jirovecii* pneumonitis, and CMV reactivations led to widespread withdrawal of its use. However, this substance is still a later line relapse treatment option for patients being refractory to BTK inhibitors and venetoclax.

13.4.3 BCL-2 Antagonists in r/r CLL

The bcl2 inhibitor venetoclax induced an objective response in approximately 80% of patients with relapsed/refractory CLL including del(17p), 16–20% of whom demonstrate CR [38]. The M13–982 phase II trial including only patients with relapsed CLL carrying del(17p) reported an OR rate with venetoclax monotherapy of 79.4%, with CR occurring in 7.5% of patients. Among the side effects, particularly grade 3–4 neutropenia, occurring in 43% of subjects, was assessed [39]. In 2016, venetoclax gained FDA and subsequent European Medicines Agency (EMA) approval for patients with del(17p) and TP53 CLL who had been treated with at least one prior therapy.

Table 13.3 Efficacy of selected therapies in relapsed CLL

Study	Treatment	Number of patients	Median age	Previous regimens	Overall response rate	Complete response rate	Progression free survival	Overall survival
RESONATE I Byrd et al. (2014) [35]	Ibrutinib vs. ofatumumab	195 vs. 196	67 years vs. 67 years	Median (range) 3 (1–12) vs. 2 (1–13)	42.6% vs. 4.1%, $p < 0.001$	2 vs. 1	Not reached vs. 8.1 m $p < 0.001$	At 12 months 90% vs. 81% $p = 0.005$
HELIOS Chanan-Khan et al. (2016) [57]	Ibrutinib + BR vs. BR	289 vs. 289	64 years vs. 63 years	Mean (range) 2 (1–11) vs. 2 (1–9)	82.7% vs. 67.8% $p < 0.0001$	10.4 vs. 2.8	NR vs. 13.3 m $p < 0.0001$	NR vs. NR $p = 0.0598$
Study 116 Furman et al. (2015) [37]	Idelalisib + rituximab vs. rituximab	110 vs. 110	71 years vs. 71 years	Median no. of drugs (range) 3 (1–12) vs. 3 (1–9)	81% vs. 13% $p < 0.001$	0 vs. 0	NR vs. 5.5 m $p < 0.001$	At 12 m 92% vs. 80% $p = 0.02$
Murano Seymour et al. (2018) [25]	Venetoclax + rituximab vs. BR	194 vs. 195	64 years vs. 66 years	More than 1 prior therapy 43% vs. 40%	92% vs. 72%	27% vs. 8%	At 2 years: 85% vs. 36%	At 2 years: 92% vs. 87%

R rituximab, *B* bendamustine

Within the phase III MURANO trial, 389 patients with relapsed or refractory CLL were randomized to receive venetoclax for up to 2 years plus rituximab for the first 6 months or BR for 6 months [25]. At a median follow-up of 23.8 months, PFS was greater in the venetoclax plus rituximab arm (84.9% vs. 36.3% $p < 0.0001$), with the advantage seen in all subgroups including those with 17p deletion and higher rates of undetectable MRD in peripheral blood after 9 months of treatment (62.4% vs. 13.3%).

13.4.4 Treatment of After Therapy Discontinuation of Targeted Agents

The most common reasons for discontinuation of BCR inhibitors are toxicity, CLL progression, and Richter syndrome [29]. Mato et al. analyzed the reasons for ibrutinib (143 patients) or idelalisib (35 patients) discontinuation in 187 heavily pretreated patients who had undergone a median of three prior therapies [40]. BCR inhibitor toxicity was the reason for treatment discontinuation in 51% of the patients and CLL progression in 29%. Currently, the best option for treatment of CLL patients who fail ibrutinib or idelalisib therapy is the BCL-2 antagonist venetoclax, showing overall response rates of 65% [41].

Vice versa, registry data have demonstrated that the Btk inhibitor ibrutinib induces responses following prior treatment with venetoclax [42]. In addition, reexposure to venetoclax after treatment-free interval might also be considered as option, but more data from clinical trials are warranted here in order to determine the minimum Bcl2 inhibitor-free interval.

13.4.5 Investigational Drugs in r/r Disease

Recently, several new agents have shown promise in treating CLL, and the second-generation BTK inhibitors as acalabrutinib (ACP-196) are now under investigation [22, 43]. Second-generation PI3Kδ inhibitors that are in development to address the safety concerns observed with idelalisib by reducing the severity of associated transaminase elevations include umbralisib and duvelisib (IPI-145) [44–46]. The phase III DUO trial demonstrated higher PFS rates with duvelisib when compared to ofatumumab in relapsed or refractory CLL (13.3 vs. 9.9 months, $p < 0.0001$) [46].

The novel anti-CD20 mAb ublituximab is effective in relapsed/refractory CLL, particularly when combined with ibrutinib [47]. A phase II study evaluating combined therapy with ublituximab and ibrutinib revealed rapid and high response rates in patients with relapsed or refractory CLL. An OR rate of 88% was achieved at 6 months in the total population, and this rate grew to 95% including 15% MRD negativity in 20 patients with 17p or 11q deletions or *TP53* mutation.

Otlertuzumab (TRU-016) is a humanized anti-CD37 protein therapeutic that induces ADCC and triggers direct caspase-independent apoptosis of malignant B-cells. A randomized study compared bendamustine plus otlertuzumab therapy with the use of bendamustine alone in patients with relapsed CLL [48]. Median PFS was also longer in the otlertuzumab combination arm than with bendamustine alone (15.9 vs. 10.2 months $p = 0.0192$).

Another anti-CD37 antibody (BI 836826) administered as monotherapy induced a 45% ORR in a very-high-risk patient population carrying del(17p) or *Tp53* mutation [49].

13.4.6 Allogenic Stem Cell Transplantation in r/r Disease

Allogeneic hematopoietic stem cell transplantation (allo-HCT) is currently still the only curative therapy of CLL. The CLL3X trial based on long-term observation of allografted patients found that reduced intensity conditioning (RIC) allo-HCT can provide sustained disease control in patients with high-risk CLL, independent of TP53 status [50]. In this study, 33 of 44 patients (75%) with available long-term observation data were alive at the 6-year follow-up.

Patients with del(17p) or *TP53* mutation may still be candidates for allo-HCT after at least one previous line of therapy. Allo-HCT should be considered for patients who did not achieve OR or who progressed after BCR inhibitor administration but receive BCL-2 inhibitors or vice versa [51]. However, with several different types of targeted therapy being available and more coming up, allo-HCT is currently mainly performed in patients being refractory to two targeted agents or having transformed into a diffuse large B-cell lymphoma, defined as Richter transformation.

13.5 Conclusion of Relapse Treatment

Despite recent progress in the treatment of CLL, almost all patients are destined to relapse. Actual guidelines recommend kinase inhibitor or bcl2 inhibitor therapy before repeat chemotherapy or chemoimmunotherapy in all patient subgroups. Novel combinations based on targeted agents might particularly be beneficial for patients with very-high-risk profile or being refractory to targeted agents. Allo-HCT can be considered in fit patients, especially those with a *del(17p)/TP53* mutation and who are refractory to BCR or bcl2 inhibitors. Patients with refractory disease should be treated within clinical trials whenever possible.

13.6 Outlook to Future Combinations

The combination therapy with ibrutinib plus venetoclax, without a CD20 antibody, was evaluated in a phase II trial in relapsed CLL [52]. After 8 weeks of ibrutinib monotherapy, venetoclax was added and gradually ramped up. Fifty patients showed good tolerance to this regimen. Despite the presence of high-risk factors, all 25 evaluable patients responded; 60% had a complete response and 76% had less than 1% CLL cells in the bone marrow, leading to venetoclax plus ibrutinib being added as an additional arm to the UK FLAIR trial [52]. Similar combinations based on BCR inhibitors and venetoclax with or without CD20 antibodies have already been tested in phase II trials in frontline [53, 54] and are now undergoing evaluation in randomized settings.

Conflicts of Interest B. Eichhorst was speaker for Abbvie, Janssen, Novartis, Roche, Gilead, and Celgene; she participated at advisory boards of Janssen, Abbvie, Novartis, AstraZeneca, Gilead, and Arqule and received research funding from Roche, Abbvie, Janssen, Gilead, and BeiGene.

References

1. Hallek M, et al. iwCLL guidelines for diagnosis, indications for treatment, response assessment, and supportive management of CLL. Blood. 2018;131(25):2745–60.
2. Döhner H, et al. Genomic aberrations and survival in chronic lymphocytic leukemia. N Engl J Med. 2000;343(26):1910–6.
3. Rossi D, et al. The prognostic value of TP53 mutations in chronic lymphocytic leukemia is independent of Del17p13: implications for overall survival and chemorefractoriness. Clin Cancer Res. 2009;15(3):995–1004.
4. Landau DA, et al. Mutations driving CLL and their evolution in progression and relapse. Nature. 2015;526(7574):525–30.
5. Baliakas P, et al. Recurrent mutations refine prognosis in chronic lymphocytic leukemia. Leukemia. 2014;29:329–36.
6. Extermann M, et al. Comorbidity and functional status are independent in older cancer patients. J Clin Oncol. 1998;16(4):1582–7.
7. Goede V, et al. Interactions between comorbidity and treatment of chronic lymphocytic leukemia: results of German Chronic Lymphocytic Leukemia Study Group trials. Haematologica. 2014;99(6):1095–100.
8. Bottcher S, et al. Minimal residual disease quantification is an independent predictor of progression-free and overall survival in chronic lymphocytic leukemia: a multivariate analysis from the randomized GCLLSG CLL8 trial. J Clin Oncol. 2012;30(9):980–8.
9. Hallek M, et al. Addition of rituximab to fludarabine and cyclophosphamide in patients with chronic lymphocytic leukemia: a randomised, open-label, phase III trial. Lancet. 2010;376:1164–74.
10. Fischer K, et al. Long-term remissions after FCR chemoimmunotherapy in previously untreated patients with CLL: updated results of the CLL8 trial. Blood. 2016;127(2):208–15.
11. Fischer K, et al. Bendamustine in combination with rituximab for previously untreated patients with chronic lymphocytic leukemia: a multicenter phase II

trial of the German Chronic Lymphocytic Leukemia Study Group. J Clin Oncol. 2012;30(26):3209–16.
12. Eichhorst B, et al. First-line chemoimmunotherapy with bendamustine and rituximab versus fludarabine, cyclophosphamide, and rituximab in patients with advanced chronic lymphocytic leukaemia (CLL10): an international, open-label, randomised, phase 3, non-inferiority trial. Lancet Oncol. 2016;17(7):928–42.
13. Burger JA, et al. Ibrutinib as initial therapy for patients with chronic lymphocytic leukemia. N Engl J Med. 2015;373(25):2425–37.
14. Shanafelt TD, et al. Ibrutinib-rituximab or chemoimmunotherapy for chronic lymphocytic leukemia. N Engl J Med. 2019;381(5):432–43.
15. Goede V, et al. Obinutuzumab plus chlorambucil in patients with CLL and coexisting conditions. N Engl J Med. 2014;370(12):1101–10.
16. Michallet AS, et al. Rituximab plus bendamustine or chlorambucil for chronic lymphocytic leukemia: primary analysis of the randomized, open-label MABLE study. Haematologica. 2018;103(4):698–706.
17. Woyach JA, et al. Ibrutinib regimens versus chemoimmunotherapy in older patients with untreated CLL. N Engl J Med. 2018;379(26):2517–28.
18. Moreno C, et al. Ibrutinib plus obinutuzumab versus chlorambucil plus obinutuzumab in first-line treatment of chronic lymphocytic leukaemia (iLLUMINATE): a multicentre, randomised, open-label, phase 3 trial. Lancet Oncol. 2019;20(1):43–56.
19. Leong DP, et al. The risk of atrial fibrillation with ibrutinib use: a systematic review and meta-analysis. Blood. 2016;128(1):138–40.
20. Dickerson T, et al. Hypertension and incident cardiovascular events following ibrutinib initiation. Blood. 2019;134(22):1919–28.
21. Ghia P, et al. ASCEND: phase III, randomized trial of acalabrutinib versus idelalisib plus rituximab or bendamustine plus rituximab in relapsed or refractory chronic lymphocytic leukemia. JCO. 2020;38(25): 2849–61.
22. Awan FT, et al. Acalabrutinib monotherapy in patients with chronic lymphocytic leukemia who are intolerant to ibrutinib. Blood Adv. 2019;3(9):1553–62.
23. Tam CS, et al. A head-to-head phase III study comparing zanubrutinib versus ibrutinib in patients with Waldenstrom macroglobulinemia. Future Oncol. 2018;14(22):2229–37.
24. Stilgenbauer S, et al. Venetoclax for patients with chronic lymphocytic leukemia with 17p deletion: results from the full population of a phase II pivotal trial. J Clin Oncol. 2018;36(19):1973–80.
25. Seymour JF, et al. Venetoclax-rituximab in relapsed or refractory chronic lymphocytic leukemia. N Engl J Med. 2018;378(12):1107–20.
26. Fischer K, et al. Venetoclax and obinutuzumab in patients with CLL and coexisting conditions. N Engl J Med. 2019;380(23):2225–36.
27. Zenz T, et al. TP53 mutation and survival in chronic lymphocytic leukemia. J Clin Oncol. 2010;28(29):4473–9.
28. Stilgenbauer S, et al. Gene mutations and treatment outcome in chronic lymphocytic leukemia: results from the CLL8 trial. Blood. 2014;123(21):3247–54.
29. Jain P, et al. Outcomes of patients with chronic lymphocytic leukemia after discontinuing ibrutinib. Blood. 2015;125(13):2062–7.
30. Ahn IE, et al. Clonal evolution leading to ibrutinib resistance in chronic lymphocytic leukemia. Blood. 2017;129(11):1469–79.
31. Cramer P, et al. Outcome of advanced chronic lymphocytic leukemia following different first-line and relapse therapies: a meta-analysis of five prospective trials by the German CLL Study Group (GCLLSG). Haematologica. 2015;100(11):1451–9.
32. Herling CD, et al. Clonal dynamics towards the development of venetoclax resistance in chronic lymphocytic leukemia. Nat Commun. 2018;9(1):727.
33. Gribben JG, et al. Optimising outcomes for patients with chronic lymphocytic leukaemia on ibrutinib therapy: European recommendations for clinical practice. Br J Haematol. 2018;180(5):666–79.
34. Robak T, et al. Rituximab plus fludarabine and cyclophosphamide prolongs progression-free survival compared with fludarabine and cyclophosphamide alone in previously treated chronic lymphocytic leukemia. J Clin Oncol. 2010;28(10):1756–65.
35. Byrd JC, et al. Ibrutinib versus ofatumumab in previously treated chronic lymphoid leukemia. N Engl J Med. 2014;371:213–23.
36. Ryan CE, et al. Ibrutinib efficacy and tolerability in patients with relapsed chronic lymphocytic leukemia following allogeneic HCT. Blood. 2016;128(25):2899–908.
37. Furman RR, et al. Idelalisib and rituximab in relapsed chronic lymphocytic leukemia. N Engl J Med. 2014;370(11):997–1007.
38. Roberts AW, et al. Targeting BCL2 with venetoclax in relapsed chronic lymphocytic leukemia. N Engl J Med. 2016;374(4):311–22.
39. Stilgenbauer S, et al. Venetoclax in relapsed or refractory chronic lymphocytic leukaemia with 17p deletion: a multicentre, open-label, phase 2 study. Lancet Oncol. 2016;17(6):768–78.
40. Mato AR, et al. Outcomes of CLL patients treated with sequential kinase inhibitor therapy: a real world experience. Blood. 2016;128(18):2199–205.
41. Jones JA, et al. Venetoclax for chronic lymphocytic leukaemia progressing after ibrutinib: an interim analysis of a multicentre, open-label, phase 2 trial. Lancet Oncol. 2018;19(1):65–75.
42. Mato AR, et al. Toxicities and outcomes of 616 ibrutinib-treated patients in the United States: a real-world analysis. Haematologica. 2018;103(5):874–9.
43. Byrd JC, et al. Acalabrutinib (ACP-196) in relapsed chronic lymphocytic leukemia. N Engl J Med. 2016;374(4):323–32.
44. Lampson BL, Brown JR. PI3Kdelta-selective and PI3Kalpha/delta-combinatorial inhibitors in clinical development for B-cell non-Hodgkin lymphoma. Expert Opin Investig Drugs. 2017;26(11):1267–79.

45. Nastoupil LJ, et al. Tolerability and activity of ublituximab, umbralisib, and ibrutinib in patients with chronic lymphocytic leukaemia and non-Hodgkin lymphoma: a phase 1 dose escalation and expansion trial. Lancet Haematol. 2019;6(2):e100–9.
46. Flinn IW, et al. The phase 3 DUO trial: duvelisib vs ofatumumab in relapsed and refractory CLL/SLL. Blood. 2018;132(23):2446–55.
47. Sharman JP, et al. Ublituximab (TG-1101), a novel glycoengineered anti-CD20 antibody, in combination with ibrutinib is safe and highly active in patients with relapsed and/or refractory chronic lymphocytic leukaemia: results of a phase 2 trial. Br J Haematol. 2017;176(3):412–20.
48. Robak T, et al. Randomized phase 2 study of otlertuzumab and bendamustine versus bendamustine in patients with relapsed chronic lymphocytic leukaemia. Br J Haematol. 2017;176(4):618–28.
49. Stilgenbauer S, et al. Phase 1 first-in-human trial of the anti-CD37 antibody BI 836826 in relapsed/refractory chronic lymphocytic leukemia. Leukemia. 2019;33(10):2531–5.
50. Kramer I, et al. Allogeneic hematopoietic cell transplantation for high-risk CLL: 10-year follow-up of the GCLLSG CLL3X trial. Blood. 2017;130(12):1477–80.
51. Dreger P, et al. High-risk chronic lymphocytic leukemia in the era of pathway inhibitors: integrating molecular and cellular therapies. Blood. 2018;132(9):892–902.
52. Hillmen P, et al. Ibrutinib plus venetoclax in relapsed/refractory chronic lymphocytic leukemia: the CLARITY study. J Clin Oncol. 2019;37(30):JCO1900894.
53. Jain N, et al. Ibrutinib and venetoclax for first-line treatment of CLL. N Engl J Med. 2019;380(22):2095–103.
54. Woyach JA, et al. Acalabrutinib plus obinutuzumab in treatment-naive and relapsed/refractory chronic lymphocytic leukemia. Cancer Discov. 2020;10(3):394–405.
55. Keating MJ, et al. Early results of a chemoimmunotherapy regimen of fludarabine, cyclophosphamide, and rituximab as initial therapy for chronic lymphocytic leukemia. J Clin Oncol. 2005;23:4079–88.
56. Tam CS, et al. Long-term results of the fludarabine, cyclophosphamide, and rituximab regimen as initial therapy of chronic lymphocytic leukemia. Blood. 2008;112(4):975–80.
57. Chanan-Khan A, et al. Ibrutinib combined with bendamustine and rituximab compared with placebo, bendamustine, and rituximab for previously treated chronic lymphocytic leukaemia or small lymphocytic lymphoma (HELIOS): a randomised, double-blind, phase 3 study. Lancet Oncol. 2016;17(2):200–11.

Part II

T-Cell Lymphoma

Indolent Cutaneous T-Cell Lymphomas

14

Rein Willemze, Sebastian Theurich, and Max Schlaak

Mycosis fungoides (MF)

Clinical outline
MF manifests in adulthood as erythematous (or, less frequently, hyper-/hypopigmented) patches, which slowly progress to plaques, tumoral lesions and/or to erythroderma. Ultimately, peripheral blood and lymph nodes become involved. Clinic-pathologic variants appear as follicular papules with alopecia (folliculotropic MF), solitary, scaled plaques (Woringer-Kolopp type MF / pagetoid reticulosis) or pendulous skin folds (granulomatous slack skin).

Cytology	Small to medium sized cells with convoluted, cerebriform nuclei. Large transformed cells in advanced stages.	Mycosis fungoides, cytology 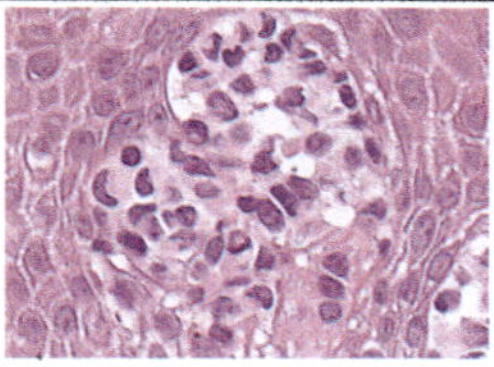
Histology	Variable picture, dependent on presentation. Typical MF at patch/plaque stage with intraepidermal lining the basal layer, intraepidermal aggregates (microabscesses of Pautrier). Tumoral stage features mass forming lesions, which may ulcerate. Folliculotropic MF with dilated infiltrated follicles and mucinosis. Pagetoid reticulosis with striking epidermotropism within a hyperplastic epidermis. Foreign body reaction-like giant multinucleated cells and features of elastolysis in granulomatous slack skin, which can be only clinically distinguished from granulomatous MF.	Mycosis fungoides, hystology 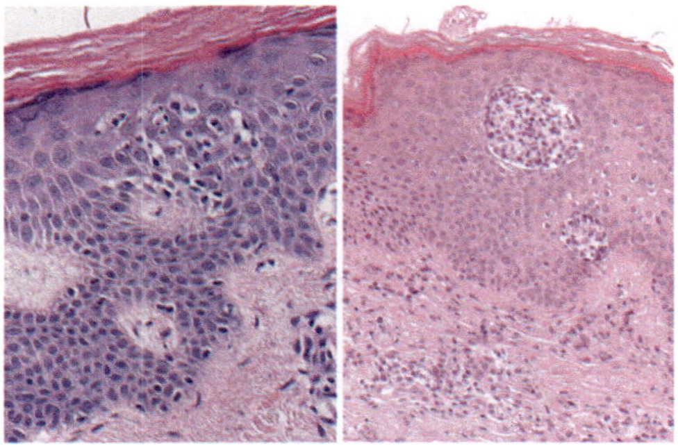

	CD20	CD3	CD5[1]	CD4[2]	CD8[2]	CD71	CD53	TCR[4]	CD57	CD30[1]
notes	[1]variable loss/expression of each marker. CD30 expression increased at progression/transformation [2]most cases CD4+/CD8-, rarer: CD4-/CD8+ or CD4-/CD8-, [3]rare cases reported, [4]most cases of $\alpha\beta$ type									
other marker	PD1 positive in a subset of cases.									

■ = majority of cases positive ▒ = variable fraction of cases positive □ = negative

M. Dreyling, M. Ladetto (eds.), *Indolent Lymphomas*, Hematologic Malignancies,
https://doi.org/10.1007/978-3-030-55989-2_14

Main differential diagnosis	Inflammatory lesions/dermatitis (should be polyclonal), Tumor-stage appears undistinguishable from cutaneous CD30+ lymphoproliferation (clinical presentation/history needed to distinguish), CD8+ epidermotropic lymphoma (should show epidermal necrosis) or cutaneous γ/δ-lymphoma (phenotype and clinical presentation).

Key molecular features

Clonally rearranged T-cell receptor (TCR) genes.

Frequent translocations: *CTLA4-CD28*, involvement of PDL1.

Frequent copy number alterations: *TNFRSF1B* gain.

Frequent mutations: *TNFR2, PLCG1*

Precursor lesions

Whether parapsoriasis en plaque as a chronic dermatitis represents an early MF /MF-precursor or whether it is a non-neoplastic independent disease is a matter of debate.

Progression

Histologic transformation (defined by by >25% large cells) and progression to tumor stage (clinically defined by tumor of >=1cm) are often associated

Clinically relevant pathologic features	Relevance	Evidence
Extent of dermal involvement (stage)	Prognostic: larger involved areas=higher stage (unfavourable)	**A**
Large cell transformation	Prognostic: correlates with lower OS	**B**
CD30 expression	Prognostic: predicts transformation to higher stage Predictive: anti-CD30 immunotherapy	**C** **B**
TCR clonality	Prognostic: detection of clone in skin and peripheral blood correlates with lower OS	**C**
Histologic variant	Prognostic: folliculotropic MF and granulomatous MF carry a more aggressive behavior	**B**
Legend: A= verified in multiple studies, randomized trials and/or integrated in guidelines; B= variable between studies/ needs definitive validation; C= preliminary / discrepant results		

R. Willemze (✉)
Department of Dermatology, Leiden University Medical Centre, Leiden, The Netherlands

S. Theurich
Department of Medicine III, LMU Hospital, Munich, Germany
e-mail: Sebastian.Theurich@med.uni-muenchen.de

M. Schlaak
Department of Dermatology and Allergology, LMU Hospital, Munich, Germany
e-mail: Max.Schlaak@med.uni-muenchen.de

14.1 Introduction

The term cutaneous T-cell lymphoma (CTCL) refers to T-cell lymphomas that present in the skin with no evidence of extracutaneous disease at the time of diagnosis. CTCL represent approximately 75–80% of all primary cutaneous lymphomas, whereas primary cutaneous B-cell lymphomas account for approximately 20–25% and are not a focus of this chapter [1, 2]. CTCL constitute a heterogeneous group of lymphomas that show considerable variation in clinical presentation, histologic appearance, immunophenotype, and prognosis. The relative frequency and prognosis of the different types of CTCL that are recognized in the 2018 update of the World Health Organization—European Organization for Research and Treatment of Cancer (WHO-EORTC) classification for primary cutaneous lymphomas and the 2016 revision of the WHO classification are presented in Table 14.1 [1, 2]. In this chapter, the clinicopathologic characteristics, prognosis, prognostic factors, and treatment options of indolent types of CTCL are discussed.

Table 14.1 Relative frequency and prognosis of cutaneous T-cell lymphomas included in the 2018 update of the WHO-EORTC classification (modified from [1])

WHO-EORTC classification 2018	Frequency (%)[a]	5-year DSS (%)[a]
Mycosis fungoides	52	88
Mycosis fungoides variants		
• Folliculotropic MF	6	75
• Pagetoid reticulosis	<1	100
• Granulomatous slack skin	<1	100
Sézary syndrome	3	36
Adult T-cell leukemia/ lymphoma	<1	NDA
Primary cutaneous CD30-positive lymphoproliferative disorders		
• Primary cutaneous anaplastic large cell lymphoma	11	95
• Lymphomatoid papulosis	16	99
Subcutaneous panniculitis-like T-cell lymphoma	1	87
Extranodal NK/T-cell lymphoma, nasal type	<1	16
Chronic active EBV infection	<1	NDA
Primary cutaneous peripheral T-cell lymphoma, rare subtypes		
• Primary cutaneous γ/δ T-cell lymphoma	<1	11
• Primary cutaneous aggressive epidermotropic CD8-positive T-cell lymphoma (provisional)	<1	31
• Primary cutaneous CD4+ small/medium T-cell lymphoproliferative disorder (provisional)	8	100
• Primary cutaneous acral CD8+ T-cell lymphoma (provisional)	<1	100
Primary cutaneous peripheral T-cell lymphoma, not otherwise specified	3	15

DSS disease-specific survival, *NDA* no data available
[a]Based on data included in Dutch and Austrian cutaneous lymphoma registries between 2002 and 2017

14.2 Mycosis Fungoides

Mycosis fungoides (MF) is the most common type of CTCL and accounts for more than 50% of all cases (Table 14.1). It is defined as an epidermotropic CTCL characterized by a proliferation of small- to medium-sized T-lymphocytes with cerebriform nuclei. The term MF should be used only for the classical "Alibert–Bazin" type characterized by the evolution of patches, plaques, and tumors or for variants showing a similar clinical course.

14.2.1 Clinical Features

MF typically affects older adults (median age at diagnosis: 55–60 years) but may occur in children and adolescents as well. Men are affected more often than women, with a male-to-female ratio of 1.6–2.0:1 [3–6]. Patients with classical MF present with patches and plaques that are preferentially located on the buttocks and other covered sites of the trunk and limbs (sun-protected areas) (Fig. 14.1a). Most patients have a protracted clinical course over years or even decades without progression beyond early patch/plaque stage disease. However, a proportion of patients may develop nodules or tumors and eventually progress to extracutaneous disease. Skin tumors may be solitary, localized, or widespread and often show ulceration (Fig. 14.2a).

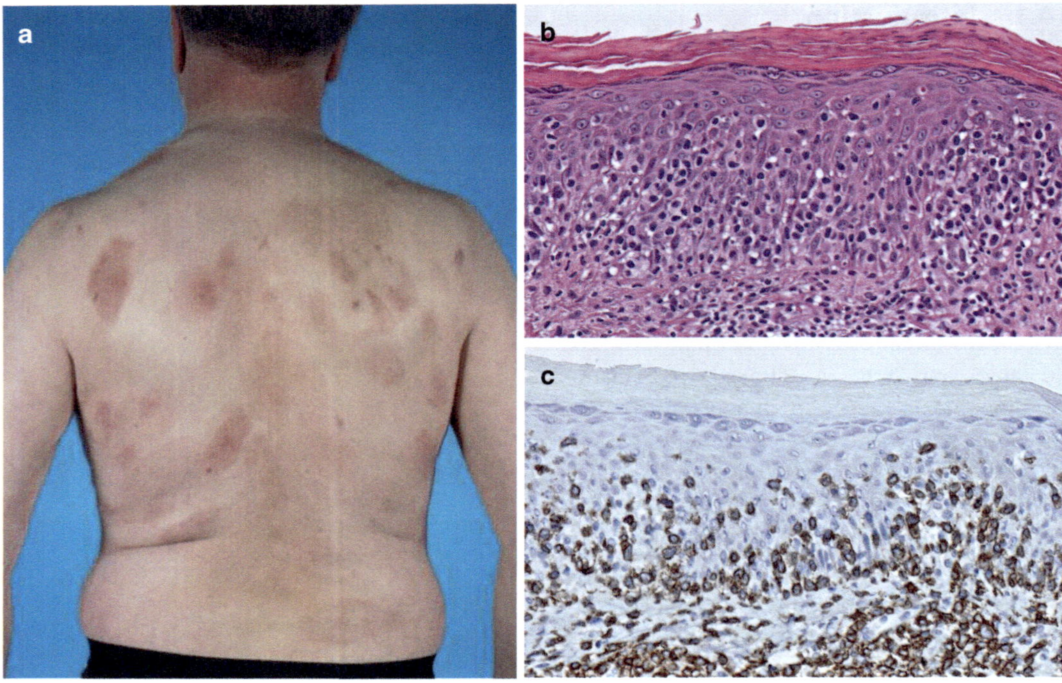

Fig. 14.1 Mycosis fungoides, plaque stage. Generalized patches and thin plaques on the trunk (**a**); histopathologic examination shows extensive infiltration of the epidermis by atypical T-cells (epidermotropism) (**b**); CD3 expression by dermal and intraepidermal T-cells (**c**)

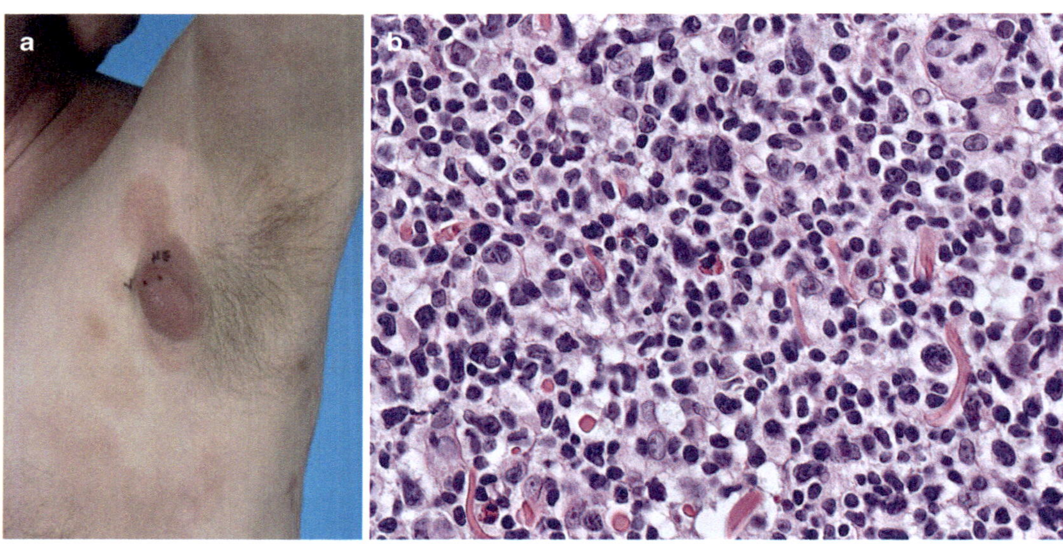

Fig. 14.2 Mycosis fungoides, tumor stage. Patches and a solitary tumor in the left armpit (**a**); histopathologic examination of the tumor shows a diffuse dermal infiltrate of small- and medium-sized and large neoplastic T-cells (**b**)

Extracutaneous dissemination most commonly first involves the regional lymph nodes draining areas of extensive skin involvement. Visceral involvement may develop subsequently and can involve any organ. The risk of developing extracutaneous disease correlates with the extent and stage of disease. The revised TNMB classification and clinical staging system used for MF and Sézary syndrome is presented in Table 14.2 [7]. Development of extracutaneous disease is exceedingly rare in patients with limited patch/plaque stage disease (stage IA), relatively uncommon in patients with generalized patches and/or plaques (stage IB), and much more common in patients with skin tumors (stage IIB) or erythroderma (stage III) [3–6].

Table 14.2 Revised TNMB classification and clinical staging system for MF/SS [7]

T (skin)	
T_1	Limited patch/plaque (involving <10% of total skin surface)
T_2	Generalized patch/plaque (involving ≥10% of total skin surface)
T_3	Tumor(s)
T_4	Erythroderma
N (lymph node)	
N_0	No clinically abnormal peripheral lymph nodes
N_1	Clinically abnormal peripheral lymph nodes; histologically uninvolved
N_2	Clinically abnormal peripheral lymph nodes; histologically involved (nodal architecture uneffaced)
N_3	Clinically abnormal peripheral lymph nodes; histologically involved (nodal architecture (partially) effaced)
Nx	Clinically abnormal peripheral lymph nodes; no histological confirmation
M (viscera)	
M_0	No visceral involvement
M_1	Visceral involvement
B (blood)	
B_0	No circulating atypical (Sézary) cells (or <5% of lymphocytes)
B_1	Low blood tumor burden (≥5% of lymphocytes are Sézary cells, but not B2)
B_2	High blood tumor burden (positive clone and either ≥1000/μL Sézary cells or CD4/CD8 ratio>10 or CD4+CD7- cells more than 40% or CD4+CD26- cells more than 30%

Clinical stage				
IA	T_1	N_0	M_0	B_{0-1}
IB	T_2	N_0	M_0	B_{0-1}
IIA	T_{1-2}	N_{1-2}	M_0	B_{0-1}
IIB	T_3	N_{0-2}	M_0	B_{0-1}
III	T_4	N_{0-2}	M_0	B_{0-1}
IVA_1	T_{1-4}	N_{0-2}	M_0	B_2
IVA_2	T_{1-4}	N_3	M_0	B_{0-2}
IVB	T_{1-4}	N_{0-3}	M_1	B_{0-2}

MF mycosis fungoides, *SS* Sézary syndrome

14.2.2 Histopathology

Histopathologically, early patch/plaque stage disease is characterized by the presence of superficial band-like or lichenoid infiltrates of small- to medium-sized atypical T-cells with cerebriform and sometimes hyperchromatic nuclei, which characteristically infiltrate into the epidermis (epidermotropism). They characteristically colonize the basal layer of the epidermis either as single often haloed cells or in a linear configuration [8, 9]. The presence of intraepidermal nests of atypical cells (Pautrier's microabscesses) is a highly characteristic feature but is observed in only a minority of cases (Fig. 14.1b). With progression to tumor stage, the dermal infiltrates become more diffuse and epidermotropism may no longer be present. The tumor cells increase in number and size, showing variable proportions of small, medium-sized or large cells with cerebriform nuclei, blast cells with prominent nuclei, and intermediate forms (Fig. 14.2b). Large cell transformation, defined by the presence of CD30-negative or CD30-positive large cells exceeding 25% of the infiltrate or forming microscopic nodules, may occur and is generally associated with a poor prognosis [10, 11].

The neoplastic cells in MF have a mature CD3+, CD4+, CD45RO+, CD8− phenotype and represent the so-called skin resident memory T-cells [12]. In a minority of cases of otherwise classical MF, a CD4−, CD8+ mature T-cell phenotype or more rarely a γ/δ T-cell phenotype (βF1−, TCR γ/δ+, CD3+, CD4−, CD8+) may be seen [13, 14]. Such cases have the same clinical behavior and prognosis as CD4+ cases and should not be considered separately. Demonstration of an aberrant phenotype (e.g., loss of pan-T-cell antigens such as CD2, CD3, and CD5) is an important adjunct in the diagnosis of MF but is uncommon in the early stages of MF.

Demonstration of clonal T-cell receptor gene rearrangement is also used as an adjunct to differentiate between MF and benign inflammatory dermatoses. However, caution is warranted, since clonal T-cell populations can occasionally also be found in benign skin conditions. Demonstration of an identical T-cell clone in skin biopsies from different anatomical sites is however highly specific for MF and rarely found in benign dermatoses [15, 16]. Although not a clinical standard method so far, high-throughput gene sequencing has been shown to have higher detection sensitivity for clonal T-cell populations and might in the future complement the diagnostic instrumentarium in uncertain cases [17].

14.2.3 Treatment

The choice of an initial treatment in MF depends on the stage of the disease and the general condition and age of the patient. Given the chronic and recurrent nature of MF, treatment should be aimed at improving symptoms while limiting toxicity. Therefore, a stage-adapted conservative therapeutic approach is recommended for MF and its variants [18–20].

In general, as long as the disease is confined to the skin, patients should be treated with skin-directed therapies including topical or intralesional steroids, phototherapy such as psoralens plus ultraviolet A (PUVA) or narrowband UVB (nb-UVB), topical cytostatic agents such as mechlorethamine (nitrogen mustard), and radiotherapy (Table 14.3). In patients with stage IA disease, even an expectant policy with careful monitoring can be followed. The efficacy of skin-directed therapies in MF is explained by the preferential localization of the neoplastic skin-homing T-cells to the epidermis and superficial dermis. Systemic multi-agent chemotherapy is not useful in these early stages, since it does not improve survival and is associated with considerable morbidity [21].

Topical steroids may be effective in controlling disease activity in patients with only patches and very thin plaques. In the more advanced stages, they continue to be an important adjuvant therapy. PUVA treatment has become a standard therapy for the early stages of MF with complete response rates of 80–90% in patients with stage IA–IIA disease. Nb-UVB should only be used in patients with patches or very thin plaques. Topical application of mechlorethamine, either in aqueous solution or in an ointment-based preparation, has been used successfully for decades in the treatment of early-stage MF. Recently, a commercial 0.02% gel preparation was approved by the EMA as an orphan drug for the treatment of early-stage MF [22]. In patients developing one or few infiltrated plaques or tumors (stage IIB), additional low-dose local radiotherapy (2 × 4 Gy) may suffice [23, 24].

For patients with more extensive infiltrated plaques and tumors or patients refractory to skin-directed therapies, a combination of PUVA and interferon alpha or PUVA and retinoids, includ-

Table 14.3 Recommendations for the treatment of mycosis fungoides

Stage	First-line treatment	Second-line treatment
Stage IA–IIA	Expectant policy Topical steroids Nb-UVB PUVA Topical mechlorethamine Local RT	PUVA + retinoids PUVA + IFNα Retinoids IFNα Retinoids + IFNα TSEBI
Stage IIB	PUVA + local RT PUVA + retinoids PUVA + IFNα TSEBI	Gemcitabine Liposomal doxorubicin Brentuximab vedotin Combination chemotherapy Allo-SCT
Stage III	PUVA + retinoids PUVA + IFNα ECP −/+ IFNα −/+ retinoids Low-dose MTX	TSEBI
Stage IV	Gemcitabine Liposomal doxorubicin Brentuximab vedotin	Combination chemotherapy Allo-SCT

MF mycosis fungoides, *PUVA* psoralens plus ultraviolet A, *Nb-UVB* narrow-band ultraviolet B, *RT* radiotherapy, *IFNα* interferon alpha, *TSEBI* total skin electron beam irradiation, *allo-SCT* allogeneic stem cell transplantation, *MTX* methotrexate, *ECP* extracorporeal photopheresis ing bexarotene, and a combination of interferon alpha and retinoids or total skin electron beam irradiation can be considered [18–20, 25]. Total skin electron beam irradiation (TSEBI) is a highly effective treatment in patients with skin-limited MF. TSEBI was often given to total doses of 30–36 Gy in fractions of 1.5–2 Gy over an 8–10-week period. Recently, lower doses (10–12 Gy) have been employed with the advantages of briefer duration, fewer side effects, and opportunity for re-treatment [26, 27].

In patients with advanced and refractory disease, gemcitabine or liposomal doxorubicin may be considered, but responses are generally short-lived [28, 29]. Recent studies also report high response rates of brentuximab vedotin (BV; a monoclonal anti-CD30 antibody coupled to the anti-tubulin agent monomethyl auristatin E) in patients with advanced MF/SS expressing CD30 [30–32]. Other agents like histone deacetylase (HDAC) inhibitors, such as vorinostat and romidepsin, have been approved in the United States by the Food and Drug Administration for patients with relapsed and refractory CTCL but have not yet been registered for CTCL in Europe [33–35]. Recently, the CCR-4 monoclonal antibody mogamulizumab has been approved by registration authorities. Mogamulizumab showed clinical activity with an overall response rate of app. 28% but is particularly effective in clearing tumor cells from the peripheral blood [36, 37].

Multi-agent chemotherapy, including CHOP and CHOP-like courses, is only indicated in patients with effaced lymph nodes or visceral involvement (stage IV) or in patients with widespread tumor stage MF, which cannot be controlled with skin-targeted and immunomodulating therapies, but—similar to single-agent chemotherapy—responses are generally short-lived.

In relatively young patients with refractory, progressive MF or with SS, an allogeneic stem cell transplantation (allo-SCT) should be considered. Using nonmyeloablative reduced-intensity conditioning regimens, durable responses have been reported, but experience is still limited and the optimal conditioning regimen and timing for an allogeneic transplant are currently unknown [38, 39]. Recent studies suggest that patients may benefit from tumor debulking with TSEBI or immunochemotherapy with BV prior to transplantation [40–42]. Results with autologous stem cell transplantation in MF and SS have been disappointing [43], suggesting the need for a graft-versus-lymphoma response.

14.2.4 Prognosis and Predictive Factors

The prognosis of patients with MF is dependent on the stage and in particular the type and extent of skin lesions and the presence of extracutaneous disease [3–6]. The disease-related 10-year survival is 96% for stage IA, 77–83% for stage IB, and 42% for stage IIB but only 20% for patients with stage IV [4, 6]. Patients with effaced lymph nodes, visceral involvement, and transformation into a large T-cell lymphoma generally run an aggressive clinical course. Patients usually die of systemic involvement or infections.

14.3 Variants of MF

Apart from classical MF, many clinical and/or histopathologic variants of MF mimicking a wide variety of inflammatory skin diseases have been described [44, 45]. Most variants have a clinical behavior similar to that of classic MF and have therefore not been classified separately. In recent classifications, only folliculotropic MF (FMF), pagetoid reticulosis, and granulomatous slack skin are recognized as distinct variants of MF, because of their distinctive clinicopathologic features, clinical behavior, and/or prognosis [1, 2]. Whereas FMF is not uncommon and accounts for approximately 10% of all cases of MF, pagetoid reticulosis and granulomatous slack skin are extremely rare conditions (Table 14.1).

14.4 Folliculotropic MF

Folliculotropic MF (FMF) is a distinct variant of MF characterized by the presence of folliculotropic infiltrates, often with sparing of the interfollicular epidermis and preferential involvement of the head and neck region [1, 2]. In large series, FMF accounts for approximately 10% of all patients with MF [4, 6]. Most cases show mucinous degeneration of the hair follicles (follicular mucinosis) and were originally designated as MF-associated follicular mucinosis. Similar cases, but without follicular mucinosis, have been reported as pilotropic MF [46].

14.4.1 Clinical Features

FMF mostly presents in adults but has also been reported in children and adolescents. [47–52] Men are affected more often than women. Patients may present with (grouped) follicular papules, acneiform lesions, indurated plaques, or tumors [47–50, 53]. Infiltrated plaques or tumors in the eyebrow region with concurrent hair loss are a highly characteristic feature (Fig. 14.3a). Some patients may show keratosis pilaris-like lesions that are mainly localized on trunk and extremities (Fig. 14.3b) [54]. The skin lesions are often associated with alopecia. Pruritus is often severe and may represent a reliable parameter of disease activity. Secondary bacterial infections are frequently observed [53]. In rare cases, FMF may present with a solitary skin lesion (solitary or unilesional FMF) or with erythroderma [55–57].

14.4.2 Histopathology

Histopathologically, FMF is characterized by the presence of perifollicular to diffuse infiltrates with variable infiltration of the follicular epithelium by small, medium-sized or sometimes large T-cells with cerebriform and hyperchromatic nuclei (Fig. 14.3c) [47–50, 53]. Many cases show mucinous degeneration of the follicular epithelium (follicular mucinosis), which can be visualized by Alcian blue or colloidal iron staining, but cases without follicular mucinosis have been described as well [46]. Infiltration of the follicular epithelium may be accompanied by infiltration of the eccrine sweat glands (syringotropism),

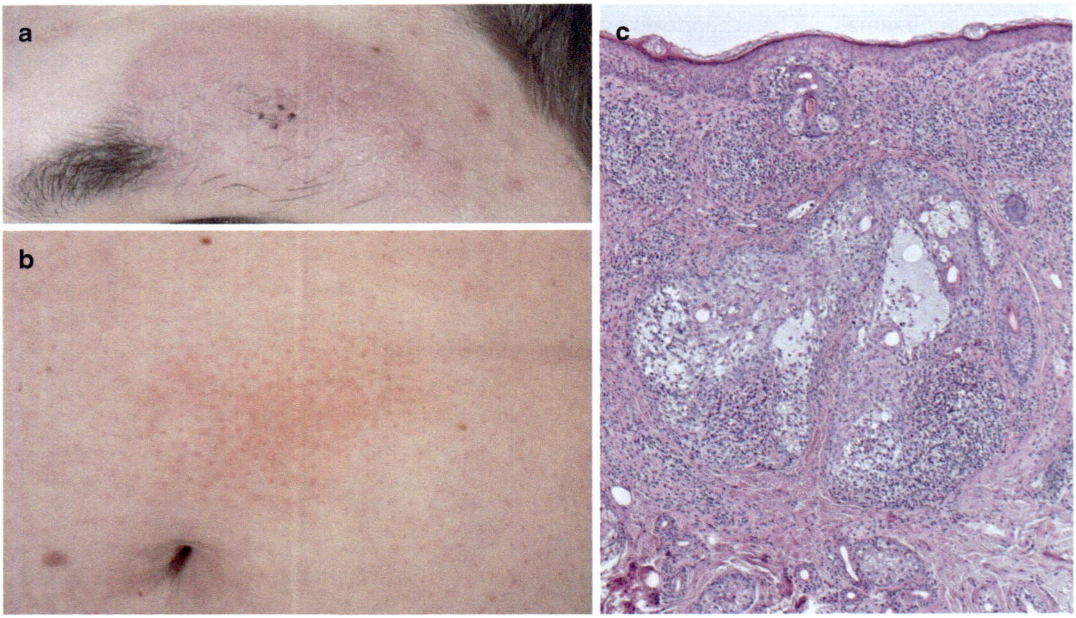

Fig. 14.3 Folliculotropic mycosis fungoides. Slightly infiltrated plaque with associated alopecia in the left eyebrow (**a**); keratosis pilaris-like lesions on the abdomen (**b**); histopathologic examination shows perifollicular infiltrates with infiltration of the follicular epithelium and extensive follicular mucinosis (**c**)

a combination that is often referred to as adnexotropic MF [57–59]. However, concurrent infiltration of the interfollicular epidermis (epidermotropism) characteristic of early-stage classic MF is uncommon. In early-stage lesions, clinically characterized by follicle-based patches or acneiform or keratosis pilaris-like lesions, the perifollicular infiltrates are generally sparse and contain, apart from atypical T-cells, variable numbers of small reactive T-cells, histiocytes, and occasional eosinophils. With progression of the skin lesions to more infiltrated plaques or tumors, the dermal infiltrates become more diffuse and may contain increasing numbers of blast cells. There is often a considerable admixture with eosinophils and, in particular in cases with secondary bacterial infection, plasma cells. In some cases, clusters of small B-cells may be present. In cases with destruction of the hair follicle epithelium, a granulomatous reaction can be observed [58]. Large cell transformation, defined by the presence of more than 25% of blast cells or the presence of clusters of blast cells, has been reported in more than 20% of FMF cases and is more common than in classical MF [48, 50, 53].

In virtually all cases, the neoplastic cells in FMF have a CD3+, CD4+, CD8− T-cell phenotype as in classic MF [58]. Admixed blast cells are often CD30-positive. Most cases show clonal T-cell receptor gene rearrangements [58].

14.4.3 Treatment and Prognosis

Previous studies emphasized that FMF is generally less responsive to several skin-directed therapies and runs a more aggressive clinical course similar to that of tumor stage classic MF and should therefore be treated accordingly [47, 48]. However, more recent studies defined a subgroup of FMF patients with an indolent clinical behavior and an excellent prognosis, with a 5- and 10-year survival similar to that of early-stage classic MF [53, 54, 60]. Recognition of indolent and aggressive subgroups of FMF is also important from a therapeutic point of view, since it implies that early- and advanced-stage FMF require a different therapeutic approach. Recent studies suggest a stepwise, stage-adapted therapeutic approach, similar as in early- and advanced-stage classic MF [61]. Patients with early-stage FMF may benefit very well from non-aggressive skin-directed therapies (SDT), such as topical steroids, psoralen plus ultraviolet A (PUVA), or topical nitrogen mustard. In patients with advanced-stage FMF, these SDTs are less effective. For these patients, PUVA combined with local radiotherapy and PUVA combined with interferon alpha and/or retinoids or total skin electron beam irradiation have been recommended [48, 50, 61]. For rare FMF patients presenting with a solitary plaque or tumor, local radiotherapy is highly effective and is the preferred mode of treatment [55–57]. Apart from stage, advanced age, large cell transformation, and extensive secondary bacterial infection have been reported to be associated with reduced survival [50, 53].

14.5 Pagetoid Reticulosis (Woringer–Kolopp Disease)

Pagetoid reticulosis is a rare unilesional variant of MF, clinically characterized by the presence of a solitary, slowly progressive, psoriasiform, or hyperkeratotic patch or plaque, which is usually localized on an extremity, particularly hands or feet, and histologically by an intraepidermal proliferation of neoplastic T-cells [1, 2, 62]. The term pagetoid reticulosis should only be used for the localized type (Woringer–Kolopp type) and not for the disseminated type (Ketron–Goodman type). Nowadays, most patients with generalized disease would be classified as primary cutaneous CD8+ aggressive epidermotropic cytotoxic T-cell lymphoma, primary cutaneous gamma/delta T-cell lymphoma, or tumor stage MF [1, 63].

Histologically, these lesions show a hyperplastic epidermis with marked infiltration by small- to medium-sized atypical pagetoid cells, arranged singly or in nests or clusters. The superficial dermis may have an infiltrate of mostly small lymphocytes but rarely contains neoplastic

T-cells. The neoplastic T-cells may show either a CD3+, CD4−, and CD8+ or less commonly a CD3+, CD4+, CD8−, or CD3+, CD4−, CD8− phenotype. Cases with a CD8+ or CD4−, CD8− phenotype express cytotoxic proteins. CD30 is often expressed [62].

The preferred mode of treatment is radiotherapy or surgical excision. The prognosis of pagetoid reticulosis is excellent; extracutaneous dissemination or disease-related deaths have never been reported [63].

14.6 Granulomatous Slack Skin

Granulomatous slack skin (GSS) is a very rare variant of MF, clinically characterized by the slow development of pendulous folds of lax skin in the major skin folds (axilla and groins) and histologically by the presence of dense infiltrates of small clonal CD4-positive T-cells admixed with numerous macrophages and many scattered multinucleated giant cells [1, 64]. The presence of multinucleated giant cells containing more than ten nuclei per cell is considered as a characteristic feature but has also been observed in cases of granulomatous MF [65]. Loss of elastic tissue, elastophagocytosis, and emperipolesis (engulfment of lymphocytes) by multinucleated cells are commonly observed. The epidermis may be infiltrated by small atypical T-cells with cerebriform nuclei, as in classic MF. Most cases have a $CD3^{+}$, $CD4^{+}$, $CD8^{-}$ T-cell phenotype and show clonal T-cell receptor gene rearrangement [65]. Extracutaneous dissemination is rare, but in approximately one-third of patients, an association with other malignant lymphomas, particularly MF and Hodgkin lymphoma, has been reported [66]. Treatment of GSS is unsatisfactory. Patients have been treated with PUVA, radiotherapy, surgical excision, interferon alpha, and other systemic therapies, but complete responses have never been reported [67]. Because of the increased risk of a second malignant lymphoma, long-term follow-up is mandatory in patients with GSS [65].

14.7 Primary Cutaneous CD30-Positive T-Cell Lymphoproliferative Disorders

Primary cutaneous CD30-positive lymphoproliferative disorders (LPD) are the second most common group of the cutaneous T-cell lymphomas (CTCL), accounting for more than 25% of all CTCL (Table 14.1) [1]. This group includes primary cutaneous anaplastic large lymphoma (C-ALCL) and lymphomatoid papulosis (LyP), which show overlapping clinical, histologic, and phenotypic features and form a spectrum of disease. The clinical appearance and clinical course are used as decisive criteria for the definite diagnosis and choice of treatment.

14.8 Lymphomatoid Papulosis

Lymphomatoid papulosis (LyP) is a chronic, recurrent, and self-healing skin disease, which combines a usually benign clinical course with histologic features of a (CD30-positive) CTCL [1].

14.8.1 Clinical Features

LyP most often occurs in adults (median age, 45 years), but children may also be affected. The youngest patient published to date is an 8-month-old child. The male-to-female ratio is 2–3:1 [68–71]. Characteristically, patients show papular, papulonecrotic, and/or nodular skin lesions in different stages of evolution (Fig. 14.4a). The number of lesions may vary from a few to more than a hundred. In very rare cases, concurrent oral mucosal lesions may be present. Individual skin lesions disappear within 3–12 weeks and may leave behind superficial scars. The duration of the disease may vary from several months to decades. In up to 20% of patients, LyP may be preceded by, associated with, or followed by another type of malignant lymphoma, most commonly MF or C-ALCL [68, 70, 72–74].

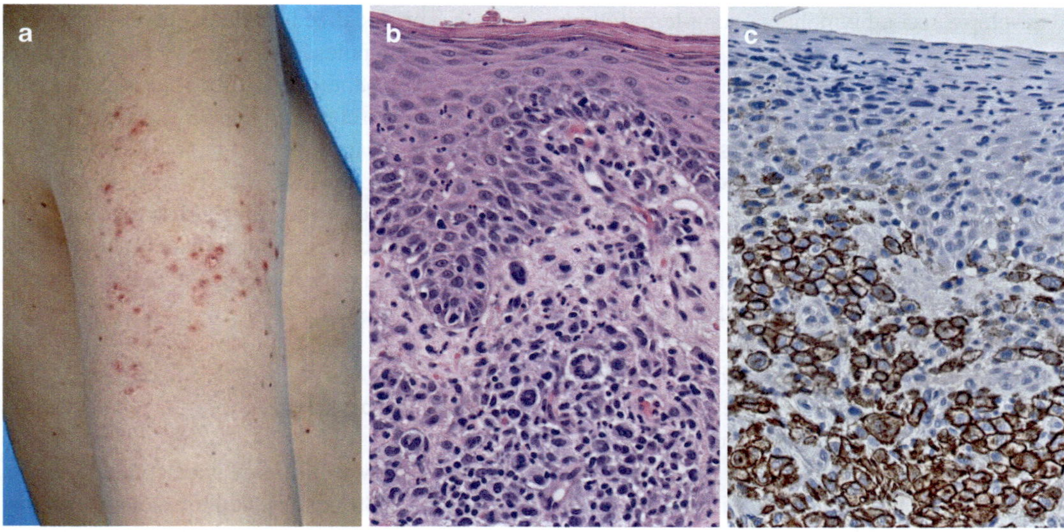

Fig. 14.4 Lymphomatoid papulosis. Clustered papules in various stages of evolution on the right upper arm (**a**); histopathologic examination shows a dense inflammatory infiltrate with many large atypical blast cells (**b**); CD30 expression by large atypical cells (**c**)

14.8.2 Histopathology

The histologic picture of LyP is extremely variable, which in part correlates with the age of the biopsied skin lesion (Fig. 14.4b, c). In recent classifications, six histologic subtypes are recognized: five histologic subtypes resembling different types of CTCL, including C-ALCL (types A and C), plaque stage MF (type B), primary cutaneous CD8+ aggressive epidermotropic cytotoxic T-cell lymphoma (type D), and angiocentric lymphomas (type E), and a new subtype characterized by the presence of chromosomal rearrangements involving the *DUSP-IRF4* locus on 6p25.3 [75, 76]. The same rearrangement is found in approximately 25% of C-ALCL [77]. Recognition of these different types of LyP is important to avoid misdiagnosis of other often more aggressive types of CTCL but has no therapeutic or prognostic implications. The atypical cells are predominantly CD4+ in LyP types A, B, and C; CD8+ in LyP types D and E; and either CD8+ or double negative for CD4 and CD8 in *DUSP22/IRF4* translocated cases [76].

14.8.3 Treatment and Prognosis

Treatment of LyP is unsatisfactory. Since a curative therapy is not available and none of the available treatment modalities affects the natural course of the disease, the short-term benefits of active treatment should be balanced carefully against potential side effects [68, 78]. In patients with relatively few non-scarring lesions, an expectant policy can be followed. In the case of cosmetically disturbing lesions (e.g., scarring or many papulonodules), low-dose oral MTX (5–20 mg/week) is the most effective therapy for reducing the number of skin lesions [79]. PUVA therapy is also effective but is less attractive in case maintenance treatment is required. LyP has an excellent prognosis in the vast majority of patients. However, because of the risk to develop a second lymphoma, long-term follow-up is advised.

14.9 Primary Cutaneous Anaplastic Large Cell Lymphoma

Primary cutaneous anaplastic large cell lymphoma (C-ALCL) is composed of large cells with an anaplastic, pleomorphic, or immunoblastic cytomorphology and expression of the CD30 antigen by the majority (more than 75%) of tumor cells [1, 2]. Patients should not have clinical evidence or a history of MF. In such cases, a diagnosis of tumor stage MF with blastic transformation is more likely.

14.9.1 Clinical Features

C-ALCL affects mainly adults with a male-to-female ratio of 2–3:1. Most patients present with solitary or localized nodules or tumors, and sometimes papules, and often show ulceration (Fig. 14.5a) [68, 69]. Multifocal lesions are seen in about 20% of the patients. The skin lesions may show partial or complete spontaneous regression, as in LyP. These lymphomas frequently relapse in the skin. Extracutaneous dissemination occurs in approximately 10% of the patients and mainly involves the regional lymph nodes [68].

14.9.2 Histopathology

Histology shows infiltrates with cohesive sheets of large CD30-positive tumor cells. In most cases, the tumor cells have the characteristic morphology of anaplastic cells, showing round, oval, or irregularly shaped nuclei, prominent eosinophilic nucleoli, and abundant cytoplasm (Fig. 14.5b, c). Less commonly (20–25%), they have a non-anaplastic (pleomorphic or immunoblastic) appearance [68, 80]. Reactive lympho-

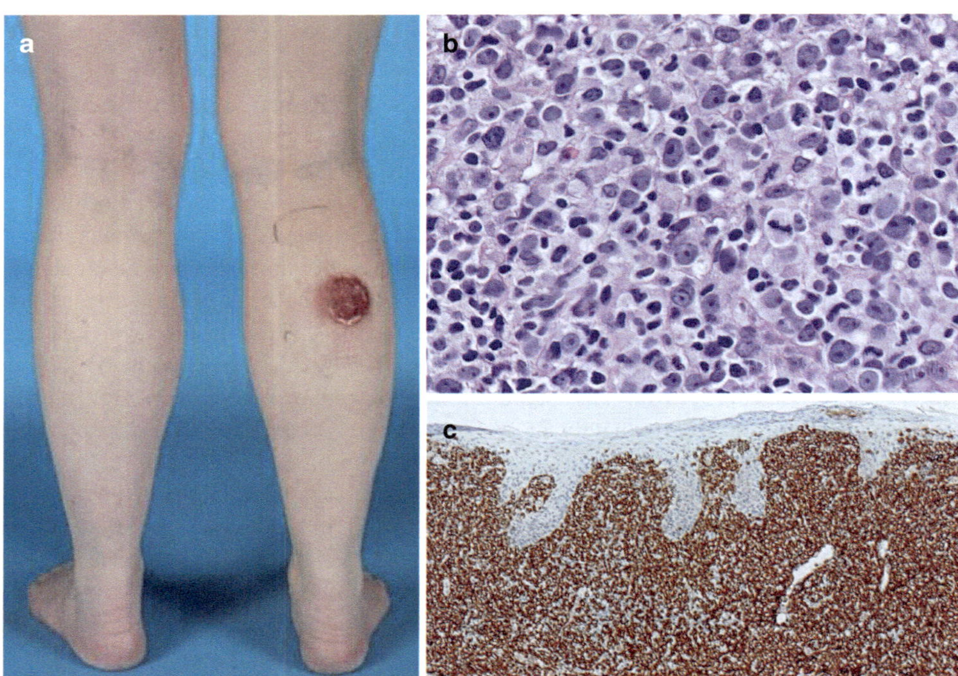

Fig. 14.5 Primary cutaneous anaplastic large cell lymphoma. Solitary tumor on right calf (**a**); histopathologic examination shows a monotonous infiltrate of large cells with anaplastic morphology (**b**); expression of CD30 by the tumor cells (**c**)

cytes are often present at the periphery of the lesions. Ulcerating lesions may show a LyP-like histology with an abundant inflammatory infiltrate of reactive T-cells, histiocytes, eosinophils, neutrophils, and relatively few CD30-positive cells. In such cases, epidermal hyperplasia may be prominent. The neoplastic cells show an activated CD4+ T-cell phenotype with variable loss of CD2, CD5, CD7, and/or CD3 and frequent expression of cytotoxic proteins (granzyme B, TIA-1, perforin). Some cases may have a CD4-, CD8+ or CD4+, CD8+ T-cell phenotype. CD30 is by definition expressed by a majority (>75%) of the neoplastic cells (Fig. 14.5b) [81–83].

Unlike systemic ALCL, the vast majority of C-ALCL does not carry translocations involving the *ALK* gene at chromosome 2 and does not express ALK (anaplastic lymphoma kinase), indicative of the 2;5 chromosomal translocation or its variants [84]. Expression of ALK protein therefore strongly suggests secondary cutaneous involvement of a systemic ALK-positive ALCL. However, unusual cases of ALK+ C-ALCL, including both cases showing strong nuclear and cytoplasmic staining characteristic of the t(2;5) chromosomal translocation, and cases expressing cytoplasmic ALK protein, indicative of a variant translocation, have been reported [85–88]. Many of these cases had an excellent prognosis. However, rapid progression to systemic ALCL has been reported as well. It is at present impossible to predict whether such ALK+ C-ALCL presenting with only skin lesions will run an indolent or aggressive course. Rearrangements of the *DUSP22-IRF4* locus are found in approximately 25% of C-ALCL and in a small subset of LyP but do not have prognostic significance [77].

14.9.3 Treatment and Prognosis

Radiotherapy or surgical excision is the first choice of treatment in patients presenting with a solitary or few localized nodules or tumors. In case of complete spontaneous resolution, an expectant policy is justified. Patients presenting with multifocal skin lesions can best be treated with radiotherapy in case of only a few lesions or with low-dose methotrexate as in LyP [68, 78, 89, 90]. Recent studies suggest a total radiation dose of 20 Gy for patients presenting with solitary or localized skin lesions and dose of 8 Gy (2 × 4 Gy) for patients with multifocal or relapsing skin lesions [91, 92]. Recent studies report high response rates of brentuximab vedotin (BV) in patients with primary cutaneous CD30+ lymphoproliferations, and BV should therefore be considered in cases with multifocal skin lesions refractory to conventional therapies and patients developing extracutaneous disease [30–32]. Multi-agent chemotherapy is only indicated in patients presenting with or developing extracutaneous disease and in rare patients with rapidly progressive skin disease not responsive to BV.

The prognosis is usually favorable with a 10-year disease-related survival exceeding 90% [68, 69]. Patients presenting with extensive skin lesions on the leg have a reduced survival [69, 93, 94].

14.10 Subcutaneous Panniculitis-Like T-Cell Lymphoma

SPTCL is a cytotoxic T-cell lymphoma of α/β T-cell receptor-positive T-cells that preferentially infiltrates the subcutaneous tissue [1, 2]. In past classifications, cases with a γ/δ T-cell phenotype were included in this group. However, these cases expressing the γ/δ T-cell receptor have different clinicopathologic features and usually a much more aggressive clinical course than cases with an α/β T-cell phenotype and are reclassified as primary cutaneous gamma/delta T-cell lymphoma (PCGD-TCL). Differentiation is important, since PCGD-TCL with panniculitis-like features generally have a poor prognosis and require systemic chemotherapy [95, 96].

14.10.1 Clinical Features

SPTCL occur slightly more common in females than in males and may affect both children and adults [96, 97]. Patients present with solitary but

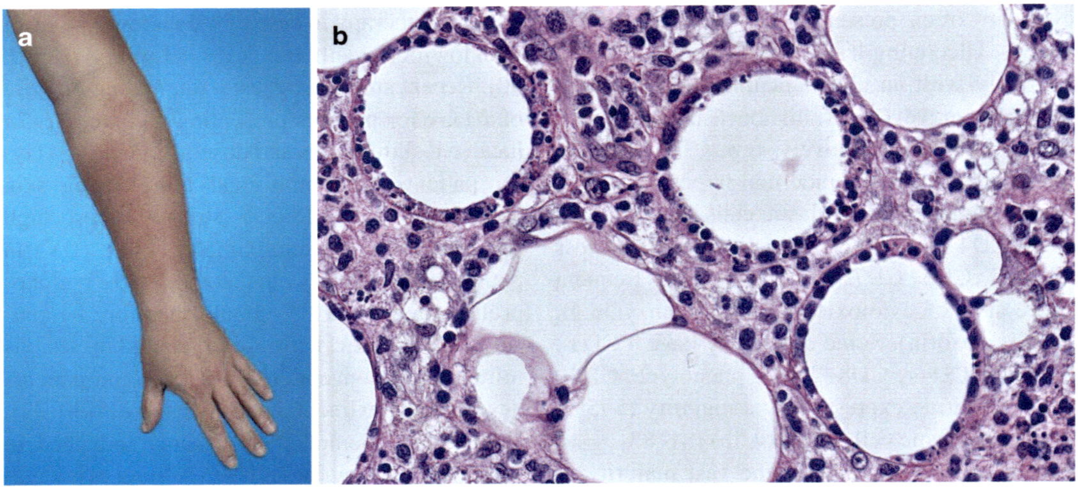

Fig. 14.6 Subcutaneous panniculitis-like T-cell lymphoma. Deeply seated plaques on the left arm (**a**); histopathologic examination shows a subcutaneous infiltrate with rimming of adipocytes by neoplastic T-cells (**b**)

more commonly multiple nodules or deeply seated plaques with a diameter varying between 1 and 20 cm. The skin lesions mainly involve the legs, the arms, and the trunk and less commonly the face and may leave areas of lipoatrophy after disappearance (Fig. 14.6a). Ulceration is uncommon. Systemic symptoms, such as fever, fatigue, and weight loss, and laboratory abnormalities, including cytopenias and elevated liver function tests, are common, but a frank hemophagocytic syndrome (HPS) is observed in only 15–20% of patients [96]. Dissemination to extracutaneous sites is rare. Hepatosplenomegaly may be seen but is generally not due to lymphomatous involvement. Up to 20% of patients may have an associated autoimmune disease, most commonly systemic lupus erythematosus [96]. The differential diagnosis with lupus panniculitis may sometimes be challenging [98].

14.10.2 Histopathology

Histologically, SPTCL reveals subcutaneous infiltrates simulating a lobular panniculitis showing small medium-sized or sometimes large pleomorphic T-cells with hyperchromatic nuclei and often many macrophages. The overlying epidermis and dermis are typically uninvolved. Rimming of individual fat cells by neoplastic T-cells is a helpful, though not completely specific diagnostic feature (Fig. 14.6b). Necrosis, karyorrhexis, cytophagocytosis, and fat necrosis are common findings [99]. In the early stages, the neoplastic infiltrates may lack significant atypia, and a heavy inflammatory infiltrate may predominate [100, 101]. In contrast to lupus panniculitis clusters of B-cells, plasma cells and plasmacytoid dendritic cells are not present.

The neoplastic cells have a mature CD3+, CD4−, CD8+ T-cell phenotype, with expression of cytotoxic proteins [96, 99, 102, 103]. The neoplastic T-cells express βF1, but not TCR γ/TCRδ, and are negative for CD56, facilitating differentiation from cutaneous gamma/delta T-cell lymphoma [95, 96]. CD30 is rarely, if ever, expressed. The proliferation rate is usually high. The neoplastic T-cells show clonal TCR gene rearrangements. EBV is absent.

14.10.3 Treatment and Prognosis

Traditionally, patients with SPTCL have been treated with combination chemotherapy. However, more recent studies indicate that in SPTCL without associated HPS, systemic steroids or other immunosuppressive agents (ciclosporin, MTX) should be considered first, whereas in cases of solitary skin lesions radiotherapy with electrons is advised. Bexarotene may be also effective in SPTCL [104]. Only in cases with progressive disease not responding to immunosuppressive therapy and in cases with HPS, multi-agent chemotherapy is required. Most cases of SPTCL have a favorable prognosis, particularly if not associated with an HPS. One study reported 5-year overall survival (OS) rates of 91% and 46% in SPTCL patients without and with an HPS, respectively [96].

14.11 Primary Cutaneous Acral CD8+ T-Cell Lymphoma

Primary cutaneous acral CD8+ T-cell lymphoma is a newly described entity histologically characterized by a diffuse infiltrate of medium-sized CD8+ cytotoxic T-cells suggesting an aggressive malignant lymphoma but clinically with usually a solitary skin lesion at acral sites and an indolent clinical behavior [1, 2]. This condition, initially designated "indolent CD8-positive lymphoid proliferation of the ear," has been included as a new provisional entity in the updated WHO-EORTC classification [105].

14.11.1 Clinical Features

This condition has only been reported in adult patients and shows a male-to-female ratio of 1.7:1. Patients typically present with a solitary, slowly progressive papule or nodule, preferentially located on the ear or less commonly on other acral sites including the nose and the foot (Fig. 14.7a) [105, 106]. Occasionally, lesions are bilateral, in particular on the ears.

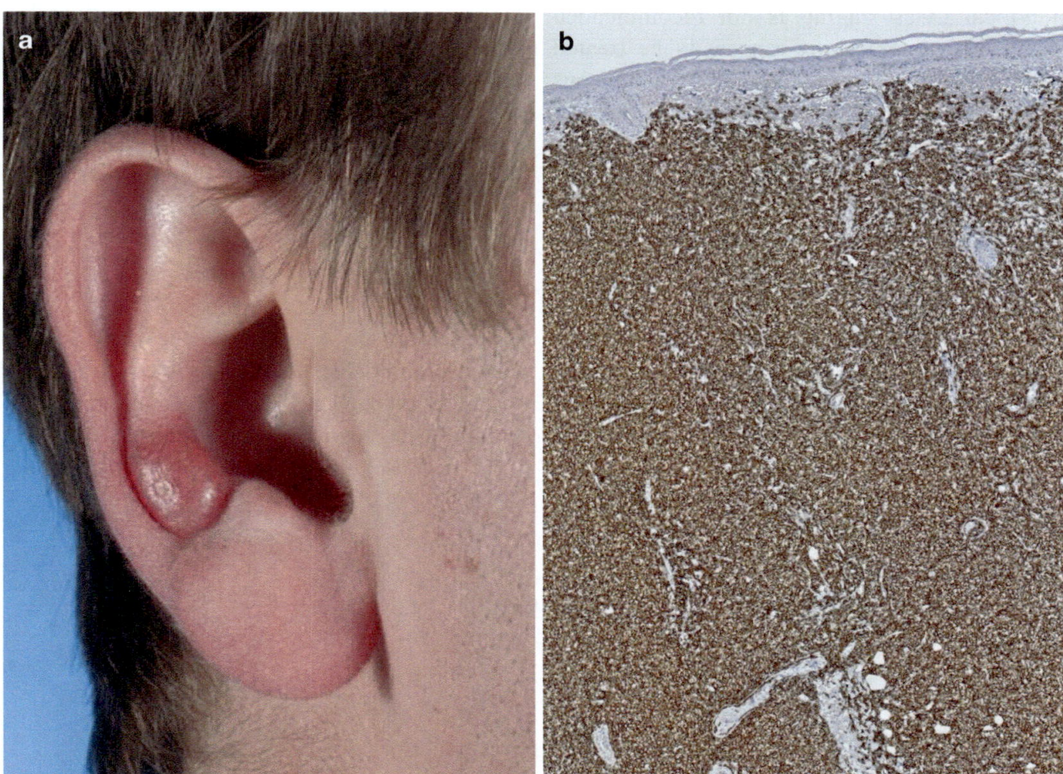

Fig. 14.7 Primary cutaneous CD8-positive acral T-cell lymphoma. Presenting with small tumor on the right ear (**a**); histopathologic examination shows a diffuse infiltrate of atypical CD8+ T-cells throughout the dermis (**b**)

14.11.2 Histopathology

These lesions show a diffuse proliferation of clonal medium-sized blast cells throughout the dermis, separated from the epidermis by a clear grenz zone. The atypical cells show a CD3+, CD4−, CD8+, CD30− T-cell phenotype with variable loss of pan-T-cell antigens (CD2, CD5, CD7) (Fig. 14.7b). They are positive for TIA-1 but, unlike other types of CD8+ CTCL, negative for other cytotoxic proteins (granzyme B, perforin) [107]. CD68 often shows a positive Golgi dot-like staining [108]. In almost all cases, the proliferation rate is very low (<10%). Epstein–Barr virus is negative. Most cases show clonal rearrangement of T-cell receptor genes.

14.11.3 Treatment and Prognosis

The prognosis of this condition is excellent, and in typical cases staging is not recommended [105, 106]. Skin lesions can easily be treated with surgical excision or radiotherapy. Cutaneous relapses may occur, but dissemination to extracutaneous sites is exceptional [109]. Whether this condition should be labeled lymphoproliferative disorder or lymphoma has been a matter of debate. However, recognition that these lesions have an indolent clinical behavior, despite an aggressive histology, is most important to prevent unnecessarily aggressive treatment. Clinicopathologic correlation is essential to differentiate these cases from other types of CD8+ CTCL, such as primary cutaneous aggressive epidermotropic CD8+ T-cell lymphoma and cases of CD8+ MF.

14.12 Primary Cutaneous CD4-Positive Small/Medium T-Cell Lymphoproliferative Disorder

In the 2005 WHO-EORTC classification, primary cutaneous CD4-positive small/medium T-cell lymphoma was included as a provisional type of CTCL, defined by a predominance of small- to medium-sized CD4+ pleomorphic T-cells, presentation with a solitary skin lesion without prior or concurrent patches and plaques typical of MF [110]. These cases have the same clinicopathologic and immunophenotypic features and the same clinical presentation and benign clinical course as cases previously referred to as nodular cutaneous pseudo-T-cell lymphomas, and it is highly uncertain if they represent a frank malignancy [111, 112]. In the 2016 revision of the WHO classification and in the updated WHO-EORTC classification, the term "primary cutaneous CD4+ small/medium T-cell lymphoproliferative disorder" rather than lymphoma is therefore preferred.

14.12.1 Clinical Features

Characteristically, patients present with a solitary plaque or tumor, generally on the face, the neck, or the upper trunk (Fig. 14.8a). Less commonly, they present with generalized skin lesions [113–116].

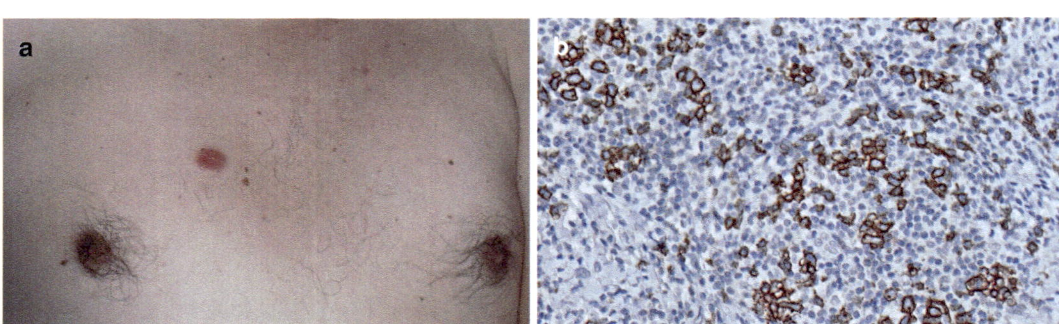

Fig. 14.8 Primary cutaneous CD4-positive small/medium T-cell lymphoproliferative disorder. Clinical presentation with solitary plaque on the chest (**a**). Expression of CD279 (PD-1) by atypical cells, partly arranged in clusters (**b**)

14.12.2 Histopathology

These lesions show nodular to diffuse dermal infiltrates, which often extend into the subcutaneous fat. Epidermotropism may be present focally. There is a predominance of small-/medium-sized pleomorphic T-cells. A small proportion (<30%) of large pleomorphic cells may be present [117]. Almost all cases have a considerable admixture with reactive CD8+ T-cells and B-cells, including some centroblasts, plasma cells, and histiocytes, including multinucleated giant cells. Eosinophils are generally few or absent.

These lesions have a CD3+, CD4+, CD8−, CD30- phenotype, sometimes with loss of pan T-cell markers. Recent studies showed that the medium-sized to large atypical CD4+ T-cells consistently express the follicular helper T-cell markers PD-1, BCL6, and CXCL13 (Fig. 14.8b) [87, 112, 118]. The proliferation rate is low, varying between less than 5% and at most 20%. Cytotoxic proteins are not expressed [113, 116]. EBV is negative. The TCR genes are clonally rearranged.

14.12.3 Treatment and Prognosis

Patients presenting with a solitary lesion have an excellent prognosis with a 5-year survival of almost 100%. In typical cases, staging procedures are not required. Skin lesions, if not resolved spontaneously after skin biopsy, should be treated primarily with intralesional steroids or surgical excision and only by exception with radiotherapy [112].

Rare cases presenting with generalized skin lesions, large, rapidly growing tumors, more than 30% large pleomorphic T-cells and/or a high proliferative fraction do not belong to this category [115, 116]. Such cases usually have a more aggressive clinical behavior and should be classified as peripheral T-cell lymphoma, NOS.

14.13 Conclusion

CTCL represent a heterogeneous group of extranodal malignant lymphomas which show a wide variation in clinical behavior and prognosis. Because of overlapping clinical and histopathological features, differentiation between different types of CTCL may be challenging. Clinicopathologic correlation with integration of immunophenotypical and genetic data and a multidisciplinary approach with close collaboration between dermatologists, pathologists, hematologists, and radiation oncologists are the best guarantee for correct diagnosis and adequate treatment.

References

1. Willemze R, Cerroni L, Kempf W, et al. The 2018 update of the WHO-EORTC classification for primary cutaneous lymphomas. Blood. 2019;133(16):1703–14.
2. Swerdlow SH, Campo E, Harris NL, et al. World Health Organization classification of tumours of hematopoietic and lymphoid tissue (revised 4th edition). Lyon: IARC Press; 2017.
3. Zackheim HS, Amin S, Kashani-Sabet M, McMillan A. Prognosis in cutaneous T-cell lymphoma by skin stage: long-term survival in 489 patients. J Am Acad Dermatol. 1999;40:418–25.
4. van Doorn R, van Haselen CW, van Voorst Vader PC, et al. Mycosis fungoides: disease evolution and prognosis of 309 Dutch patients. Arch Dermatol. 2000;136:504–10.
5. Kim YH, Liu HL, Mraz-Gernhard S, Varghese A, Hoppe RT. Long-term outcome of 525 patients with mycosis fungoides and Sezary syndrome: clinical prognostic factors and risk for disease progression. Arch Dermatol. 2003;139:857–66.
6. Agar NS, Wedgeworth E, Crichton S, et al. Survival outcomes and prognostic factors in mycosis fungoides/Sezary syndrome: validation of the revised International Society for Cutaneous Lymphomas/European Organisation for Research and Treatment of Cancer staging proposal. J Clin Oncol. 2010;28:4730–9.
7. Olsen E, Vonderheid E, Pimpinelli N, et al. Revisions to the staging and classification of mycosis fungoides and Sezary syndrome: a proposal of the International Society for Cutaneous Lymphomas (ISCL) and the cutaneous lymphoma task force of the European Organization of Research and Treatment of Cancer (EORTC). Blood. 2007;110:1713–22.
8. Pimpinelli N, Olsen EA, Santucci M, et al. Defining early mycosis fungoides. J Am Acad Dermatol. 2005;53:1053–63.
9. Smoller BR, Bishop K, Glusac E, Kim YH, Hendrickson M. Reassessment of histologic parameters in the diagnosis of mycosis fungoides. Am J Surg Pathol. 1995;19:1423–30.
10. Benner MF, Jansen PM, Vermeer MH, Willemze R. Prognostic factors in transformed mycosis fun-

goides: a retrospective analysis of 100 cases. Blood. 2012;119:1643–9.
11. Diamandidou E, Colome-Grimmer M, Fayad L, Duvic M, Kurzrock R. Transformation of mycosis fungoides/Sezary syndrome: clinical characteristics and prognosis. Blood. 1998;92:1150–9.
12. Campbell JJ, Clark RA, Watanabe R, Kupper TS. Sezary syndrome and mycosis fungoides arise from distinct T-cell subsets: a biologic rationale for their distinct clinical behaviors. Blood. 2010;116:767–71.
13. Massone C, Crisman G, Kerl H, Cerroni L. The prognosis of early mycosis fungoides is not influenced by phenotype and T-cell clonality. Br J Dermatol. 2008;159:881–6.
14. Rodriguez-Pinilla SM, Ortiz-Romero PL, Monsalvez V, et al. TCR-gamma expression in primary cutaneous T-cell lymphomas. Am J Surg Pathol. 2013;37:375–84.
15. Vega F, Luthra R, Medeiros LJ, et al. Clonal heterogeneity in mycosis fungoides and its relationship to clinical course. Blood. 2002;100:3369–73.
16. Thurber SE, Zhang B, Kim YH, Schrijver I, Zehnder J, Kohler S. T-cell clonality analysis in biopsy specimens from two different skin sites shows high specificity in the diagnosis of patients with suggested mycosis fungoides. J Am Acad Dermatol. 2007;57:782–90.
17. Kirsch IR, Watanabe R, O'Malley JT, et al. TCR sequencing facilitates diagnosis and identifies mature T cells as the cell of origin in CTCL. Sci Transl Med. 2015;7:308ra158.
18. Trautinger F, Eder J, Assaf C, et al. European Organisation for Research and Treatment of Cancer consensus recommendations for the treatment of mycosis fungoides/Sezary syndrome—update 2017. Eur J Cancer. 2017;77:57–74.
19. Whittaker S, Hoppe R, Prince HM. How I treat mycosis fungoides and Sezary syndrome. Blood. 2016;127:3142–53.
20. Willemze R, Hodak E, Zinzani PL, Specht L, Ladetto M. Primary cutaneous lymphomas: ESMO clinical practice guidelines for diagnosis, treatment and follow-up. Ann Oncol. 2018;29:iv30–40.
21. Kaye FJ, Bunn PA Jr, Steinberg SM, et al. A randomized trial comparing combination electron-beam radiation and chemotherapy with topical therapy in the initial treatment of mycosis fungoides. N Engl J Med. 1989;321:1784–90.
22. Lessin SR, Duvic M, Guitart J, et al. Topical chemotherapy in cutaneous T-cell lymphoma: positive results of a randomized, controlled, multicenter trial testing the efficacy and safety of a novel mechlorethamine, 0.02%, gel in mycosis fungoides. JAMA Dermatol. 2013;149:25–32.
23. Neelis KJ, Schimmel EC, Vermeer MH, Senff NJ, Willemze R, Noordijk EM. Low-dose palliative radiotherapy for cutaneous B- and T-cell lymphomas. Int J Radiat Oncol Biol Phys. 2009;74:154–8.
24. Specht L, Dabaja B, Illidge T, Wilson LD, Hoppe RT. Modern radiation therapy for primary cutaneous lymphomas: field and dose guidelines from the International Lymphoma Radiation Oncology Group. Int J Radiat Oncol Biol Phys. 2015;92:32–9.
25. Quaglino P, Maule M, Prince HM, et al. Global patterns of care in advanced stage mycosis fungoides/Sezary syndrome: a multicenter retrospective follow-up study from the Cutaneous Lymphoma International Consortium. Ann Oncol. 2018;28(10):2517–25.
26. Kamstrup MR, Gniadecki R, Iversen L, et al. Low-dose (10-Gy) total skin electron beam therapy for cutaneous T-cell lymphoma: an open clinical study and pooled data analysis. Int J Radiat Oncol Biol Phys. 2015;92:138–43.
27. Hoppe RT, Harrison C, Tavallaee M, et al. Low-dose total skin electron beam therapy as an effective modality to reduce disease burden in patients with mycosis fungoides: results of a pooled analysis from 3 phase-II clinical trials. J Am Acad Dermatol. 2015;72:286–92.
28. Dummer R, Quaglino P, Becker JC, et al. Prospective international multicenter phase II trial of intravenous pegylated liposomal doxorubicin monochemotherapy in patients with stage IIB, IVA, or IVB advanced mycosis fungoides: final results from EORTC 21012. J Clin Oncol. 2012;30:4091–7.
29. Marchi E, Alinari L, Tani M, et al. Gemcitabine as frontline treatment for cutaneous T-cell lymphoma: phase II study of 32 patients. Cancer. 2005;104:2437–41.
30. Prince HM, Kim YH, Horwitz SM, et al. Brentuximab vedotin or physician's choice in CD30-positive cutaneous T-cell lymphoma (ALCANZA): an international, open-label, randomised, phase 3, multicentre trial. Lancet. 2017;390:555–66.
31. Kim YH, Tavallaee M, Sundram U, et al. Phase II investigator-initiated study of brentuximab vedotin in mycosis fungoides and Sezary syndrome with variable CD30 expression level: a multi-institution collaborative project. J Clin Oncol. 2015;33:3750–8.
32. Duvic M, Tetzlaff MT, Gangar P, Clos AL, Sui D, Talpur R. Results of a phase II trial of brentuximab vedotin for CD30+ cutaneous T-cell lymphoma and lymphomatoid papulosis. J Clin Oncol. 2015;33:3759–65.
33. Olsen E, Duvic M, Frankel A, et al. Pivotal phase III trial of two dose levels of denileukin diftitox for the treatment of cutaneous T-cell lymphoma. J Clin Oncol. 2001;19:376–88.
34. Prince HM, Duvic M, Martin A, et al. Phase III placebo-controlled trial of denileukin diftitox for patients with cutaneous T-cell lymphoma. J Clin Oncol. 2010;28:1870–7.
35. Whittaker SJ, Demierre MF, Kim EJ, et al. Final results from a multicenter, international, pivotal study of romidepsin in refractory cutaneous T-cell lymphoma. J Clin Oncol. 2010;28:4485–91.

36. Duvic M, Pinter-Brown LC, Foss FM, et al. Phase 1/2 study of mogamulizumab, a defucosylated anti-CCR4 antibody, in previously treated patients with cutaneous T-cell lymphoma. Blood. 2015;125:1883–9.
37. Kim YH, Bagot M, Pinter-Brown L, et al. Mogamulizumab versus vorinostat in previously treated cutaneous T-cell lymphoma (MAVORIC): an international, open-label, randomised, controlled phase 3 trial. Lancet Oncol. 2018;19:1192–204.
38. Virmani P, Zain J, Rosen ST, Myskowski PL, Querfeld C. Hematopoietic stem cell transplant for mycosis fungoides and Sezary syndrome. Dermatol Clin. 2015;33:807–18.
39. Schlaak M, Pickenhain J, Theurich S, Skoetz N, von Bergwelt-Baildon M, Kurschat P. Allogeneic stem cell transplantation versus conventional therapy for advanced primary cutaneous T-cell lymphoma. Cochrane Database Syst Rev. 2013;CD008908.
40. Duvic M, Donato M, Dabaja B, et al. Total skin electron beam and non-myeloablative allogeneic hematopoietic stem-cell transplantation in advanced mycosis fungoides and Sezary syndrome. J Clin Oncol. 2010;28:2365–72.
41. Schneeweiss M, Porpaczy E, Koch M, et al. Transformed mycosis fungoides: bridging to allogeneic stem cell transplantation with brentuximab vedotin. Leuk Lymphoma. 2016;57:206–8.
42. Mahevas T, Ram-Wolff C, Battistella M, et al. Dramatic response to brentuximab vedotin in refractory nontransformed CD30(-) mycosis fungoides allowing allogeneic stem cell transplant and long-term complete remission. Br J Dermatol. 2018;180(6):1517–20.
43. Duarte RF, Schmitz N, Servitje O, Sureda A. Haematopoietic stem cell transplantation for patients with primary cutaneous T-cell lymphoma. Bone Marrow Transplant. 2008;41:597–604.
44. Nashan D, Faulhaber D, Stander S, Luger TA, Stadler R. Mycosis fungoides: a dermatological masquerader. Br J Dermatol. 2007;156:1–10.
45. Martinez-Escala ME, Gonzalez BR, Guitart J. Mycosis fungoides variants. Surg Pathol Clin. 2014;7:169–89.
46. Vergier B, Beylot-Barry M, Beylot C, et al. Pilotropic cutaneous T-cell lymphoma without mucinosis. A variant of mycosis fungoides? French Study Group of Cutaneous Lymphomas. Arch Dermatol. 1996;132:683–7.
47. van Doorn R, Scheffer E, Willemze R. Follicular mycosis fungoides, a distinct disease entity with or without associated follicular mucinosis: a clinicopathologic and follow-up study of 51 patients. Arch Dermatol. 2002;138:191–8.
48. Gerami P, Rosen S, Kuzel T, Boone SL, Guitart J. Folliculotropic mycosis fungoides: an aggressive variant of cutaneous T-cell lymphoma. Arch Dermatol. 2008;144:738–46.
49. Lehman JS, Cook-Norris RH, Weed BR, et al. Folliculotropic mycosis fungoides: single-center study and systematic review. Arch Dermatol. 2010;146:607–13.
50. Wieser I, Wang C, Alberti-Violetti S, et al. Clinical characteristics, risk factors and long-term outcome of 114 patients with folliculotropic mycosis fungoides. Arch Dermatol Res. 2017;309:453–9.
51. Hodak E, Amitay-Laish I, Feinmesser M, et al. Juvenile mycosis fungoides: cutaneous T-cell lymphoma with frequent follicular involvement. J Am Acad Dermatol. 2014;70:993–1001.
52. Boulos S, Vaid R, Aladily TN, Ivan DS, Talpur R, Duvic M. Clinical presentation, immunopathology, and treatment of juvenile-onset mycosis fungoides: a case series of 34 patients. J Am Acad Dermatol. 2014;71:1117–26.
53. van Santen S, Roach RE, van Doorn R, et al. Clinical staging and prognostic factors in folliculotropic mycosis fungoides. JAMA Dermatol. 2016;152:992–1000.
54. Hodak E, Amitay-Laish I, Atzmony L, et al. New insights into folliculotropic mycosis fungoides (FMF): a single-center experience. J Am Acad Dermatol. 2016;75:347–55.
55. Kempf W, Kazakov DV, Schermesser M, et al. Unilesional follicular mycosis fungoides: report of two cases with progression to tumor stage and review of the literature. J Cutan Pathol. 2012;39:853–60.
56. Amitay-Laish I, Feinmesser M, Ben-Amitai D, Fenig E, Sorin D, Hodak E. Unilesional folliculotropic mycosis fungoides: a unique variant of cutaneous lymphoma. J Eur Acad Dermatol Venereol. 2016;30(1):25–9.
57. van Santen S, Jansen PM, Vermeer MH, Willemze R. Folliculotropic mycosis fungoides presenting with a solitary lesion: clinicopathological features and long-term follow-up data in a series of nine cases. J Cutan Pathol. 2018;45(2):122–8.
58. Gerami P, Guitart J. The spectrum of histopathologic and immunohistochemical findings in folliculotropic mycosis fungoides. Am J Surg Pathol. 2007;31:1430–8.
59. de Masson A, Battistella M, Vignon-Pennamen MD, et al. Syringotropic mycosis fungoides: clinical and histologic features, response to treatment, and outcome in 19 patients. J Am Acad Dermatol. 2014;71:926–34.
60. Tomasini C, Kempf W, Novelli M, et al. Spiky follicular mycosis fungoides: a clinicopathologic study of 8 cases. J Cutan Pathol. 2015;42:164–72.
61. van Santen S, van Doorn R, Neelis KJ, et al. Recommendations for treatment in folliculotropic mycosis fungoides: report of the Dutch Cutaneous Lymphoma Group. Br J Dermatol. 2017;177:223–8.
62. Haghighi B, Smoller BR, LeBoit PE, Warnke RA, Sander CA, Kohler S. Pagetoid reticulosis (Woringer-Kolopp disease): an immunophenotypic, molecular, and clinicopathologic study. Mod Pathol. 2000;13:502–10.

63. Steffen C. Ketron-Goodman disease, Woringer-Kolopp disease, and pagetoid reticulosis. Am J Dermatopathol. 2005;27:68–85.
64. LeBoit PE. Granulomatous slack skin. Dermatol Clin. 1994;12:375–89.
65. Kempf W, Ostheeren-Michaelis S, Paulli M, et al. Granulomatous mycosis fungoides and granulomatous slack skin: a multicenter study of the Cutaneous Lymphoma Histopathology Task Force Group of the European Organization for Research and Treatment of Cancer (EORTC). Arch Dermatol. 2008;144(12):1609–17.
66. van Haselen CW, Toonstra J, van der Putte SJ, van Dongen JJ, van Hees CL, van Vloten WA. Granulomatous slack skin. Report of three patients with an updated review of the literature. Dermatology. 1998;196:382–91.
67. Clarijs M, Poot F, Laka A, Pirard C, Bourlond A. Granulomatous slack skin: treatment with extensive surgery and review of the literature. Dermatology. 2003;206:393–7.
68. Bekkenk MW, Geelen FA, van Voorst Vader PC, et al. Primary and secondary cutaneous CD30(+) lymphoproliferative disorders: a report from the Dutch Cutaneous Lymphoma Group on the long-term follow-up data of 219 patients and guidelines for diagnosis and treatment. Blood. 2000;95:3653–61.
69. Liu HL, Hoppe RT, Kohler S, Harvell JD, Reddy S, Kim YH. CD30+ cutaneous lymphoproliferative disorders: the Stanford experience in lymphomatoid papulosis and primary cutaneous anaplastic large cell lymphoma. J Am Acad Dermatol. 2003;49:1049–58.
70. de Souza A, el-Azhary RA, Camilleri MJ, Wada DA, Appert DL, Gibson LE. In search of prognostic indicators for lymphomatoid papulosis: a retrospective study of 123 patients. J Am Acad Dermatol. 2012;66:928–37.
71. Wieser I, Wohlmuth C, Nunez CA, Duvic M. Lymphomatoid papulosis in children and adolescents: a systematic review. Am J Clin Dermatol. 2016;17:319–27.
72. Wieser I, Oh CW, Talpur R, Duvic M. Lymphomatoid papulosis: treatment response and associated lymphomas in a study of 180 patients. J Am Acad Dermatol. 2016;74:59–67.
73. Cordel N, Tressieres B, D'Incan M, et al. Frequency and risk factors for associated lymphomas in patients with lymphomatoid papulosis. Oncologist. 2016;21:76–83.
74. Melchers RC. Willemze R, Bekkenk MW, et al. Frequency and prognosis of associated malignancies in 504 patients with lymphomatoid papulosis. J Eur Acad Dermatol Venereol 2020;34:260–66.
75. Karai LJ, Kadin ME, Hsi ED, et al. Chromosomal rearrangements of 6p25.3 define a new subtype of lymphomatoid papulosis. Am J Surg Pathol. 2013;37:1173–81.
76. Kempf W. A new era for cutaneous CD30-positive T-cell lymphoproliferative disorders. Semin Diagn Pathol. 2017;34:22–35.
77. Wada DA, Law ME, Hsi ED, et al. Specificity of IRF4 translocations for primary cutaneous anaplastic large cell lymphoma: a multicenter study of 204 skin biopsies. Mod Pathol. 2011;24:596–605.
78. Kempf W, Pfaltz K, Vermeer MH, et al. EORTC, ISCL, and USCLC consensus recommendations for the treatment of primary cutaneous CD30-positive lymphoproliferative disorders: lymphomatoid papulosis and primary cutaneous anaplastic large-cell lymphoma. Blood. 2011;118:4024–35.
79. Bruijn MS, Horvath B, van Voorst Vader PC, Willemze R, Vermeer MH. Recommendations for treatment of lymphomatoid papulosis with methotrexate: a report from the Dutch Cutaneous Lymphoma Group. Br J Dermatol. 2015;173:1319–22.
80. Massone C, El-Shabrawi-Caelen L, Kerl H, Cerroni L. The morphologic spectrum of primary cutaneous anaplastic large T-cell lymphoma: a histopathologic study on 66 biopsy specimens from 47 patients with report of rare variants. J Cutan Pathol. 2008;35:46–53.
81. Kummer JA, Vermeer MH, Dukers D, Meijer CJ, Willemze R. Most primary cutaneous CD30-positive lymphoproliferative disorders have a CD4-positive cytotoxic T-cell phenotype. J Invest Dermatol. 1997;109:636–40.
82. Boulland ML, Wechsler J, Bagot M, Pulford K, Kanavaros P, Gaulard P. Primary CD30-positive cutaneous T-cell lymphomas and lymphomatoid papulosis frequently express cytotoxic proteins. Histopathology. 2000;36:136–44.
83. Massone C, Cerroni L. Phenotypic variability in primary cutaneous anaplastic large T-cell lymphoma: a study on 35 patients. Am J Dermatopathol. 2014;36:153–7.
84. DeCoteau JF, Butmarc JR, Kinney MC, Kadin ME. The t(2;5) chromosomal translocation is not a common feature of primary cutaneous CD30+ lymphoproliferative disorders: comparison with anaplastic large-cell lymphoma of nodal origin. Blood. 1996;87:3437–41.
85. Kadin ME, Pinkus JL, Pinkus GS, et al. Primary cutaneous ALCL with phosphorylated/activated cytoplasmic ALK and novel phenotype: EMA/MUC1+, cutaneous lymphocyte antigen negative. Am J Surg Pathol. 2008;32:1421–6.
86. Oschlies I, Lisfeld J, Lamant L, et al. ALK-positive anaplastic large cell lymphoma limited to the skin: clinical, histopathological and molecular analysis of 6 pediatric cases. A report from the ALCL99 study. Haematologica. 2013;98:50–6.
87. Quintanilla-Martinez L, Jansen PM, Kinney MC, Swerdlow SH, Willemze R. Non-mycosis fungoides cutaneous T-cell lymphomas: report of the 2011 Society for Hematopathology/European Association for Haematopathology workshop. Am J Clin Pathol. 2013;139:491–514.
88. Melchers RC, Willemze R, van de Loo M, et al. Clinical, histologic and molecular characteristics of anaplastic lymphoma kinase-positive primary cuta-

neous anaplastic large cell lymphoma. Am J Surg Pathol. 2020;44:776–81.
89. Vonderheid EC, Sajjadian A, Kadin ME. Methotrexate is effective therapy for lymphomatoid papulosis and other primary cutaneous CD30-positive lymphoproliferative disorders. J Am Acad Dermatol. 1996;34:470–81.
90. Melchers RC, Willemze R, Bekkenk MW, et al. Evaluation of treatment results in multifocal primary cutaneous anaplastic large cell lymphoma: report of the Dutch Cutaneous Lymphoma Group. Br J Dermatol. 2018;179(3):724–31.
91. Melchers RC, Willemze R, Daniels LA, et al. Recommendations for the optimal radiation dose in patients with primary cutaneous anaplastic large cell lymphoma: a report of the Dutch Cutaneous Lymphoma Group. Int J Radiat Oncol Biol Phys. 2017;99(5):1279–85.
92. Million L, Yi EJ, Wu F, et al. Radiation therapy for primary cutaneous anaplastic large cell lymphoma: an International Lymphoma Radiation Oncology Group multi-institutional experience. Int J Radiat Oncol Biol Phys. 2016;95:1454–9.
93. Benner MF, Willemze R. Applicability and prognostic value of the new TNM classification system in 135 patients with primary cutaneous anaplastic large cell lymphoma. Arch Dermatol. 2009;145:1399–404.
94. Woo DK, Jones CR, Vanoli-Storz MN, et al. Prognostic factors in primary cutaneous anaplastic large cell lymphoma: characterization of clinical subset with worse outcome. Arch Dermatol. 2009;145:667–74.
95. Toro JR, Liewehr DJ, Pabby N, et al. Gamma-delta T-cell phenotype is associated with significantly decreased survival in cutaneous T-cell lymphoma. Blood. 2003;101:3407–12.
96. Willemze R, Jansen PM, Cerroni L, et al. Subcutaneous panniculitis-like T-cell lymphoma: definition, classification, and prognostic factors: an EORTC Cutaneous Lymphoma Group Study of 83 cases. Blood. 2008;111:838–45.
97. Huppmann AR, Xi L, Raffeld M, Pittaluga S, Jaffe ES. Subcutaneous panniculitis-like T-cell lymphoma in the pediatric age group: a lymphoma of low malignant potential. Pediatr Blood Cancer. 2013;60:1165–70.
98. Pincus LB, LeBoit PE, McCalmont TH, et al. Subcutaneous panniculitis-like T-cell lymphoma with overlapping clinicopathologic features of lupus erythematosus: coexistence of 2 entities? Am J Dermatopathol. 2009;31:520–6.
99. Massone C, Chott A, Metze D, et al. Subcutaneous, blastic natural killer (NK), NK/T-cell, and other cytotoxic lymphomas of the skin: a morphologic, immunophenotypic, and molecular study of 50 patients. Am J Surg Pathol. 2004;28:719–35.
100. Hoque SR, Child FJ, Whittaker SJ, et al. Subcutaneous panniculitis-like T-cell lymphoma: a clinicopathological, immunophenotypic and molecular analysis of six patients. Br J Dermatol. 2003;148:516–25.
101. Marzano AV, Berti E, Paulli M, Caputo R. Cytophagic histiocytic panniculitis and subcutaneous panniculitis-like T-cell lymphoma: report of 7 cases. Arch Dermatol. 2000;136:889–96.
102. Salhany KE, Macon WR, Choi JK, et al. Subcutaneous panniculitis-like T-cell lymphoma: clinicopathologic, immunophenotypic, and genotypic analysis of alpha/beta and gamma/delta subtypes. Am J Surg Pathol. 1998;22:881–93.
103. Santucci M, Pimpinelli N, Massi D, et al. Cytotoxic/natural killer cell cutaneous lymphomas. Report of EORTC Cutaneous Lymphoma Task Force Workshop. Cancer. 2003;97:610–27.
104. Mehta N, Wayne AS, Kim YH, et al. Bexarotene is active against subcutaneous panniculitis-like T-cell lymphoma in adult and pediatric populations. Clin Lymphoma Myeloma Leuk. 2012;12:20–5.
105. Petrella T, Maubec E, Cornillet-Lefebvre P, et al. Indolent CD8-positive lymphoid proliferation of the ear: a distinct primary cutaneous T-cell lymphoma? Am J Surg Pathol. 2007;31:1887–92.
106. Greenblatt D, Ally M, Child F, et al. Indolent CD8(+) lymphoid proliferation of acral sites: a clinicopathologic study of six patients with some atypical features. J Cutan Pathol. 2013;40:248–58.
107. Li JY, Guitart J, Pulitzer MP, et al. Multicenter case series of indolent small/medium-sized CD8+ lymphoid proliferations with predilection for the ear and face. Am J Dermatopathol. 2014;36:402–8.
108. Wobser M, Roth S, Reinartz T, Rosenwald A, Goebeler M, Geissinger E. CD68 expression is a discriminative feature of indolent cutaneous CD8-positive lymphoid proliferation and distinguishes this lymphoma subtype from other CD8-positive cutaneous lymphomas. Br J Dermatol. 2015;172:1573–80.
109. Alberti-Violetti S, Fanoni D, Provasi M, Corti L, Venegoni L, Berti E. Primary cutaneous acral CD8 positive T-cell lymphoma with extracutaneous involvement: a long-standing case with an unexpected progression. J Cutan Pathol. 2017;44:964–8.
110. Willemze R, Jaffe ES, Burg G, et al. WHO-EORTC classification for cutaneous lymphomas. Blood. 2005;105:3768–85.
111. Beltraminelli H, Leinweber B, Kerl H, Cerroni L. Primary cutaneous CD4+ small-/medium-sized pleomorphic T-cell lymphoma: a cutaneous nodular proliferation of pleomorphic T lymphocytes of undetermined significance? A study of 136 cases. Am J Dermatopathol. 2009;31:317–22.
112. Cetinozman F, Jansen PM, Willemze R. Expression of programmed death-1 in primary cutaneous CD4-positive small/medium-sized pleomorphic T-cell lymphoma, cutaneous pseudo-T-cell lymphoma, and other types of cutaneous T-cell lymphoma. Am J Surg Pathol. 2012;36:109–16.
113. Bekkenk MW, Vermeer MH, Jansen PM, et al. Peripheral T-cell lymphomas unspecified presenting

in the skin: analysis of prognostic factors in a group of 82 patients. Blood. 2003;102:2213–9.
114. Fink-Puches R, Zenahlik P, Back B, Smolle J, Kerl H, Cerroni L. Primary cutaneous lymphomas: applicability of current classification schemes (European Organization for Research and Treatment of Cancer, World Health Organization) based on clinicopathologic features observed in a large group of patients. Blood. 2002;99:800–5.
115. Garcia-Herrera A, Colomo L, Camos M, et al. Primary cutaneous small/medium CD4+ T-cell lymphomas: a heterogeneous group of tumors with different clinicopathologic features and outcome. J Clin Oncol. 2008;26(20):3364–71.
116. Grogg KL, Jung S, Erickson LA, McClure RF, Dogan A. Primary cutaneous CD4-positive small/medium-sized pleomorphic T-cell lymphoma: a clonal T-cell lymphoproliferative disorder with indolent behavior. Mod Pathol. 2008;21:708–15.
117. Beljaards RC, Meijer CJ, Van der Putte SC, et al. Primary cutaneous T-cell lymphoma: clinicopathological features and prognostic parameters of 35 cases other than mycosis fungoides and CD30-positive large cell lymphoma. J Pathol. 1994;172:53–60.
118. Rodriguez Pinilla SM, Roncador G, Rodriguez-Peralto JL, et al. Primary cutaneous CD4+ small/medium-sized pleomorphic T-cell lymphoma expresses follicular T-cell markers. Am J Surg Pathol. 2009;33:81–90.

15 Large Granular Lymphocyte Leukemia

Antonella Teramo, Cristina Vicenzetto, Gregorio Barilà, Giulia Calabretto, Vanessa Rebecca Gasparini, Gianpietro Semenzato, and Renato Zambello

T-cell large granular lymphocyte leukemia (T-LGL)

Clinical outline
Adults with large granulated lymphocytes in peripheral blood, bone marrow and spleen and liver. Usually no lymphadenopathy. Severe neutropenia and anemia. Frequent associated with autoimmune conditions, such as rheumatoid arthritis or hematological malignancies. May arise in the post-transplant setting.

Cytology	Medium to large lymphoid cells with condensed chromatin and abundant cytoplasm with azurophilic granules.	T-large granular lymphocytes leukemia, cytology	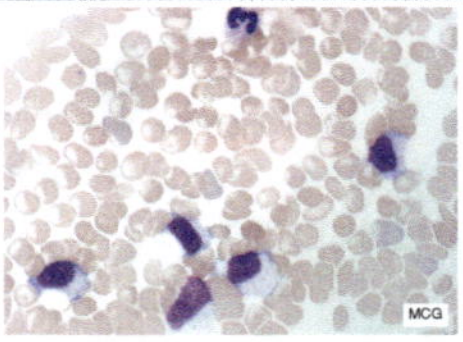
Histology	Sinusoidal and interstitial pattern in bone marrow. Associated reactive lymphoid aggregates. Left-shifted and/or reduced hematopoiesis. In spleen expanding the cords and the sinusoids of the red pulp, sparing the whit pulp.	T-large granular lymphocytes leukemia, hystology	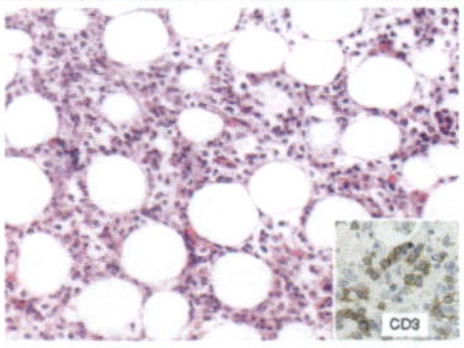

	CD20	CD3	CD5[1]	CD4[2]	CD8[2]	CD7[1]	CD56[3]	TCR[4]	CD57	CD30
notes	[1]weak/dim, [2]small subset is CD4+ and CD8-, [3]small subset CD56+ and CD57-, [4]Tcell receptor usually $\alpha\beta$, rarely $\gamma\delta$- phenotype									
other marker	Consistent with its activated cytotoxic nature, expression of TIA-1, perforin, granzyme-B and granzyme-M is commonly observed.									

■ = majority of cases positive ▒ = variable fraction of cases positive □ = negative

Main differential diagnosis	Reactive T-cell expansion (should be polyclonal); chronic lymphoproliferative disorder of NK cells (should be CD3-, CD57-, CD56+; no TCR rearrangement); hepatosplenic T-cell lymphoma (should be CD56+, majority TCRγ+, TCR$\alpha\beta$- (with some exceptions expressing TCR$\alpha\beta$) CD4-, CD8-/+, CD57-, granzyme B-, perforin-).

M. Dreyling, M. Ladetto (eds.), *Indolent Lymphomas*, Hematologic Malignancies,
https://doi.org/10.1007/978-3-030-55989-2_15

Key molecular features
Clonally rearranged T-cell receptor (TCR) genes, restricted TCR repertoire.
Frequent translocations: not reported.
Frequent copy number alterations: not reported.
Frequent mutations: *STAT3*, less common *STAT5b*
Precursor lesions
Not known.
Progression
Only anecdotic reports of transformation to other T-cell lymphoma

Clinically relevant pathologic features	Relevance	Evidence
***STAT3* mutation**	Predictive: better response to first line, immunosuppressive therapy; may be suitable for target therapy	B
***STAT5b* mutation**	Prognostic: identifies cases with more aggressive course	C
Legend: A= verified in multiple studies, randomized trials and/or integrated in guidelines; B= variable between studies/ needs definitive validation; C= preliminary / discrepant results.		

15.1 Introduction

The 2017 WHO classification reports large granular lymphocyte (LGL) leukemia in the category of cytotoxic T and NK cell lymphoma and leukemia. LGL leukemia is a lymphoproliferative disorder, defined by the presence of a high percentage of circulating LGLs in peripheral blood. The lymphocytosis is chronic and is sustained by clonal mature T or NK cells, thus configuring T-LGL leukemia (T-LGLL) or chronic lymphoproliferative disease of NK cells (CLPD-NK), respectively. T-LGLL is the most frequent form, accounting for about 85% of cases, whereas NK form is less represented with 10% of cases. In this scenario, also rare cases (incidence 5%) of aggressive LGL disorders of T or NK lineage are included, with very poor prognosis. Among these latter, the T-related type is described in the literature, but it is not yet included in the WHO classification that actually recognizes only the NK form, referred to as aggressive NK cell lymphoma (ANKL), more frequently found in oriental populations and usually associated with Epstein-Barr virus (EBV) infection. The etiopathogenesis of LGL leukemia has not been established, but it is hypothesized that a viral or autologous antigen triggers the initial lymphocytosis whose survival over the time is then maintained by the activation of many cell pathways. Among these, JAK/STAT3 axis is claimed as the principal signal involved in cell imbalance toward cell survival, the signal transducer and activator of transcription 3 (STAT3) activation being the hallmark of LGL disease. Moreover, in about 40% of patients, mutations on *STAT3* have been recognized that further sustain the activation of this pathway.

A. Teramo · C. Vicenzetto · G. Barilà · G. Calabretto
V. R. Gasparini · G. Semenzato · R. Zambello (✉)
Padova University School of Medicine, Department of Medicine, Hematology and Clinical Immunology, Padova, Italy

Veneto Institute of Molecular Medicine (VIMM), Padova, Italy
e-mail: antonella.teramo@unipd.it; cristina.vicenzetto@phd.unipd.it; g.semenzato@unipd.it; r.zambello@unipd.it

T and NK cell disorders share several biological and clinical features. Both entities are characterized by STAT3 activation, and both types of patients show clinical manifestations due to cytopenia. Furthermore, the treatment of T-LGLL and CLPD-NK patients is very similar, entailing an immunosuppressive regimen or careful observation of chronic lymphocytosis.

15.1 LGL Leukemia: Clinical Aspects

15.1.1 Leukemic LGL Cytology and Immunophenotype

On blood films, the LGL nucleus is typically round with condensed, mature chromatin; the cytoplasm is pale and abundant with randomly distributed azurophilic granules containing perforins and granzyme conferring its cell lytic ability [1] (Fig. 15.1). Leukemic LGLs do not show morphologic difference with LGLs in healthy individuals.

The immunophenotype is central to identify LGLs among lymphocytes. The presence/absence of CD3 expression on cell surface distinguishes LGL belonging to T or NK lineage, respectively.

CD3+ LGL leukemia cells usually express the TCR αβ+, CD4−, CD8+ phenotype, and the disease may be also referred to as CD8+ T-LGLL. Less frequently, in 10–15% of cases, the disorder is sustained by TCR αβ+, CD4+, CD8+/− LGLs, often expressing TCR Vβ13.1 [2], defining the CD4+ T-LGLL. T-LGLs are also typically equipped with CD16, CD56, and CD57. CD57 is almost always present, and it is considered a specific marker of LGL, whereas CD16 and CD56 may be present or absent in different combinations. The rare cases with T-LGLs CD57 negative are usually characterized by the expression of CD16. In T-LGLL, CD5 and CD7 are weakly expressed, and LGLs usually display a cytotoxic phenotype corresponding to that of a fully differentiated mature cytotoxic T lymphocyte (CD45RA+, CD27−, CD28−, CD62L−, CCR7−). Leukemic LGLs are constitutively equipped with IL-2Rβ (CD122), but not IL-2Rα (CD25), and can variably express NK receptors as CD94/NKG2 (A or C) and killer immunoglobulin-like receptors (KIRs) [3].

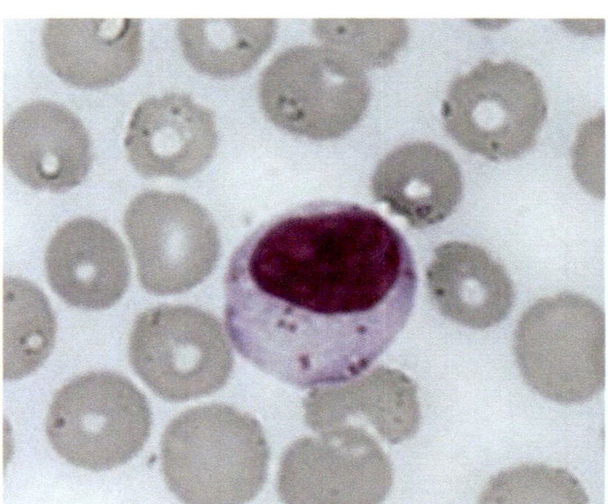

Fig. 15.1 May-Grünwald-Giemsa staining of a large granular lymphocyte in peripheral blood

Beyond the expansions of T cells bearing the TCR αβ+, there is a minority of cases derived from TCRγδ+ cells, presenting a Vγ9+/Vδ2+ or, less frequently, a Vγ9−/Vδ1+ phenotypic profile with TCRγ monoclonal restriction [4].

Some cases of a rare aggressive form of T-LGLL were reported, and these cases are usually equipped with a phenotype CD3+, CD8+, and CD56+ but devoid of CD16 and CD57 expression [5].

CLPD-NK are characterized by the lack of TCR and the CD16+, CD56+, CD45RA+, CD122+, CD25− phenotype. CD57 antigen is usually weakly detectable. CD56 antigen is normally expressed by LGL, although some negative cases are reported. CD94 antigen is found at high density on patients' NK cells; this antigen is usually associated with the inhibitory subunit NKG2A, although in some cases the association CD94/NKG2C has been reported [6]. Patients' NK cells characteristically express functional β and γ chains of IL-2/IL-15 receptor, which are strictly related to the role of these cytokines in the pathogenesis of disease [7]. Expression of NK receptors, mostly represented by KIR, is altered in patients with CLPD-NK. A restricted pattern of KIR expression is currently used in these patients to define the clonal nature of NK cell proliferation [6, 8, 9].

The aggressive and rare ANKL is not provided by an immunophenotype specifically distinguishable from CLPD-NK, and clinical evaluation is necessary to make the diagnosis. The presence of large nucleoli in NK cells strongly supports the diagnosis of ANKL, associated with age <40 years, systemic symptoms, lymph node swelling, and hepatosplenomegaly [10, 11].

Some representative cytometer panels of the most frequent immunophenotype for each LGLL subtype are reported in Fig. 15.2.

15.1.2 Diagnosis

Historically, the evidence of a lymphocytosis greater than 2 x 10^9 LGL/L, lasting for more than 6 months and clonal, was requested for the diag-

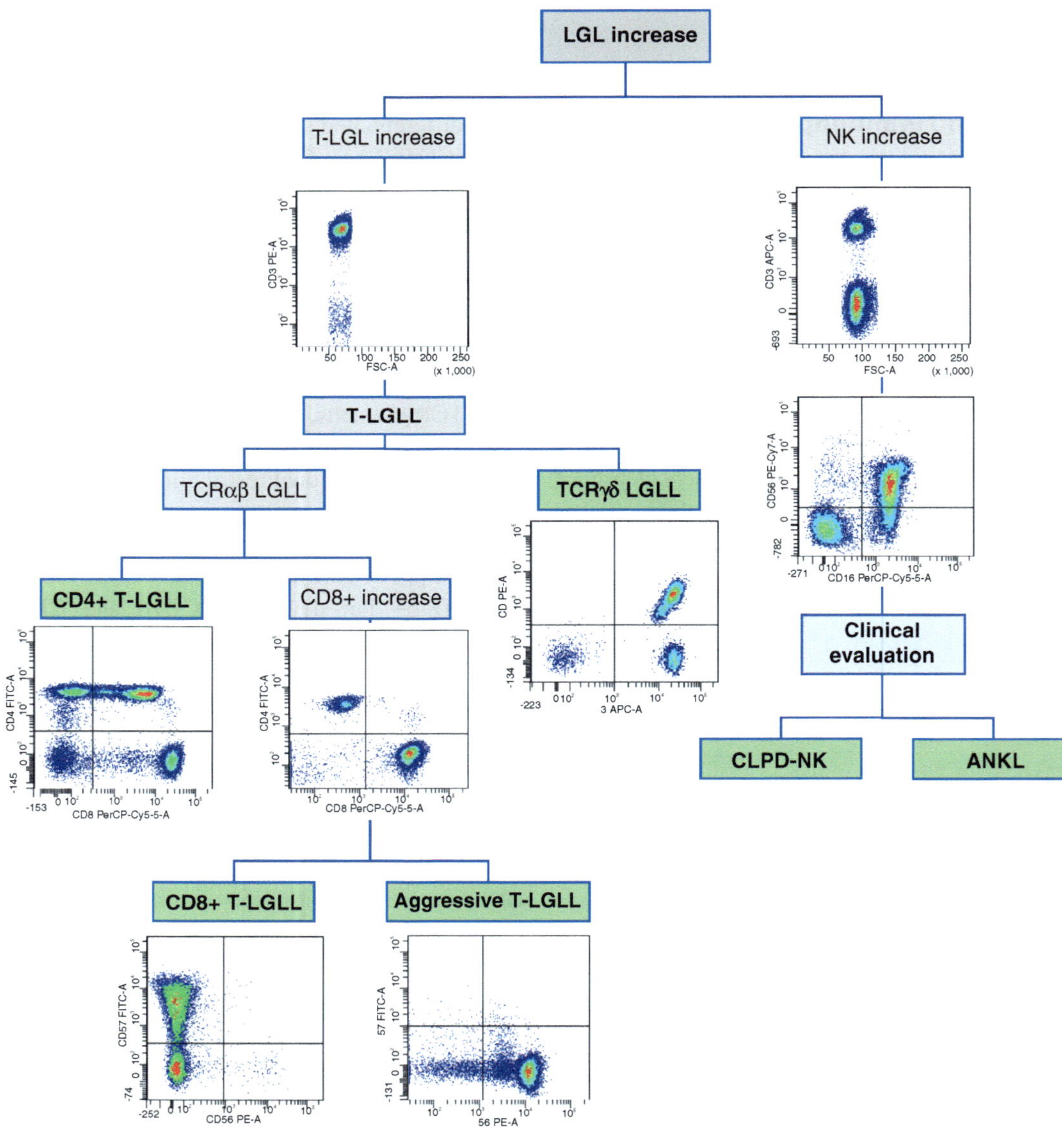

Fig. 15.2 Algorithm of the flow cytometer evaluation of the immunophenotypic features on LGL leading to the different types of LGL disorders

nosis of disease [1], considering that normally circulating LGL count is 0.25×10^9/L. However, the demonstration of clonal restriction of LGL proliferation can often be provided even in the presence of less than 2×10^9 LGL/L, particularly in symptomatic disease. For this reason, the threshold actually accepted for diagnosis is 0.5×10^9 LGL/L [12]. Additionally, the lymphocytosis must be characterized by immunophenotyping and molecular analyses.

As detailed in the previous paragraph, a proper definition of LGL immunophenotype is mandatory to recognize LGL lymphoproliferation and to define LGL leukemia subtypes: Tαβ LGLL including CD8+ T-LGLL, CD4+ T-LGLL, and aggressive T-LGLL; Tγδ LGLL; and CLPD-NK.

The molecular analysis is critical to distinguish reactive LGL proliferation from true LGL leukemic clonal expansion. Polyclonal expansions of LGLs are usually transient and due to a viral infection, such as EBV or cytomegalovirus (CMV), neoplasms, or autoimmune diseases [13–16]. Sometimes, this condition may develop after splenectomy. In contrast, clonal LGL proliferations are stably maintained for time, whether or not the patients are symptomatic.

The T-LGL leukemia can be tested for clonality by TCR rearrangement study. TCR gamma polymerase chain reaction analysis is a routine and easy technique to assess T-LGL clonality in both Tαβ and Tγδ LGLL. Showing the preferential use of one or two TCR-Vβ segments, flow cytometry analysis with monoclonal antibodies against the various Vβ regions of the TCR allows to suggest, and then used as a surrogate marker, the clonality of the LGLs [17]. The current Vβ monoclonal antibody panel covers 75% of the Vβ spectrum, with a high correlation between Vβ flow cytometry and TCRγ-polymerase chain reaction results. No prevalence of any of Vβ was reported in T-LGLL but Vβ13.1 in CD4+ T-LGLL [2]. These techniques should be applied to all suspected cases and are useful in those patients in whom the absolute LGL count is not significantly increased. To these routinely used investigations, deep sequencing (NGS) of TCR has recently emerged to be a useful tool to demonstrate restricted diversity of TCR repertoire [18], not only supplying information about the clonal nature of LGL expansion but also providing the number and the entity of clones included in LGL increase and the identification of the CDR3 sequence. NGS analysis has been proven to be also useful to monitor therapy response and minimal residual disease.

The clonality of CLPD-NK is more difficult to assess, NK-LGLs being not equipped with the TCR. In this case, chromosomal abnormalities or the restriction fragment polymorphism of X-linked gene analysis can provide the proof of clonality. A KIR-restricted expression pattern, demonstrated by flow cytometry analysis, has been accepted as a surrogate marker of monoclonal expansion [8].

At the diagnosis, when the criteria are difficult to be satisfied, histologic bone marrow (BM) immunochemistry analysis is requested. LGLs in BM appear as individual cells or small clusters localized in sinusoids. Since the amount of infiltrating cells is usually low, BM involvement by leukemic LGLs is often difficult to identify, even when LGL expansion is apparent in peripheral blood [19, 20].

15.1.3 Clinical Features

LGL leukemia is an extremely rare disease representing 2–5% of chronic lymphoproliferative disorders in North America and Europe and 5–6% in Asia. Two registries, one Dutch and one American, report the incidence of LGL leukemia as 0.72 and 0.2 cases per one million of individuals per year, respectively [21, 22]. T-LGL leukemia patients have reduced survival compared with general population, with a median overall survival of 9 years [12].

The disease usually affects old people (mean 60 years), men or women with the same proportion. The disease runs asymptomatic in nearly 40% of cases, with lymphocytosis representing the only observed hematological abnormality [23, 24]. The definition of T-cell clonopathy of unknown significance (TCUS) has also been suggested to designate these asymptomatic patients [25]. Disease may run asymptomatic for many years; however, during the course of disease in 60% of cases, therapy is needed, mostly for cytopenia-related manifestations. Symptomatic patients show clinical complications more frequently due to neutropenia, as fever caused by infections or mouth lesions. Recurrent infections are reported in 15–39% of cases [26]. Neutropenia is defined as an absolute neutrophil count (ANC) less than 1.5×10^9/L and severe neutropenia with ANC $<0.5 \times 10^9$/L. However, some patients with severe and persistent neutropenia can be also devoid of infections for a long period of time; in these cases, therapy can be delayed. Weakness due to anemia represents another relevant finding, with 10–30% of cases being transfusion-dependent. B-related symptoms (fever, night sweats, weight loss) are observed in nearly 25% of cases. Thrombocytopenia is generally moderate and is found in less than 25% of cases, whereas pure red cell aplasia (PRCA) occurs in 8–19% of the cases [27].

Frequently, patients may have other associated conditions; among these, rheumatoid arthritis (RA) is the most commonly reported comorbidity condition [12, 28], but several other connective tissue diseases, including systemic lupus erythematosus, vasculitis, and polymyositis, have been reported [29–32]. Hematological disorders are another well-represented group including monoclonal gammopathies, multiple myeloma, myelodysplastic syndromes, myelofibrosis, and Hodgkin's and non-Hodgkin's lymphomas [12, 28]. An association has been established between LGL disorders and pulmonary hypertension, with documented infiltration of the lung by LGLs, and inclusion body myositis has occasionally been reported [32]. From 20% up to a half of the patients have splenomegaly, around 20% of cases present skin lesions, and only a minority have hepatomegaly; lymphadenopathy is rare [33]. Diseases associated with LGL leukemia are listed in Table 15.1.

Table 15.1 Conditions associated with the lymphoproliferative disease of granular lymphocytes

Associated disease	Frequency
Autoimmune disease	15–40%
Rheumatoid arthritis	25%
Systemic lupus erythematosus	<5%
Still disease	<5%
Systemic sclerosis	<5%
Vasculitis	<5%
Polymyositis	<5%
Poly/multineuritis	<5%
Autoimmune cytopenia	5–10%
Pure red cell aplasia	5%
Autoimmune hemolytic anemia	<5%
Idiopathic thrombocytopenic purpura	<5%
Hematological malignancies	<10%
MGUS/multiple myeloma	<5%
Myelodysplasia	<5%
Myelofibrosis	<5%
Hodgkin's and non-Hodgkin's lymphomas	<5%
Pulmonary arterial hypertension	<5%
Chronic viral infection (EBV, HTLV, CMV, HIV, HCV)	<5%

MGUS monoclonal gammopathy of undetermined significance, *EBV* Epstein-Barr virus, *HTLV* human T-lymphotropic virus, *CMV* cytomegalovirus, *HIV* human immunodeficiency virus, *HCV* hepatitis C virus

15.1.4 The Predicting Value of the Immunophenotype

Intriguingly, a correlation between immunophenotype and clinical and genetic features has been reported [34, 35], even if the nature of this relationship needs to be elucidated. In CD8+ T-LGLL, it has been demonstrated that CD16+/CD56− phenotype, with or without CD57, is strongly linked to patients characterized by neutropenia and the presence of *STAT3* mutation [35]. The association between *STAT3* mutation and symptomatic disease has been further reported in several papers [36–38]. The rare aggressive form of T-LGLL is characterized by proliferations of CD8+/CD56+/CD16−/CD57− LGLs, and patients are frequently mutated in *STAT5b* [39]. Interestingly, CD4+ T-LGLL patients are always CD8±/CD56+ and include patients carrying *STAT5b* mutations, but they never show to carry *STAT3* mutations, and they are almost always characterized by an indolent clinical course [35, 40].

In 2017 WHO classification, *STAT3* and *STAT5b* mutations are introduced to be considered for the identification of a subset of patients, *STAT5b* mutations being associated with a more aggressive disease. Anyway, this consideration will need to be updated with the discovery of *STAT5b* genetic lesions also in indolent CD4+ T-LGLL [40].

Similar to T-LGLL, discrete subtypes of CLPD-NK can be identified by flow analysis depending on the intensity of CD56 and CD16 expression and on CD57 presence or absence. Interestingly, patients characterized by $CD56^{-/dim}/CD16^{high}/CD57^{-}$ cytotoxic NK cell expansion include a unique phenotypic subgroup characterized by a more symptomatic disease and the presence of *STAT3* mutation [41].

The dominant LGL immunophenotypes indicative for clinical presentation are schematically reported in Fig. 15.3.

15.1.5 Therapy

The percentage of patients requiring therapy during the natural history of the disease ranges from 30% to 70%, according to different series [12, 28]. Indications for treatment include severe and symptomatic neutropenia (associated with recurrent infections), transfusion-dependent anemia, or thrombocytopenia as far as progressive disease (i.e., appearance of organomegaly, B symptoms, and rapidly LGL raising counts). Correction of cytopenias with therapy may be achieved without eradication of the clone, which often persists even after treatment. Given that LGLs are activated cytotoxic lymphocytes, therapy is based on immunomodulatory drugs. Methotrexate (MTX, 10 mg/m^2/weekly), low-dose cyclophosphamide (CTX, 50–100 mg/day), or cyclosporine A (CyA, 3–5 mg/kg/day) are commonly used [42, 43]. Corticosteroids may be useful as part of the initial treatment to accelerate response, and growth factors are often used as supportive care. Splenectomy may be considered as an adjuvant in patients with relevant splenomegaly and refractory cytopenias [44].

The first-line therapy relies on the use of single immunosuppressive oral agent, and up to now MTX or CTX have been considered as the best first-line choice. Moreover, MTX is reported to be more efficient for neutropenic and *STAT3* Y640F mutated patients [42, 45].

Once patients with LGL leukemia start treatment, the regimen should be continued for a period of at least 4 months, and they should be closely observed through complete blood counts [43]. After this time point, a hematological complete response is considered achieved when blood counts reveal platelets $>150 \times 10^9$/L, ANC $>1.5 \times 10^9$/L, lymphocytes $<4 \times 10^9$/L, and hemoglobin >12 g/dL. Complete molecular remission is reached when the T-cell clone is no longer detectable through PCR analysis [43]. Partial response is considered when overall blood counts improve, but the ANC has not achieved levels

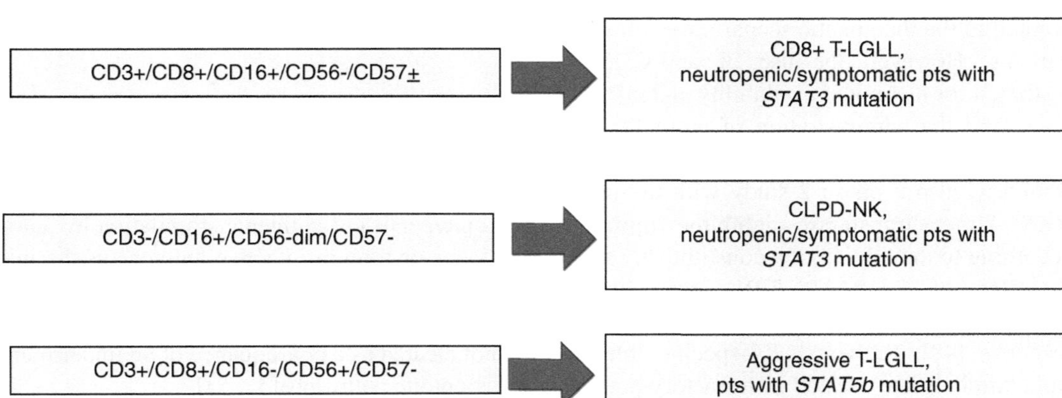

Fig. 15.3 The LGL immunophenotypes indicative for clinical and biological presentations

> 0.5 x 10^9 cells/L, still leaving the patient at potential risk for secondary infections. If an improvement is not achieved after 4 months of continued treatment, one of the alternative therapies described above must be taken into account. However, evidence is accumulating for continuing treatment once established for a longer period of time (usually 1 year), before changing therapy.

The overall response rate (ORR) ranges from 21% to 85%, with similar responses to each of the three drugs. The complete response (CR) rate is 21% for MTX, 33% for CTX, and 5% for CyA [43]. Unfortunately, when the clinical response occurs, patients frequently relapse, and new therapeutic strategies are needed.

Chemotherapeutic agents, such as gemcitabine, liposomal doxorubicin, and bendamustine, and the purine analogs, such as fludarabine, cladribine, and nelarabine, represent possible new agents to be considered for symptomatic LGL disorders [26, 28]. These molecules have been reported to be promising but only in few patients. The use of these agents should be considered for young patients as they allow the achievement of good remissions, including the reduction of bone marrow infiltration.

In some patients with refractory disease, stem cell therapy may be considered. In a series of 15 patients receiving auto- or allogeneic stem cell therapy for LGL leukemia, six patients remained disease-free after transplantation [46].

Monoclonal antibodies anti-CD52 (Campath-1H) and anti-CD122 have been incorporated in the therapeutic scenario for refractory patients. However, the use of anti-CD52 is restricted for its limited availability and infection risks, and the administration of anti-CD122 to patients did not show any response [26, 47]. Similarly, also a phase 2 study with the use of RAS farnesyltransferase inhibitor tipifarnib, according to the finding of a constitutively active signaling of Ras/MAPK/ERK pathway, has unfortunately led to unsatisfactory clinical response [48]. Rather, JAK3-specific inhibitor (tofacitinib citrate), tested in refractory patients, and the multicytokine inhibitor BNZ-1, tested in phase 1 trial, showed promising responses [49]. In addition, the proteasome inhibitor bortezomib has been reported to display anticancer activity against aggressive NK leukemia and extranodal NK/T cell lymphoma *in vitro* and *in vivo*, opening new therapeutic perspectives for LGL patients [50, 51]. Recent data support this approach [52].

Treatment of the rare forms of aggressive LGL leukemia includes polychemotherapy based on CHOP-like (CTX, doxorubicin, vincristine, and prednisone) or cytosine arabinoside-containing regimens [26], usually with unsatisfactory results.

15.2 LGL Leukemia: Molecular Aspects

15.2.1 Pathogenesis

The etiology of LGL leukemia remains still unknown, but some crucial cornerstones for disease development have been identified. It is supposed that no single, specific agent can finally trigger the LGL proliferation. In fact, the proliferation and accumulation of a transformed T or NK cell might represent the expression of a dysregulation of cytotoxic LGL homeostasis because of persistent antigenic drive in combination with immunogenetic factors favoring persistent cell expansions [53]. Moreover, the recognized role in LGL survival, played by some inflammatory cytokines and monocytes, dendritic cells, and mesenchymal stromal cells (MSC), supports the involvement of an inflammatory environment in the pathogenesis of the disease (Fig. 15.4).

15.2.2 The Inciting Event

Many reports strongly support the role of a chronic/persistent antigenic stimulation by auto-antigens or foreign infective antigens as the initial step. This would lead to the expansion of a fully differentiated effector cytotoxic LGL which is not cleared as a consequence of an impairment of apoptotic pathways [53, 54].

Supporting the involvement of auto-antigens, dysregulated autoimmune responses are fre-

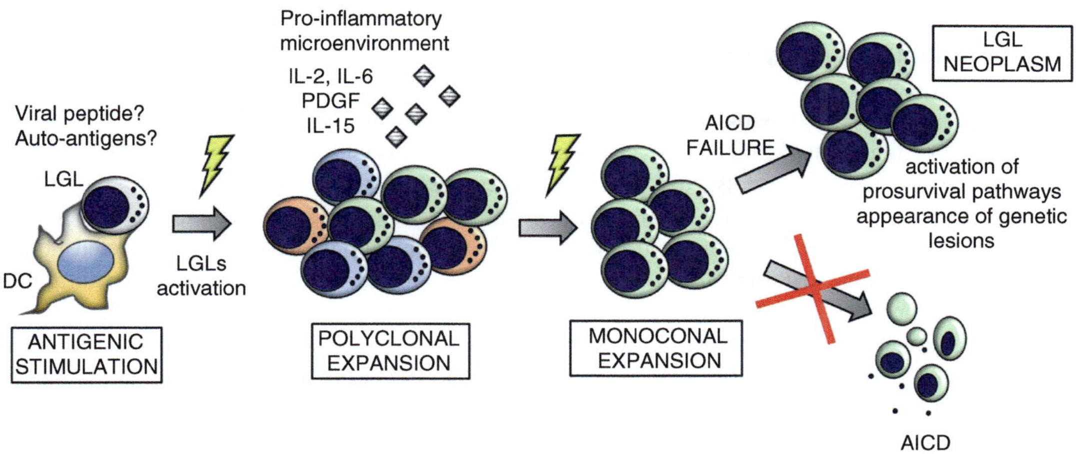

Fig. 15.4 Schematic representation of the pathogenetic hypothesis of large granular lymphocytes leukemia. *LGL* large granular lymphocyte, *DC* dendritic cell, *AICD* activation-induced cell death

quently demonstrated in LGLL patients [15, 55], such as the presence of rheumatoid factors and antinuclear antibodies, rheumatic diseases being commonly associated with LGL leukemia (Table 15.1).

Several reports support a possible role of viral antigens. The pathogenic role of EBV or human T-cell leukemia viruses (HTVL) in some cases of LGL disorder has been reported [14, 16, 56]. Although no prototypic HTLV infection was demonstrated, the evidence that sera from a series of cases from Europe and USA react with the recombinant HTLV env protein p21E, specifically in BA21 epitope, indicates that exposure to a protein containing homology to BA21 may be important in the pathogenesis of this lymphoproliferative disorder [57]. Similarly, evidence has been provided that chronic stimulation of T cells by CMV leads to a persistent clonal expansion of CD4+/CD8−/+dim LGLs, with a predominance of TCR Vb13.1 usage in individuals with an HLADRB1*0701 haplotype [58]. The hypothesis has been formulated that a persistent CMV stimulation can trigger and maintain the LGL clone in patients with a genetic predisposition.

All these data show that not an exclusive and unique factor may be responsible for the initial event causing LGL expansion but rather that multiple factors, referred to auto/viral antigens, may be alternatively involved.

15.2.3 Bone Marrow Involvement

As stated before, LGLL patients usually present leukemic infiltration in bone marrow, where clonal LGLs cluster in small lymphoid aggregates or in microvascular structures [19]. LGLL patients' bone marrow was also demonstrated to be fibrotic for the induction of high collagen (types I, III, and V) deposition by MSC, finally leading to an impaired hematopoietic stem cell proliferation. Together with LGL infiltration, fibrosis has been reported to correlate with the presence of cytopenia [59].

It has been proposed that bone marrow represents the setting in which the putative antigen presentation takes place. Furthermore, dendritic cells (DCs) have been suggested to represent the target of infection in these patients [60]. In fact, a co-localization of DCs and leukemic LGLs has been identified both in T-LGLL and in CLPD-NK. Moreover, bone marrow-derived DCs induced a strong proliferation of autologous purified LGLs from T-LGLL patients pointing that DCs pulsed with a specific antigen might be the putative-inciting agent responsible for T-LGL proliferation [60]. On the contrary, the clonal expansion of NK cells might be due to an impairment in NK/DC equilibrium in the bone marrow, because leukemic NK cells failed to induce DC maturation due to a NKp30 down-modulation [61].

15.2.4 Peripheral Blood Inflammatory Cytokines

Several proinflammatory cytokines have been identified to be higher in LGLL patients' plasma in comparison to healthy controls, such as IL-1β, IL-1Rα, IFNγ, CCL5, CCL4, IL-18, IL-8, CXCL10, CXCL9, and IL-6. Most of them can be related to immune cytotoxic response after viral infection or to RA, which is often associated with LGLL [62–66]. The role of IL-6 was demonstrated: IL-6 and its specific receptor, IL-6Rα, were found to be higher in patients' plasma, and they were released by the non-leukemic fraction of the mononuclear cells; IL-6 contributed to the survival by stimulating STAT3, a key protein in LGLL development [66].

IL-15 is another cytokine that was proven to be important in LGLL pathogenesis both *in vitro* and *in vivo*. IL-15 was shown to induce LGL cytotoxicity and proliferation through proteasomal degradation of the pro-apoptotic protein Bid [7, 67]. The pathogenetic role was demonstrated by the generation of IL-15 transgenic mice (IL-15tg) as they developed a fatal clonal NK and memory CD8+ expansion [68]. IL-15 induced chromosomal instability and DNA hypermethylation via repression of *mir*-29b and the induction of a Myc/NF-kB/DNMT3a axis [51]. Nevertheless, the lethal expansion was induced only when there was a *cis* activation by IL15Rα. In fact, the specific receptor IL-15Rα was expressed by LGLs, and it was detectable in high amounts in patients' plasma [7, 69]. Further supporting the role of IL-15 in the pathogenesis, a systematic biology approach identified IL-15 and PDGF as master survival signaling switches that may have a profound effect on all known deregulations in T-LGL leukemia [70].

15.2.5 Clonal Drift

The phenomenon of clonal drift supports the theory that the emergence of LGL clone might be caused by the recognition of different epitopes of the same chronic antigen. This phenomenon is characterized by the change of the dominant LGL clone over the time. It has been reported that 37% of T-LGLL patients displayed a change in the dominant clone, developing a different Vβ clone instead of the original one owned at diagnosis as demonstrated by Vβ typing [71]. In another series of 42 patients with KIR-restricted CLPD-NK, the presence of monoclonal T cell populations in 48% of cases was also demonstrated. These T monoclonal populations can be detected at the time of diagnosis or occur during the natural history of disease, indicating that the association of T and NK proliferations is more frequent than initially thought. The T cell clone can eventually become so relevant to be dominant, leading to the shift from CLPD-NK to T-LGLL [72]. Similarly, also a T-LGLL patient who developed CLPD-NK over time has been described [73] (Fig. 15.5). All these observations indicate that cells are under antigenic pressure, suggesting that the putative antigen is likely to persist for many years and possibly for the lifelong of patients.

15.2.6 AICD Failure

Physiologically, during infection exposure or antigen stimulation, LGLs undergo proliferation and, after antigen clearance, are eliminated by a process called activation-induced cell death (AICD). This process leads to cell death through the induction of a death-inducing signaling complex (DISC). In LGLL patients, LGLs do not undergo apoptosis for a dysfunctional AICD mechanism, leading to the increase of leukemic cells in the peripheral blood. In detail, LGLs are not sensitive to Fas-induced apoptosis [74], a process essential for AICD [75], and possess high levels of c-FLIP, a DISC inhibitory protein [53].

15.2.7 JAK/STAT Pathway

In addition to the deregulation of apoptosis mechanism, in leukemic LGLs, multiple cell survival pathways have been found to be constitutively activated. Among these, JAK/STAT3 is the main involved axis. In fact, the activated (phosphorylated) form of STAT3 characterizes all leukemic LGLs, and it is currently considered the disease hallmark. The finding that the JAK-

Fig. 15.5 Schematic representation of the main mechanisms leading to the phenomenon of clonal drift. *TCR* T cell receptor, *KIR* killer immunoglobulin-like receptor, *CLPD-NK* chronic lymphoproliferative disease of NK cells, *T-LGLL* T-large granular lymphocyte leukemia

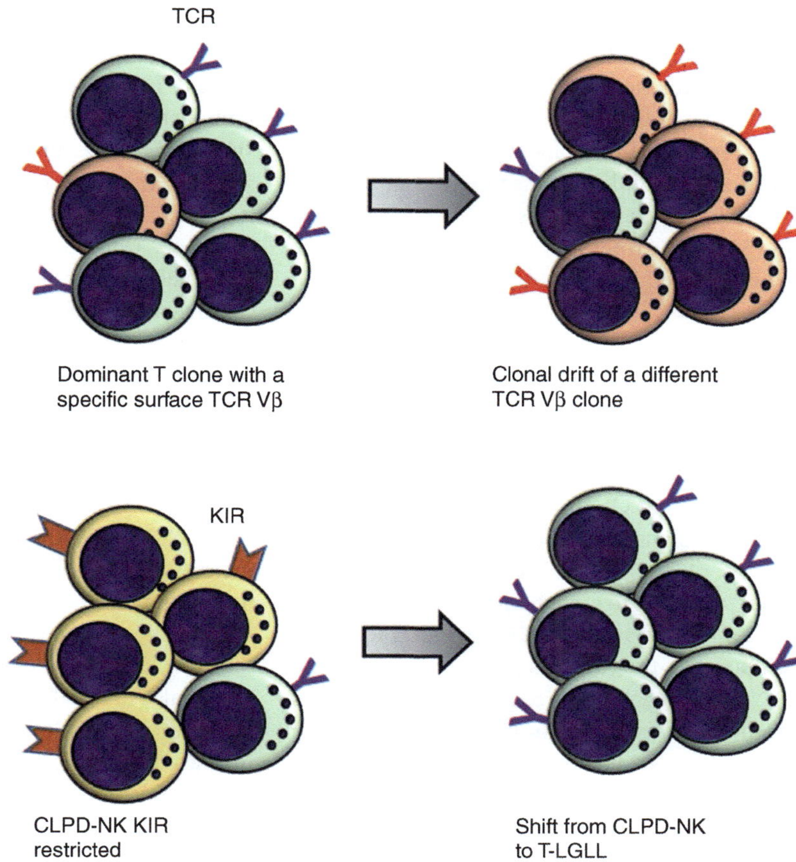

selective tyrosine kinase inhibitor AG-490 or the STAT3-specific inhibitor, Stattic, *in vitro* induces LGL apoptosis highlights the role of STAT3 in LGL clonal expansion [66, 76]. In 2012, recurrent somatic mutations in the Src homology 2 (SH2) domain of the *STAT3* gene have been discovered. These gain-of-function mutations increase the stability of STAT3 dimers resulting in an enhanced transcriptional activity of the mutated proteins. Their frequency is 27–40% in T-LGLL patients [34, 77] and 9-30% in CLPD-NK [77, 90]. In the T-LGLL, *STAT3* mutations characterize the CD8+ T-LGLL and have never been observed in the CD4+ T-LGLL [35, 40, 89]. Patients with *STAT3* mutations present with neutropenia more frequently than patients without these mutations [35]. The association between PRCA and neutropenia with *STAT3* gene mutations was also reported in Asia [78, 79]. The most frequent *STAT3* mutations are Y640F and D661Y, representing 60% of the recognized mutations. Although almost all *STAT3* lesions are located in SH2 domain, very rare activating mutations were described also in DNA-binding and coiled-coil domains [80]. Another member of STAT protein family has been reported carrying activating mutations in the SH2 domain, *STAT5B*. *STAT5b* mutations were identified in 2% of the CD8+ T-LGLL, specifically affecting the rare aggressive form of LGL leukemia [39], and were also found in 15–55% of CD4+ T-LGLL, whereas indolent CD8+ T-LGLL and CLPD-NK seemed to be devoid of these genetic lesions [35, 40].

Since *in vitro* inhibition of STAT3 was observed to restore the apoptosis of LGL independently from *STAT3* mutational status and that STAT3 is activated also in *STAT3* wild-type LGLL patients, *STAT3* mutation cannot represent the only factor or be itself mandatory to trigger LGL clonal expansion. In unmutated LGLL patients, a high amount of the proinflammatory cytokine IL-6 is able to activate the STAT3 axis [66], and the inhibition of this cytokine restores LGL apoptosis. Moreover, in LGLL the physiological negative feedback loop carried out by the suppressor of cytokine signaling (SOCS3) protein on the activated STAT3 is downregulated [66].

15.2.8 Other Cell Survival Dysregulated Pathways

Although STAT3 activation plays the most significant role in LGL disorders, other multiple cell survival pathways have been described. Increased activity of the PI3K-AKT signaling axis in T-LGLs appears to operate in conjunction with or parallel to increased STAT3 activation to inhibit the apoptotic program [81]. Sustaining this axis, RANTES, MIP-1beta, and IL-18 are high in serum LGLL patients [64]. Acting downstream of the PI3K-AKT pathway to prevent apoptosis through Mcl-1 independently of STAT3, a crucial role is played by NF-kB. Leukemic LGLs express high levels of c-Rel, a member of the NF-kB family, and exhibit higher NF-kB activity than normal PBMCs [70]. A pathogenetic role for NF-kB signaling is also proved by the finding of a recurrent (8%) mutation of TNFAIP3, a NFkB inhibitor [82]. In CLPD-NK, the activation of Ras/MEK/ERK pathway contributes to the accumulation of NK cells caused by a constitutive stimulation of both ERK and Ras. Consistently, Ras and ERK inhibition causes the reduction of the survival of patient NK cells [83]. In addition, ERK1/2 signaling can be activated also by a dysregulation of sphingolipid rheostat [84, 85].

15.2.9 Neutropenia Molecular Mechanism

The pathogenesis of neutropenia in these patients is probably multifactorial, including humoral and cytotoxic mechanisms. However, the most important mechanism accounting for neutropenia is myeloid progenitor and neutrophil destruction via Fas-mediated apoptosis [86, 87]. T-LGLs express Fas ligand (FasL), and mature neutrophils express Fas. There is high surface expression of Fas/FasL in LGL, and large amounts of soluble FasL have been detected in sera of neutropenic T-LGL patients [35, 86]. FasL and other inhibitory cytokines produced by LGL may lead to hematopoietic suppression through apoptosis of neutrophil precursors in the bone marrow or result in direct killing of neutrophils that express a high concentration of Fas on their surface. The correction of cytopenias in T-LGL leukemia has been associated with a disappearance or reduction of serum FasL levels [86]. Intriguingly, it has been reported that FasL expression can be driven by STAT3 activation (higher in *STAT3*-mutated patients) [35]. In addition, it was recently shown that a microRNA(miR)-146b is downregulated specifically in neutropenic patients so allowing the translation of human antigen R (HuR), an essential FasL mRNA stabilizer. HuR protein mediates FasL mRNA stabilization, leading to increased FasL production and, consequently, to neutropenia development [88].

15.3 Concluding Remarks

Further knowledge of developmental pathways of normal LGLs is crucial to get insights into the characteristics of LGL disorders. This would allow to face the urgent unmet need to develop better therapeutics for LGL leukemia, because this disease still remains incurable. The knowledge of the precise mechanism through which mutated STAT5b can mediate an aggressive disease in CD8+ T-LGLL whereas the same mutation when present in CD4+ T-LGLL does not induce detrimental effects is central to design targeted therapies for these patients. Due to the rarity of disease, well-designed prospective comparative clinical trials are up to now lacking. Only the results from a randomized clinical trial from the USA recruiting 55 patients are available showing a still unsatisfactory overall response rate [42]. In addition, the results of an important prospected randomized clinical trial from France are coming (#NCT01976182). In the lack of this relevant information, the decision on which immunotherapy should be first started is still related to arbitrary medical decision. Finally, the possibility to know the biological mechanisms switching on and off in responding patients as compared to non-responding ones would certainly contribute to design more precisely targeted therapies.

References

1. Semenzato G, Zambello R, Starkebaum G, Oshimi K, Loughran TP Jr. The lymphoproliferative disease of granular lymphocytes: updated criteria for diagnosis. Blood. 1997;89:256–60.
2. Zambello R, Trentin L, Facco M, Cerutti A, Sancetta R, Milani A, et al. Analysis of the T cell receptor in the lymphoproliferative disease of granular lymphocytes: superantigen activation of clonal CD3+ granular lymphocytes. Cancer Res. 1995;55:6140–5.
3. Baesso I, Pavan L, Boscaro E, Miorin M, Facco M, Trentin L, et al. T-cell type lymphoproliferative disease of granular lymphocytes (LDGL) is equipped with a phenotypic pattern typical of effector cytotoxic cells. Leuk Res. 2007;31:371–7.
4. Bourgault-Rouxel AS, Loughran TP Jr, Zambello R, Epling-Burnette PK, Semenzato G, Donadieu J, et al. Clinical spectrum of gammadelta+ T cell LGL leukemia: analysis of 20 cases. Leuk Res. 2008;32:45–8.
5. Gentile TC, Uner AH, Hutchison RE, Wright J, Ben-Ezra J, Russell EC, et al. CD3+, CD56+ aggressive variant of large granular lymphocyte leukemia. Blood. 1994;84:2315–21.
6. Zambello R, Falco M, Della Chiesa M, Trentin L, Carollo D, Castriconi R, et al. Expression and function of KIR and natural cytotoxicity receptors in NK-type lymphoproliferative diseases of granular lymphocytes. Blood. 2003;102:1797–805.
7. Zambello R, Facco M, Trentin L, Sancetta R, Tassinari C, Perin A, et al. Interleukin-15 triggers the proliferation and cytotoxicity of granular lymphocytes in patients with lymphoproliferative disease of granular lymphocytes. Blood. 1997;89:201–11.
8. Barcena P, Jara-Acevedo M, Tabernero MD, Lopez A, Sanchez ML, Garcia-Montero AC, et al. Phenotypic profile of expanded NK cells in chronic lymphoproliferative disorders: a surrogate marker for NK-cell clonality. Oncotarget. 2015;6:42938–51.
9. Epling-Burnette PK, Painter JS, Chaurasia P, Bai F, Wei S, Djeu JY, et al. Dysregulated NK receptor expression in patients with lymphoproliferative disease of granular lymphocytes. Blood. 2004;103:3431–9.
10. Oshimi K. Progress in understanding and managing natural killer-cell malignancies. Br J Haematol. 2007;139:532–44.
11. Ishida F. Aggressive NK-cell leukemia. Front Pediatr. 2018;6:292.
12. Moignet A, Lamy T. Latest advances in the diagnosis and treatment of large granular lymphocytic leukemia. Am Soc Clin Oncol Educ Book. 2018;38:616–25.
13. Djaoud Z, David G, Bressollette C, Willem C, Rettman P, Gagne K, et al. Amplified NKG2C+ NK cells in cytomegalovirus (CMV) infection preferentially express killer cell Ig-like receptor 2DL: functional impact in controlling CMV-infected dendritic cells. J Immunol. 2013;191:2708–16.
14. Kawa-Ha K, Ishihara S, Ninomiya T, Yumura-Yagi K, Hara J, Murayama F, et al. CD3-negative lymphoproliferative disease of granular lymphocytes containing Epstein-Barr viral DNA. J Clin Invest. 1989;84:51–5.
15. Zambello R, Loughran TP Jr, Trentin L, Pontisso P, Battistella L, Raimondi R, et al. Serologic and molecular evidence for a possible pathogenetic role of viral infection in CD3-negative natural killer-type lymphoproliferative disease of granular lymphocytes. Leukemia. 1995;9:1207–11.
16. Hart DN, Baker BW, Inglis MJ, Nimmo JC, Starling GC, Deacon E, et al. Epstein-Barr viral DNA in acute large granular lymphocyte (natural killer) leukemic cells. Blood. 1992;79:2116–23.
17. Langerak AW, van Den Beemd R, Wolvers-Tettero IL, Boor PP, van Lochem EG, Hooijkaas H, et al. Molecular and flow cytometric analysis of the Vbeta repertoire for clonality assessment in mature TCRalphabeta T-cell proliferations. Blood. 2001;98:165–73.
18. Clemente MJ, Przychodzen B, Jerez A, Dienes BE, Afable MG, Husseinzadeh H, et al. Deep sequencing of the T-cell receptor repertoire in CD8+ T-large granular lymphocyte leukemia identifies signature landscapes. Blood. 2013;122:4077–85.
19. Morice WG, Kurtin PJ, Tefferi A, Hanson CA. Distinct bone marrow findings in T-cell granular lymphocytic leukemia revealed by paraffin section immunoperoxidase stains for CD8, TIA-1, and granzyme B. Blood. 2002;99:268–74.
20. Osuji N, Beiske K, Randen U, Matutes E, Tjonnfjord G, Catovsky D, et al. Characteristic appearances of the bone marrow in T-cell large granular lymphocyte leukaemia. Histopathology. 2007;50:547–54.
21. Dinmohamed AG, Brink M, Visser O, Jongen-Lavrencic M. Population-based analyses among 184 patients diagnosed with large granular lymphocyte leukemia in the Netherlands between 2001 and 2013. Leukemia. 2016;30:1449–51.
22. Shah MV, Hook CC, Call TG, Go RS. A population-based study of large granular lymphocyte leukemia. Blood Cancer J. 2016;6:e455.
23. Semenzato G, Pandolfi F, Chisesi T, De Rossi G, Pizzolo G, Zambello R, et al. The lymphoproliferative disease of granular lymphocytes. A heterogeneous disorder ranging from indolent to aggressive conditions. Cancer. 1987;60:2971–8.
24. Loughran TP Jr. Clonal diseases of large granular lymphocytes. Blood. 1993;82:1–14.

25. Dhodapkar MV, Li CY, Lust JA, Tefferi A, Phyliky RL. Clinical spectrum of clonal proliferations of T-large granular lymphocytes: a T-cell clonopathy of undetermined significance? Blood. 1994;84:1620–7.
26. Lamy T, Moignet A, Loughran TP Jr. LGL leukemia: from pathogenesis to treatment. Blood. 2017;129:1082–94.
27. Go RS, Li CY, Tefferi A, Phyliky RL. Acquired pure red cell aplasia associated with lymphoproliferative disease of granular T lymphocytes. Blood. 2001;98:483–5.
28. Zambello R, Semenzato G. Large granular lymphocyte disorders: new etiopathogenetic clues as a rationale for innovative therapeutic approaches. Haematologica. 2009;94:1341–5.
29. Zhang R, Shah MV, Loughran TP Jr. The root of many evils: indolent large granular lymphocyte leukaemia and associated disorders. Hematol Oncol. 2010;28:105–17.
30. Audemard A, Lamy T, Bareau B, Sicre F, Suarez F, Truquet F, et al. Vasculitis associated with large granular lymphocyte (LGL) leukemia: presentation and treatment outcomes of 11 cases. Semin Arthritis Rheum. 2013;43:362–6.
31. Murphy PW, Brett LK, Verla-Tebit E, Macik BG, Loughran TP Jr. Acquired inhibitors to factor VIII and fibrinogen in the setting of T-cell large granular lymphocyte leukemia: a case report and review of the literature. Blood Coagul Fibrinolysis. 2015;26:211–3.
32. Greenberg SA, Pinkus JL, Amato AA, Kristensen T, Dorfman DM. Association of inclusion body myositis with T cell large granular lymphocytic leukaemia. Brain. 2016;139:1348–60.
33. Lamy T, Loughran TP Jr. Clinical features of large granular lymphocyte leukemia. Semin Hematol. 2003;40:185–95.
34. Koskela HL, Eldfors S, Ellonen P, van Adrichem AJ, Kuusanmaki H, Andersson EI, et al. Somatic STAT3 mutations in large granular lymphocytic leukemia. N Engl J Med. 2012;366:1905–13.
35. Teramo A, Barila G, Calabretto G, Ercolin C, Lamy T, Moignet A, et al. STAT3 mutation impacts biological and clinical features of T-LGL leukemia. Oncotarget. 2017;8:61876–89.
36. Rajala HL, Olson T, Clemente MJ, Lagstrom S, Ellonen P, Lundan T, et al. The analysis of clonal diversity and therapy responses using STAT3 mutations as a molecular marker in large granular lymphocytic leukemia. Haematologica. 2015;100:91–9.
37. Rajala HL, Porkka K, Maciejewski JP, Loughran TP Jr, Mustjoki S. Uncovering the pathogenesis of large granular lymphocytic leukemia-novel STAT3 and STAT5b mutations. Ann Med. 2014;46:114–22.
38. Haapaniemi EM, Kaustio M, Rajala HL, van Adrichem AJ, Kainulainen L, Glumoff V, et al. Autoimmunity, hypogammaglobulinemia, lymphoproliferation, and mycobacterial disease in patients with activating mutations in STAT3. Blood. 2015;125:639–48.
39. Rajala HL, Eldfors S, Kuusanmaki H, van Adrichem AJ, Olson T, Lagstrom S, et al. Discovery of somatic STAT5b mutations in large granular lymphocytic leukemia. Blood. 2013;121:4541–50.
40. Andersson EI, Tanahashi T, Sekiguchi N, Gasparini VR, Bortoluzzi S, Kawakami T, et al. High incidence of activating STAT5B mutations in CD4-positive T-cell large granular lymphocyte leukemia. Blood. 2016;128:2465–8.
41. Barila G, Teramo A, Calabretto G, Ercolin C, Boscaro E, Trimarco V, et al. Dominant cytotoxic NK cell subset within CLPD-NK patients identifies a more aggressive NK cell proliferation. Blood Cancer J. 2018;8:51.
42. Loughran TP Jr, Zickl L, Olson TL, Wang V, Zhang D, Rajala HL, et al. Immunosuppressive therapy of LGL leukemia: prospective multicenter phase II study by the eastern cooperative oncology group (E5998). Leukemia. 2015;29:886–94.
43. Lamy T, Loughran TP Jr. How I treat LGL leukemia. Blood. 2011;117:2764–74.
44. Subbiah V, Viny AD, Rosenblatt S, Pohlman B, Lichtin A, Maciejewski JP. Outcomes of splenectomy in T-cell large granular lymphocyte leukemia with splenomegaly and cytopenia. Exp Hematol. 2008;36:1078–83.
45. Loughran TP Jr, Kidd PG, Starkebaum G. Treatment of large granular lymphocyte leukemia with oral low-dose methotrexate. Blood. 1994;84:2164–70.
46. Marchand T, Lamy T, Finel H, Arcese W, Choquet S, Finke J, et al. Hematopoietic stem cell transplantation for T-cell large granular lymphocyte leukemia: a retrospective study of the European Society for Blood and Marrow Transplantation. Leukemia. 2016;30:1201–4.
47. Waldmann TA, Conlon KC, Stewart DM, Worthy TA, Janik JE, Fleisher TA, et al. Phase 1 trial of IL-15 trans presentation blockade using humanized Mikbeta1 mAb in patients with T-cell large granular lymphocytic leukemia. Blood. 2013;121:476–84.
48. Epling-Burnette PK, Sokol L, Chen X, Bai F, Zhou J, Blaskovich MA, et al. Clinical improvement by farnesyltransferase inhibition in NK large granular lymphocyte leukemia associated with imbalanced NK receptor signaling. Blood. 2008;112:4694–8.
49. Wang TT, Yang J, Zhang Y, Zhang M, Dubois S, Conlon KC, et al. IL-2 and IL-15 blockade by BNZ-1, an inhibitor of selective gamma-chain cytokines, decreases leukemic T-cell viability. Leukemia. 2019;33:1243–55.
50. Shen L, Au WY, Guo T, Wong KY, Wong ML, Tsuchiyama J, et al. Proteasome inhibitor bortezomib-induced apoptosis in natural killer (NK)-cell leukemia and lymphoma: an in vitro and in vivo preclinical evaluation. Blood. 2007;110:469–70.
51. Mishra A, Liu S, Sams GH, Curphey DP, Santhanam R, Rush LJ, et al. Aberrant overexpression of IL-15 initiates large granular lymphocyte leukemia through chromosomal instability and DNA hypermethylation. Cancer Cell. 2012;22:645–55.
52. Yang J, LeBlanc FR, Dighe SA, Hamele CE, Olson TL, Feith DJ, et al. TRAIL mediates and sustains

constitutive NF-kappaB activation in LGL leukemia. Blood. 2018;131:2803–15.
53. Yang J, Epling-Burnette PK, Painter JS, Zou J, Bai F, Wei S, et al. Antigen activation and impaired Fas-induced death-inducing signaling complex formation in T-large-granular lymphocyte leukemia. Blood. 2008;111:1610–6.
54. Zambello R, Teramo A, Barila G, Gattazzo C, Semenzato G. Activating KIRs in chronic lymphoproliferative disorder of NK cells: protection from viruses and disease induction? Front Immunol. 2014;5:72.
55. Pandolfi F, Loughran TP Jr, Starkebaum G, Chisesi T, Barbui T, Chan WC, et al. Clinical course and prognosis of the lymphoproliferative disease of granular lymphocytes. A multicenter study. Cancer. 1990;65:341–8.
56. Loughran TP Jr, Zambello R, Ashley R, Guderian J, Pellenz M, Semenzato G, et al. Failure to detect Epstein-Barr virus DNA in peripheral blood mononuclear cells of most patients with large granular lymphocyte leukemia. Blood. 1993;81:2723–7.
57. Loughran TP Jr, Hadlock KG, Yang Q, Perzova R, Zambello R, Semenzato G, et al. Seroreactivity to an envelope protein of human T-cell leukemia/lymphoma virus in patients with CD3- (natural killer) lymphoproliferative disease of granular lymphocytes. Blood. 1997;90:1977–81.
58. Rodriguez-Caballero A, Garcia-Montero AC, Barcena P, Almeida J, Ruiz-Cabello F, Tabernero MD, et al. Expanded cells in monoclonal TCR-alphabeta+/CD4+/NKa+/CD8−/+dim T-LGL lymphocytosis recognize hCMV antigens. Blood. 2008;112:4609–16.
59. Mailloux AW, Zhang L, Moscinski L, Bennett JM, Yang L, Yoder SJ, et al. Fibrosis and subsequent cytopenias are associated with basic fibroblast growth factor-deficient pluripotent mesenchymal stromal cells in large granular lymphocyte leukemia. J Immunol. 2013;191:3578–93.
60. Zambello R, Berno T, Cannas G, Baesso I, Binotto G, Bonoldi E, et al. Phenotypic and functional analyses of dendritic cells in patients with lymphoproliferative disease of granular lymphocytes (LDGL). Blood. 2005;106:3926–31.
61. Balsamo M, Zambello R, Teramo A, Pedrazzi M, Sparatore B, Scordamaglia F, et al. Analysis of NK cell/DC interaction in NK-type lymphoproliferative disease of granular lymphocytes (LDGL): role of DNAM-1 and NKp30. Exp Hematol. 2009;37:1167–75.
62. Makishima H, Ishida F, Ito T, Kitano K, Ueno S, Ohmine K, et al. DNA microarray analysis of T cell-type lymphoproliferative disease of granular lymphocytes. Br J Haematol. 2002;118:462–9.
63. Choi YL, Makishima H, Ohashi J, Yamashita Y, Ohki R, Koinuma K, et al. DNA microarray analysis of natural killer cell-type lymphoproliferative disease of granular lymphocytes with purified CD3-CD56+ fractions. Leukemia. 2004;18:556–65.
64. Kothapalli R, Nyland SB, Kusmartseva I, Bailey RD, McKeown TM, Loughran TP Jr. Constitutive production of proinflammatory cytokines RANTES, MIP-1beta and IL-18 characterizes LGL leukemia. Int J Oncol. 2005;26:529–35.
65. Momose K, Makishima H, Ito T, Nakazawa H, Shimodaira S, Kiyosawa K, et al. Close resemblance between chemokine receptor expression profiles of lymphoproliferative disease of granular lymphocytes and their normal counterparts in association with elevated serum concentrations of IP-10 and MIG. Int J Hematol. 2007;86:174–9.
66. Teramo A, Gattazzo C, Passeri F, Lico A, Tasca G, Cabrelle A, et al. Intrinsic and extrinsic mechanisms contribute to maintain the JAK/STAT pathway aberrantly activated in T-type large granular lymphocyte leukemia. Blood. 2013;121:3843–54. S1
67. Hodge DL, Yang J, Buschman MD, Schaughency PM, Dang H, Bere W, et al. Interleukin-15 enhances proteasomal degradation of bid in normal lymphocytes: implications for large granular lymphocyte leukemias. Cancer Res. 2009;69:3986–94.
68. Fehniger TA, Suzuki K, VanDeusen JB, Cooper MA, Freud AG, Caligiuri MA. Fatal leukemia in interleukin-15 transgenic mice. Blood Cells Mol Dis. 2001;27:223–30.
69. Chen J, Petrus M, Bamford R, Shih JH, Morris JC, Janik JE, et al. Increased serum soluble IL-15Ralpha levels in T-cell large granular lymphocyte leukemia. Blood. 2012;119:137–43.
70. Zhang R, Shah MV, Yang J, Nyland SB, Liu X, Yun JK, et al. Network model of survival signaling in large granular lymphocyte leukemia. Proc Natl Acad Sci U S A. 2008;105:16308–13.
71. Clemente MJ, Wlodarski MW, Makishima H, Viny AD, Bretschneider I, Shaik M, et al. Clonal drift demonstrates unexpected dynamics of the T-cell repertoire in T-large granular lymphocyte leukemia. Blood. 2011;118:4384–93.
72. Gattazzo C, Teramo A, Passeri F, De March E, Carraro S, Trimarco V, et al. Detection of monoclonal T populations in patients with KIR-restricted chronic lymphoproliferative disorder of NK cells. Haematologica. 2014;99:1826–33.
73. Yan Y, Olson TL, Nyland SB, Feith DJ, Loughran TP Jr. Emergence of a STAT3 mutated NK clone in LGL leukemia. Leuk Res Rep. 2015;4:4–7.
74. Lamy T, Liu JH, Landowski TH, Dalton WS, Loughran TP Jr. Dysregulation of CD95/CD95 ligand-apoptotic pathway in CD3(+) large granular lymphocyte leukemia. Blood. 1998;92:4771–7.
75. Krueger A, Fas SC, Baumann S, Krammer PH. The role of CD95 in the regulation of peripheral T-cell apoptosis. Immunol Rev. 2003;193:58–69.
76. Epling-Burnette PK, Liu JH, Catlett-Falcone R, Turkson J, Oshiro M, Kothapalli R, et al. Inhibition of STAT3 signaling leads to apoptosis of leukemic large granular lymphocytes and decreased Mcl-1 expression. J Clin Invest. 2001;107:351–62.
77. Jerez A, Clemente MJ, Makishima H, Koskela H, Leblanc F, Peng Ng K, et al. STAT3 mutations unify the pathogenesis of chronic lymphoproliferative dis-

orders of NK cells and T-cell large granular lymphocyte leukemia. Blood. 2012;120:3048–57.
78. Qiu ZY, Fan L, Wang L, Qiao C, Wu YJ, Zhou JF, et al. STAT3 mutations are frequent in T-cell large granular lymphocytic leukemia with pure red cell aplasia. J Hematol Oncol. 2013;6:82.
79. Ishida F, Matsuda K, Sekiguchi N, Makishima H, Taira C, Momose K, et al. STAT3 gene mutations and their association with pure red cell aplasia in large granular lymphocyte leukemia. Cancer Sci. 2014;105:342–6.
80. Andersson E, Kuusanmaki H, Bortoluzzi S, Lagstrom S, Parsons A, Rajala H, et al. Activating somatic mutations outside the SH2-domain of STAT3 in LGL leukemia. Leukemia. 2016;30:1204–8.
81. Schade AE, Wlodarski MW, Maciejewski JP. Pathophysiology defined by altered signal transduction pathways: the role of JAK-STAT and PI3K signaling in leukemic large granular lymphocytes. Cell Cycle. 2006;5:2571–4.
82. Johansson P, Bergmann A, Rahmann S, Wohlers I, Scholtysik R, Przekopowitz M, et al. Recurrent alterations of TNFAIP3 (A20) in T-cell large granular lymphocytic leukemia. Int J Cancer. 2016;138:121–4.
83. Epling-Burnette PK, Bai F, Wei S, Chaurasia P, Painter JS, Olashaw N, et al. ERK couples chronic survival of NK cells to constitutively activated Ras in lymphoproliferative disease of granular lymphocytes (LDGL). Oncogene. 2004;23:9220–9.
84. LeBlanc FR, Liu X, Hengst J, Fox T, Calvert V, Petricoin EF 3rd, et al. Sphingosine kinase inhibitors decrease viability and induce cell death in natural killer-large granular lymphocyte leukemia. Cancer Biol Ther. 2015;16:1830–40.
85. Kothapalli R, Kusmartseva I, Loughran TP. Characterization of a human sphingosine-1-phosphate receptor gene (S1P5) and its differential expression in LGL leukemia. Biochim Biophys Acta. 2002;1579:117–23.
86. Liu JH, Wei S, Lamy T, Epling-Burnette PK, Starkebaum G, Djeu JY, et al. Chronic neutropenia mediated by fas ligand. Blood. 2000;95:3219–22.
87. Lamy T, Bauer FA, Liu JH, Li YX, Pillemer E, Shahidi H, et al. Clinicopathological features of aggressive large granular lymphocyte leukaemia resemble Fas ligand transgenic mice. Br J Haematol. 2000;108:717–23.
88. Mariotti B, Calabretto G, Rossato M, Teramo A, Castellucci M, Barilà G, et al. Identification of a miR-146b-Fas ligand axis in the development of neutropenia in T large granular lymphocyte leukemia. Haematologica. 2020;105:1351–1360.
89. Teramo A, Barilà G, Calabretto G, Vicenzetto C, Gasparini VR, Semenzato G, et al. Insights Into Genetic Landscape of Large Granular Lymphocyte Leukemia. Front Oncol. 2020;10:152.
90. Gasparini VR, Binatti A, Coppe A, Teramo A, Vicenzetto C, Calabretto G, et al. A high definition picture of somatic mutations in chronic lymphoproliferative disorder of natural killer cells. Blood Cancer Journal. 2020;10:42.

GPSR Compliance

The European Union's (EU) General Product Safety Regulation (GPSR) is a set of rules that requires consumer products to be safe and our obligations to ensure this.

If you have any concerns about our products, you can contact us on ProductSafety@springernature.com

In case Publisher is established outside the EU, the EU authorized representative is:

Springer Nature Customer Service Center GmbH
Europaplatz 3
69115 Heidelberg, Germany

Batch number: 10732801

Printed by Printforce, the Netherlands